DSM-5 AND THE LAW

Changes and Challenges

Edited by Charles Scott, MD

Professor of Clinical Psychiatry
Chief, Division of Psychiatry and the Law
Training Director, Forensic Psychiatry Fellowship
Department of Psychiatry and Behavioral Sciences
University of California-Davis School of Medicine, Sacramento, CA

OXFORD
UNIVERSITY PRESS

OXFORD
UNIVERSITY PRESS

Oxford University Press is a department of the University of Oxford.
It furthers the University's objective of excellence in research,
scholarship, and education by publishing worldwide.

Oxford New York
Auckland Cape Town Dar es Salaam Hong Kong Karachi
Kuala Lumpur Madrid Melbourne Mexico City Nairobi
New Delhi Shanghai Taipei Toronto

With offices in
Argentina Austria Brazil Chile Czech Republic France Greece
Guatemala Hungary Italy Japan Poland Portugal Singapore
South Korea Switzerland Thailand Turkey Ukraine Vietnam

Published in the United States of America by
Oxford University Press
198 Madison Avenue, New York, NY 10016

Library of Congress Cataloging-in-Publication Data
DSM-5 and the law : changes and challenges / editor: Charles Scott.
p. ; cm.
Diagnostic and statistical manual of mental disorders-5 and the law
Includes bibliographical references.
ISBN 978-0-19-936846-4 (alk. paper)—ISBN 978-0-19-936847-1 (alk. paper)—
ISBN 978-0-19-936848-8 (alk. paper)
I. Scott, Charles L., 1960–, editor. II. Title: Diagnostic and statistical manual of mental
disorders-5 and the law. [DNLM: 1. Diagnostic and statistical manual of mental disorders.
5th ed. 2. Mental Disorders—classification—United States. 3. Mentally Ill Persons—
legislation & jurisprudence—United States. 4. Criminal Law—United States. WM 33 AA1]
RC455.2.C4
616.89001'2—dc23
2014026158

This book is dedicated to my family, truly inspiring individuals who have given me my life and loved me throughout that life. To my parents, I am blessed to have a mother and father who sacrificed greatly throughout my childhood in the unwavering belief that I was somehow worth that sacrifice. To my brother Hal, I admire the eternal joy you find in all that's around you and your gift of sharing that joy with me. To my sister Gayden, your beauty, creativity, and selfless dedication to others remind me what is always possible when faced with the impossible. And to my brother Paul, your utter and complete courage continually teaches me the definition of dignity.

CONTENTS

PREFACE

The Diagnostic and Statistical Manual (DSM) is the most widely used and accepted scheme for diagnosing mental disorders in the United States. In 2013, DSM-5 was released with profound changes revealed in the required diagnostic process, specific criteria for previously established diagnoses, as well as the addition and deletion of specific mental disorders. The impact of these changes on patients, clinical providers, forensic evaluators, attorneys, and judges is substantial. This book succinctly highlights the consequences of the DSM-5 for mental health providers, forensic evaluators, legal professionals, and mental health administrators in criminal and civil contexts. This book consists of 11 chapters that address four critical areas important to understanding the impact and implications of the DSM-5 on issues related to mental health and the law.

Chapters 1, 2, and 3 provide an overview of DSM-5's development and implementation, DSM-5's key diagnostic changes, and practical guidelines for making a diagnosis and writing a forensic report using the new DSM-5 diagnostic approach. Chapters 4, 5, and 6 focus on DSM-5's impact on individuals who become involved in the criminal justice system, either as an individual receiving treatment in a correctional facility or as a defendant undergoing a forensic psychiatric evaluation. The third area reviewed includes DSM5's role in a wide range of civil evaluations. In particular, Chapters 7, 8, 9, and 10 review important issues related to civil competencies, personal injury and malpractice evaluations, disability assessments, and educational evaluations of school aged children. The fourth and final area is highlighted in Chapter 11 and is one that is a cornerstone of forensic diagnostic evaluations—the assessment of malingering and how DSM-5 diagnostic changes may affect these assessments. Each chapter provides an initial overview and explanation of the legal issue, how diagnostic changes may impact that issue, guidelines to address the relevant diagnostic changes, and a summary to emphasize key points. Numerous vignettes are provided throughout the book to illustrate key clinical and forensic issues that arise from DSM-5's implementation.

The evolving editions of DSM have become increasingly interwoven with the laws that govern how we provide care and how civil and criminal forensic evaluations are conducted. DSM-5 unties many of the diagnostic threads that had been tightly tethered to the fabric of how evaluators diagnose, treat, and conduct forensic evaluations. This book provides the evaluator practical recommendations on how to move forward using the DSM-5 without fears of having their forensic skills unravel and with the knowledge and skills to appropriately move forward.

ACKNOWLEDGMENTS

I would personally like to acknowledge each and every author who patiently answered all of my E-mails, politely responded to all of my reminders, and worked so diligently on their chapter.

I am very appreciative of the opportunity provided by Oxford Press to have edited this book and wish to personally thank Christopher Reid for the amazing professionalism he has demonstrated throughout the project

Finally, none of this book would have been possible without the amazing support of the UC Davis Forensic Psychiatry Case Manager, David Spagnolo. He makes all changes easily implemented and all challenges easy to overcome.

CONTRIBUTORS

Mace Beckson, MD
Health Sciences Clinical Professor of Psychiatry and Biobehavioral Sciences
University of California, Los Angeles, VA Greater Los Angeles Healthcare System
Los Angeles, CA

Jessica Ferranti, MD
Assistant Professor of Psychiatry
Training Director—General Psychiatry Residency Training Program
Division of Psychiatry and the Law
Department of Psychiatry and Behavioral Sciences
University of California-Davis Medical Center
Sacramento, CA

Richard L. Frierson, MD
Professor and Vice Chair for Education
Department of Neuropsychiatry and Behavioral Science
University of South Carolina School of Medicine
Columbia, SC

John Greene, MD
Adjunct Clinical Faculty Member
Department of Psychiatry
Stanford University
Stanford, CA

Brian Holoyda, MD, MPH
Resident in General Psychiatry
Department of Psychiatry and Behavioral Sciences
University of California-Davis Medical Center
Sacramento, CA

Gregory B. Leong, MD
Clinical Professor of Psychiatry
Department of Psychiatry and Behavioral Sciences
Keck School of Medicine
University of Southern California
Los Angeles, CA

Anne McBride, MD
Resident in Child and Adolescent Psychiatry
Department of Psychiatry and Behavioral Sciences
University of California-Davis Medical Center
Sacramento, CA

Barbara McDermott, PhD
Professor of Clinical Psychiatry
Research Director—Napa State Hospital
Division of Psychiatry and the Law
Department of Psychiatry and Behavioral Sciences
University of California-Davis Medical Center
Sacramento, CA

William Newman, MD
Assistant Professor of Psychiatry
Associate Training Director—Forensic Psychiatry Fellowship
Division of Psychiatry and the Law
Department of Psychiatry and Behavioral Sciences
University of California-Davis Medical Center
Sacramento, CA

Stephen Noffsinger, MD
Associate Professor of Psychiatry
University Hospitals of Cleveland
Cleveland, OH

Jennifer Piel, JD, MD
Staff Psychiatrist, VA Puget Sound Health Systems
Associate Training Director, Psychiatry Residency Program
Acting Assistant Professor, University of Washington
Seattle, WA

Charles Scott, MD
Professor of Clinical Psychiatry
Chief, Division of Psychiatry and the Law
Training Director, Forensic Psychiatry Fellowship
Department of Psychiatry and Behavioral Sciences
University of California-Davis Medical Center
Sacramento, CA

Ryan Wagoner, MD
Fellow in Forensic Psychiatry
Division of Psychiatry and the Law
Department of Psychiatry and Behavioral Sciences
University of California-Davis Medical Center
Sacramento, CA

Robert Weinstock, MD
Clinical Professor of Psychiatry
David Geffen School of Medicine
University of California
Los Angeles, CA

CHAPTER 1

DSM-5: Development and Implementation

INTRODUCTION

The Diagnostic and Statistical Manual of Mental Disorders (DSM) has provided the standard language used by mental health clinicians of various disciplines, public health policy makers,and mental health researchers for more than 60 years. Beginning with the first edition in 1952, the DSM has been the primary reference for the assessment and categorization of mental disorders in the United States. The DSM was originally developed as a written document to assist clinicians in more reliably communicating diagnostic concepts and criteria. Efforts to establish a nosology for psychopathology have been met with controversy and challenges with each successive edition of the DSM. With the release of DSM-5 in May of 2013, discussions and debates about the nosology of mental disorders have resurged.

The evolution of our understanding of mental illness should be reflected by changes in our diagnostic nomenclature system. Certainly, this has always been the stated goal of the DSM—to reflect prevailing theories about the etiology of mental disorders. However, the descriptive approach to psychiatry in the DSM has prioritized a classification system that creates a common language without becoming stymied by variable hypotheses about the causes of psychiatric illness. DSM-5 sought to incorporate the most current neurobiology, developmental neuroscience, and genetics to influence psychiatric classification in the first comprehensive revision of psychiatric nomenclature in two decades. From the beginning, developers of the DSM-5 promoted the need for a "paradigm shift" in psychiatric diagnosis away from descriptive categorical diagnosis to a dimensional framework. In 2002, Kupfer et al. [1] published *A Research Agenda for DSM-5*, a monograph intended to stimulate research and discussion in preparation for the start of the DSM-5 development process. This work largely identified significant gaps in the psychiatric knowledge base that tempered the call for an ambitious "paradigm shift" in psychiatry [2]. The official process to create DSM-5 started in 1999 and involved a multidisciplinary team of more than 400 individuals, in addition to numerous contributions from international conferences held during the past decade. Despite the original hope for a major paradigm shift in psychiatry, DSM-5 continued a descriptive categorical approach but added a greatly expanded dimensional component. DSM-5 was written with the intention that it will be updated at regular intervals to incorporate future advances in neuroscience, cognitive neuroscience, genetics, and clinical practice [3].

DSM-5 has brought some significant conceptual changes in psychiatric diagnosis and nomenclature that have important implications for the intersection of psychiatry and the law. The major developments that have occurred in successive editions of the DSM have affected the clinical practice of psychiatry and the delivery of mental health services within systems, and the new developments have irrevocably shaped the intellectual underpinning of the field. Among the medical specialties, psychiatry is uniquely vulnerable to the vicissitudes of the sociopolitical climate of our times. Controversies regarding the societal impact of the DSM, the medicalization of mental disorders, and the meaning of mental illness are not new. Although its use may be criticized, the utilization of the DSM by not only clinicians but also forensic evaluators, policy makers, the legal system, and third-party reimbursement entities, makes the DSM an undeniably powerful influence worldwide.

EVOLUTION OF THE DSM PRIOR TO DSM-5

The expansion of psychiatry and the DSM-I

It was not until World War II that the profession of psychiatry shifted measurably away from the insane asylums to greater prominence in the general community. Military physicians in World War I had noted a condition in soldiers they called "shell shock." The US government was interested in whether there was an inherent temperament or predisposition that could be identified during recruitment to weed out vulnerable individuals prior to military service [4]. With the United States' entry into World War II, military psychiatrists were particularly important in not only screening potential soldiers during recruitment for underlying mental disorders but also treating the psychiatric sequelae of war. After the conclusion of World War II, psychiatrists who had served in the military returned to community practice and discovered that the current diagnostic system was not adequate for psychiatric outpatients. The US Army and the US Navy independently developed their own diagnostic classification systems [5]. The Department of Veterans

Affairs then developed a third system in order to apply a consistent system to veteran populations. With so many competing diagnostic systems, the American Psychiatric Association (APA) decided to write one definitive diagnostic system for all of American psychiatry.

The Diagnostic and Statistical Manual, Mental Disorders (it was not until the second edition that the word "of" appeared in the title) was published in 1952 [6]. This first manual separated mental illness broadly into two categories: (1) disorders due to an "organic" brain disturbance and (2) those that were not considered "organic" in nature. Mental illnesses that did not have a known organic cause were diagnosed by comparison to a general description of the disorder. These nonorganic, or "functional," disorders were further divided into psychotic disorders, personality disorders, and psychoneurotic disorders. Every illness in the manual was referred to as *a reaction*, reflecting Adolf Meyer's approach that functional mental illness was on a continuum and that individual patients "react" differently only because their life histories are different. A psychodynamic etiology was implied in the manual. Many of the diagnoses included reference to defense mechanisms a patient may use such as "projection," "denial," and "retreat from reality" in psychosis. There was a hierarchy of diagnoses that prohibited certain combinations. For example, a psychotic disorder could not be diagnosed concurrently with a psychoneurotic disorder. Substance use disorders that co-occurred with other mental disorders were viewed as being derivative of the primary mental disorder and could not be diagnosed.

The World Health Organization and the DSM-II

The creation of the DSM-II was linked with the 1948 establishment of the World Health Organization (WHO) by the United Nations [7]. The WHO published the International Classification of Diseases (ICD), and the United States was required by international treaty to report its health data using ICD codes. The DSM-I was incompatible with the psychiatric section of the ICD. When the creation of the eighth edition of the ICD was initiated, the APA's Committee on Nomenclature and Statistics was tasked with updating the DSM to make it compatible with ICD [7]. By many accounts, the creation of DSM-II was a highly political process. The APA did not have the ability to include a disorder recognized in America if it was not already included in the ICD. DSM-II was published in 1968 and included 10 main divisions [8]. Significant new groupings included mental deficiency (formerly called mental retardation in the DSM-IV and renamed intellectual disability in DSM-5) and the mental illnesses of children. Overall, DSM-II continued the practice of establishing a diagnosis based on descriptions of mental disorders. DSM-II also emphasized psychodynamic explanations for many disorders.

The most radical change in the manual was the elimination of the word "reaction" from all adult disorders. Some psychiatrists viewed this shift as progress because they favored an atheoretical system that moved away from psychoanalytic predominance. However, other psychiatrists interpreted this change as an unwelcome return to a reductionist concept of descriptive categorical diagnosis.

DSM III: A revolution in American psychiatry

In 1974, the APA appointed Robert Spitzer to head the APA Task Force on Nomenclature and Statistics. In the same year, he published an article discussing the lack of reliability of psychiatric diagnoses and advocating for the use of structured interviews and diagnostic checklists [9]. From a sociopolitical perspective during that time period, insurers were increasingly limiting coverage for mental health services citing the lower reliability of psychiatric diagnoses compared with medical diagnoses. At the same time, researchers were finding it difficult to use DSM diagnoses for studies when they were linked with psychodynamic and social explanations for the disorders. In 1972, a Washington University group published an influential classification system that came to be known informally as the St. Louis "Feighner Diagnostic Criteria," named for first author John Feighner [10]. This paper was the most cited article in psychiatry for many decades. Because of its emphasis on using the medical model when making a psychiatric diagnosis, many credited this paper as heralding the most significant paradigm shift in the field of psychiatry in the 20th century [11]. The Feighner Diagnostic Criteria were expanded in the publication of the Research Diagnostic Criteria (RDC), which was supported by the National Institute of Mental Health and ultimately formed the prototypical diagnoses adopted in the DSM-III [12].

Although Spitzer was trained as a psychoanalyst, he had significant experience as a researcher, having served on the four-person United States Steering Committee for the United States-United Kingdom Diagnostic Project, a project founded in 1965 to examine statistical differences in diagnostic frequencies among patients admitted to mental hospitals in the United States and the United Kingdom. As work on the DSM-III began, Spitzer's team showed a clear interest in removing psychodynamic theory from the new DSM. Analysts from across the country were outraged. The DSM-III task force proffered several compromises including the inclusion of a separate axis for a psychodynamic formulation. There was also a significant and heated battle over the removal of the word "neurosis" from the manual. Ultimately, a compromise position was reached with the inclusion of the term "neurotic disorder" that was clarified to imply no "special etiological process" [13]. In 1980, DSM-III was published. At almost 500 pages, this edition was voluminous compared to its predecessors DSM-I (119 pages) and DSM-II (132 pages). Major changes included expansion of childhood and related disorders, affective disorders, and substance use disorders. New diagnostic categories included eating disorders, attention deficit disorders, and pervasive developmental disorders. Schizophrenia was separated into its own section, and, for the first time, "manic-depression" was renamed "bipolar disorder" and was listed as an affective disorder instead of a psychotic disorder.

DSM-III included several overarching changes. Although DSM-I and DSM-II had used comparison to descriptions to assess diagnosis, DSM-III used checklists of specified features, considerably enhancing diagnostic reliability. More importantly, DSM-III was also the first edition to provide a mental disorder definition [11]. In addition, DSM-III introduced the multiaxial system, which was designed to outline factors that should be taken into account to form a complete diagnostic picture of the patient.

DSM-III-R

Three years after DSM-III was published, the process to revise the manual began. Again, Robert Spitzer chaired the work group to revise DSM-III. The focus was to re-examine the DSM-III from the point of view of clinical utility. The team took feedback from clinicians and researchers and proposed changes were considered. DSM-III-R was published in 1987 with prominent modifications to the multiaxial system [13]. The severity of Axis I disorders could be noted with specifiers (e.g., mild, moderate, severe, in partial remission, in complete remission, etc), and Axis II was expanded to include mental retardation and developmental disorders. Axis V added a modified version of the Global Assessment of Functioning (GAF) scale. Additional changes were made in the diagnostic criteria for psychotic disorders, anxiety disorders, affective disorders, and substance use disorders. In addition, a section was added to DSM-III-R that outlined diagnoses needing further study.

DSM-IV and DSM-IV-TR

In 1988, the APA appointed a task force to prepare DSM-IV. The reason provided for revision of DSM-III-R, only one year after its publication, was to maintain consistency with ICD codes in accordance with a new WHO ICD manual (ICD-10) and the treaty binding the United States to maintain consistency with updated ICD codes [14]. The APA appointed Allen Francis, a psychoanalyst from New York who had worked on the personality disorders section of DSM-III, as the DSM-IV task force chair. Although DSM-III relied mostly on expert opinion for writing criteria for diagnoses, the DSM-IV task force adopted a new approach by examining as much research data as possible to critically review DSM diagnoses [15]. For the first time, field trials of proposed diagnostic criteria were conducted and consisted of surveys and reliability studies. The National Institute of Mental Health (NIMH) also sponsored research to examine proposed alternative diagnostic criteria [16]. In addition to DSM-IV, five Source Books were published that included the literature reviews conducted, the data reanalysis, and summarized outcomes of the field trials. Although almost every diagnosis contained some minor adjustments, DSM-IV made only a few significant changes to DSM-III-R [17]. For example, the term "cognitive disorders" was used to replace the term "organic disorders" to avoid the implication that other disorders, that is, depression and schizophrenia, were not organic in etiology. A few diagnoses were added (e.g., Rhett Disorder, Asperger's Disorder, Bipolar II Disorder, Narcolepsy, and some others), and a small number of diagnoses were removed (e.g., passive-aggressive personality disorder and some others). Modifications in the multiaxial system included removing pervasive developmental disorders and learning disorders from Axis II and placing them instead under Axis I. The GAF scale was expanded to a 100-point scale instead of ending at 90 points [15].

The APA made the decision to update the text associated with each diagnosis in DSM-IV to reflect research conducted from 1992 to 1998. To prevent DSM-IV from being considered a revision, the manual was called DSM-IV-TR for "Text Revision." Some changes were made to the "associated features" sections that included subsections on associated laboratory findings, features, and other epidemiological information. Minor changes were made to the wording of diagnostic criteria for pervasive developmental disorders, tic disorders, and paraphilias along with changes to the designation of dementias complicated by mood disorders [18].

DSM-5'S DEVELOPMENT

The revision of DSM-IV-TR began in 1999 when the DSM-5 Research Planning Conference was convened in 1999 to set research priorities. The conference was a joint initiative of the APA and the NIMH. These organizations' combined goal was to delineate the most current scientific basis for psychiatric diagnosis and taxonomy. Under their joint sponsorship, participants included experts in basic and clinical neurosciences, genetics, cognitive and behavioral science, developmental neuroscience, and psychology. Through this process, participants recognized the need for a series of white papers that could guide future research and promote further discussion, covering over-arching topic areas that cut across many psychiatric disorders. Work groups were created, including groups covering developmental issues, gaps in the current system, disability and impairment, neuroscience, nomenclature, and cross-cultural issues [19].

In 2000, the NIMH recruited Darrel A. Regier, MD, MPH, to serve as the research director for the APA and to coordinate the development of DSM-5. In July and October of 2000, conferences were held to organize the DSM-5 research agenda, nominate the work group membership, and hold the first face-to-face meetings to organize the DSM-5 drafting process. These groups, which included liaisons from the National Institutes of Health (NIH) and the international psychiatric community, published a series of six white papers in 2000: "A Research Agenda for DSM-5" [1]. A second series of white papers entitled "Age and Gender Considerations in Psychiatric Diagnosis" was commissioned and published by the APA in 2007 [20].

Preparation and planning for DSM-5

In 2002, the American Psychiatric Institute for Research and Education (APIRE), with Executive Director Darrel A. Regier, MD, MPH, as the Principal Investigator, applied for a grant from the NIMH to implement a series of research planning conferences that would focus on the scientific evidence for revisions of specific diagnostic areas in the DSM. NIMH approved a $1.1 million cooperative agreement grant with support provided by NIMH, the National Institute on Drug Abuse (NIDA), and the National Institute on Alcoholism and Alcohol Abuse (NIAAA). Under the leadership of a steering committee comprising individuals from APIRE, the three NIH institutes, and the WHO, 13 conferences were held from 2004 to 2008. A significant international contingent participated with approximately 50% of the 397 attendees coming from outside of the United States. The participants wrote papers reviewing the literature to address specific diagnostic questions, and from these papers and the conference proceedings, a research agenda was developed. Those involved also published conference findings in peer-reviewed journals and American Psychiatric Publishing, Inc. (APPI) monographs [19].

DSM-5 workgroups

In 2006, APA President Dr. Steven Sharfstein announced Dr. Kupfer as chair and Dr. Regier as vice-chair of the task force to oversee the development of DSM-5. The APA appointed additional members to the task force, including the appointment of chairs of the diagnostic work groups who were responsible for reviewing the research and literature base to form the content for DSM-5. These task force nominees were reviewed for potential conflicts of interest, approved by the APA Board of Trustees, and announced in 2007. In turn, the work group chairs, together with the task force chair and vice-chair, recommended nominees widely viewed as leading experts in their field, who were then formally nominated as members of the work groups. All work group members were also reviewed for potential conflicts of interest, approved by the APA Board, and were announced in 2008. From 2007 until the end of 2012, each work group met regularly to review DSM-IV-TR's strengths and weaknesses and to conduct thorough investigations of literature reviews and analyses of existing data. Based on their comprehensive review of scientific advancements, research analyses, and clinical expertise, the work groups developed draft DSM-5 diagnostic criteria [19].

DSM-5 field trials

DSM-5 field trials were conducted to evaluate the clinical utility and feasibility of the proposed diagnoses and dimensional measures. Where possible, the field trials also sought to estimate the reliability and the validity of the proposed diagnoses and dimensional measures in the clinical settings where they would be utilized [21]. The field trial results were intended to inform DSM-5 decision-making process, but, in and of themselves, the results alone did not determine inclusion or exclusion of diagnoses in the final manual. The trials were conducted over a 7- to 10-month time period at 11 sites (six adult and four pediatric sites) in the United States and one adult site in Canada [21].

The main objective of the field trials was to determine the degree to which two clinicians would agree on the same diagnosis for patients. In a similar process used for DSM-III field trials, DSM-5 field trials were designed, conducted, and analyzed centrally to avoid any biases associated with the work groups assessing their own work [21]. Overall, 7789 patients were screened across the 11 field trial sites during the study period (5128 in adult sites combined and 2661 in pediatric sites combined). Of these, 4110 patients were eligible and participated (N = 2791 and 1319 across the adult and pediatric sites, respectively) [21]. Participating clinicians included board-certified psychiatrists, resident psychiatrist trainees, licensed clinical and counseling psychologists and neuropsychologists (i.e., doctorate-level training), master's-level counselors, licensed clinical social workers, and advanced practice licensed mental health nurses. DSM-5 field trials attempted to recruit diverse clinical patient populations across multiple sites and used clinicians of various mental health disciplines. In reality, most of the field trial sites were large academic centers, leading some professionals to voice concerns that the field trial results would not be as applicable to community-based practice settings.

Although outlining the specific results of DSM-5 field trials is beyond the scope of this chapter, the results of the field trials were published in three major articles in the *American Journal of Psychiatry* in 2013 [21–23]. In the data from the field trials, 14 of the 23 adult or child psychiatric diagnoses had "very good" or "good" reliability. DSM-5 Field Trials were designed to obtain measures of the kappa statistic, the degree to which two clinicians could independently agree on the presence or absence of selected DSM-5 diagnoses when the same patient was interviewed on separate occasions in clinical settings. "Very good" reliability was denoted by a kappa measure of 0.60–0.79 and a "good" reliability was indicated by a kappa measure of 0.40–0.59. Autism spectrum disorder and attention deficit hyperactivity disorder (ADHD) in children and posttraumatic stress disorder and binge-eating disorder in adults were among the disorders with "very good" or "good" reliability.

Narrow et al. [23] also reported data on "cross-cutting symptoms," symptoms that appear across many psychiatric disorders. Cross-cutting symptoms were generally found to have good to excellent reliability. Six of the diagnoses had relatively low reliability scores, which the report characterized as "questionable" but acceptable; among these were two of the most common psychiatric diagnoses: major depressive disorder and generalized anxiety disorder. Responding to questions about this surprising finding, Task Force Chair David Kupfer, MD, stated

> We believe at least some of the reason why the scores were not at the level of previous field trials is the attention we devoted to new diagnoses and criteria sets that are often comorbid with depression and anxiety. Moreover, depression and anxiety represent symptom clusters that can fluctuate during several weeks, and the rigorous trial design of the field trials—employing a test-retest design requiring two separate clinicians to evaluate the same patient on different days—may have contributed to a lower reliability score than was found in previous field trials [24 (p1)].

The two diagnoses that fell into the "unacceptable" reliability category, mixed anxiety-depressive disorder and nonsuicidal self-injury, were removed or included in Section III, respectively. DSM-5 was released in May 2013 at APA's Annual Meeting.

Structural changes in DSM-5

DSM-5 made significant overarching structural changes to the nomenclature of descriptive psychiatry. The stated goal was to create a framework for the evolution of psychiatry to advance clinical practice and facilitate ongoing research of mental disorders. DSM-5 was conceptualized from the beginning as "a living document" that would have a revision infrastructure to readily incorporate new scientific evidence as it is replicated and reviewed [25]. Overarching structural changes to psychiatric nomenclature in DSM-5 included the following: integration of dimensional aspects of diagnosis; removal of the multiaxial system; removal of the Global Assessment of Functioning (GAF) scale; removal of the "Not Otherwise Specified" specifier; and the addition of cross-cutting measures [26]. There were also changes in the names of some disorders that largely reflected the interests of consumer advocate organizations and/or the need to align DSM-5 language with the anticipated ICD-11 language. For example, the term "mental retardation" was revised to the name "intellectual disability" in response to both consumer advocacy interests and to match language proposed for ICD-11 [27].

Dimensional approaches to classification

The most prominent overarching development in DSM-5 was the incorporation of dimensional measures for assessing syndromes within diagnostic categories and assessing symptoms that cross previously strict categorical diagnostic boundaries. The movement toward a dimensional approach to psychiatric diagnosis and away from a categorical, or binary, classification reflects the research methodologies of the past 30 years that have generally used dimensional measures to ascertain the severity of mental disorders and treatment response [28]. Although DSM-IV-TR states "there is no assumption that each category of mental disorder is a completely discrete entity with absolute boundaries dividing it from other disorders" [16 (p. xxxi)], the use of categorical diagnosis inevitably conveyed the idea that psychiatric disorders are discrete illnesses. Ultimately, DSM-5 continued to rely on categorical diagnosis; however, the use of specifiers, severity ratings, and cross cutting measures (discussed below) was intended to emphasize a spectrum-based concept of mental disorders beyond the strict categorical approach that dominated DSM-IV.

DSM's historical linking with the WHO's ICD in many ways reinforced the emphasis on the use of a typology of mental disorders. In other branches of medicine, classification of diseases has typically utilized typologies. This classification approach is due, in part, to the historical assumption that most diseases are discrete entities that have identifiable discrete causative factors. Driven by the biomedical model, psychiatrists have also historically assumed that mental disorders were discrete entities that could be attributed to a causative factor and teased out from each other and from normality. For a very small number of disorders (e.g., Down's syndrome, Huntington's disease, Alzheimer's disease, etc), this theory proved to be true. Nevertheless,

DSM-5 authors cited that in the past 20 years since DSM-IV, evidence has accumulated that most mental disorders are a spectrum that merge into each other and into normality with no distinct boundaries. Researchers increasingly characterized the categorical system of psychiatric diagnosis as "fundamentally flawed" [29].

Ultimately, DSM-5 adopted a modified categorical system. In a truly dimensional classification system, no discrete categories would be present. In consideration of moving to a fully dimensional approach, the drafters noted that clinical management of patients demanded prompt treatment decisions that are easier when patients are allocated to a categorical diagnosis as opposed to a more complex dimensional conceptualization. Critics early on noted that most of the strong advocates of a totally dimensional diagnostic system in the planning stage of the DSM-5 were not practicing clinicians [1]. The consideration of a new and fully dimensional system for the diagnosis of personality disorders gained the most traction but was eventually voted down. Based on feedback from a multilevel review of proposed revisions, the APA ultimately retained the categorical approach with the same 10 personality disorders. A hybrid dimensional-categorical system for diagnosing personality disorders was included as an "alternative model" in Section III of the manual under the heading "Conditions for Further Study."

Cross-cutting measures

Clinical and epidemiological research has demonstrated that a major limitation of the categorical system of psychiatric diagnosis is the failure to recognize the reality that symptoms of different diagnoses commonly cross discrete diagnostic boundaries. For example, sleep disturbance, somatic symptoms, and anxiety and mood problems are frequently seen together in various combinations regardless of categorical diagnosis [30]. DSM-5 drafters noted that the relevance of such "cross-cutting" symptoms is commonly observed in clinical practice. In this setting, clinicians use categorical diagnoses not only for treatment planning and reporting but also to treat impactful symptoms that are not reflected in the formal diagnosis. With the increased utilization of patient health questionnaires (PHQs) and patient-reported outcomes to justify diagnostic and treatment decisions for third-party payers, the systematic measurement of common cross-cutting symptoms was proposed as a first step toward assessments that incorporate levels of symptom frequency and intensity instead of psychiatric diagnoses that rely primarily on strict categorical descriptions [25].

Section III of DSM-5 includes a number of "emerging measures." These assessment measures are administered at the initial patient encounter and used to monitor treatment progress. The cross-cutting symptom measures are designed to draw clinical attention to symptoms in a variety of domains that are important across categorical diagnostic boundaries. Section III also includes disorder-specific severity measures for individuals with a diagnosis or who have clinically significant symptoms that are subthreshold for making a diagnosis. The severity assessments include both patient self-report and clinician-report measures.

DSM-5 authors suggested that the use of cross-cutting measures will promote dimensional conceptualization of psychiatric symptoms in four key areas. First, clinical care will be improved by identifying potentially missed symptoms, particularly in complicated presentations of psychiatric disorders that have important prognostic implications, for example, major depressive disorder with concurrent anxiety or insomnia. DSM-5 provides additional specifiers as one means to lower the rate of "spurious comorbidity" that resulted from the requirement of multiple diagnoses for various symptoms under DSM-IV's more strictly categorical scheme. For example, under DSM-IV diagnostic scheme, individuals with a major depressive disorder with co-occurring anxiety could be diagnosed with both a depressive and anxiety disorder or with the designation "not otherwise specified" [25]. Second, identification of cross-cutting symptoms, in addition to making a more dimensional diagnosis, is anticipated to help clinicians justify treatment decisions in the climate of measurement-based healthcare. Third, clinical research may also benefit from the assessment of cross-cutting symptoms by more specifically delineating the course and treatment of various combinations of categorical diagnoses and cross-cutting symptoms. Finally, DSM-5 cross-cutting measures represent the first systematic attempt to capture the patient's subjective experience of their symptoms in the DSM (by patient questionnaire assessments), recognizing the importance of the patient-reported experience as the foundation of psychiatry [31].

The removal of the axial system

The purpose of a multiaxial system of diagnosis is to articulate comprehensively the fundamental components of an illness and to formulate the patient's whole clinical condition. In psychiatry, these purposes motivated the earliest multiaxial diagnostic systems. Several versions of a multiaxial system of diagnosis to were published prior to the DSM but the concept did not gain widespread acceptance [32]. DSM-III introduced the widely recognized five axis system of psychiatric diagnosis. The clinical assessment was organized into five areas, or axes, addressing the different aspects and impact of disorders.

DSM-5 moved from the multiaxial system to a new assessment nomenclature that removes the boundaries among personality disorders, intellectual functioning, and other mental disorders. DSM-III introduced the multiaxial system in part to highlight certain disorders such as personality disorders that were thought to receive inadequate clinical and research focus. As a consequence, these disorders were designated to Axis II to ensure they received greater attention. Although initially conceptualized primarily as a way of distinguishing between state and trait (i.e., Axis I and Axis II), the past 20 years of research since DSM-IV revealed no clear fundamental difference in the level of distress, frequency of presentation to treatment settings, or impairment derived from disorders based on whether they were described on Axis I versus Axis II. Therefore, DSM-5 shifted to a single axis system. The new system combines the first three axes outlined in past editions of DSM into one axis with all mental and relevant medical diagnoses. Combining the mental health and medical diagnoses removes the axial distinction between medical and psychiatric conditions to theoretically facilitate clinical practice and research.

The removal of the GAF scale

The GAF scale was used on Axis V in DSM-IV for "reporting the clinician's judgment of the individual's overall level of functioning" [17 (p30)]. The addition of the GAF in DSM-IV can be seen as the DSM's first major attempt at a dimensional approach to communicating conditions or levels of severity that are conceptualized as continuous and without clear boundaries between psychopathology and normality. The GAF, numerically coded from 0 to 100, combines assessment of symptom severity, danger to self or others, and markers of self-care and social functioning into a gestalt numerical score. Many third-party payers have used the GAF score to determine medical necessity for treatment and eligibility for short- and long-term disability compensation. However, two concerns have been noted about the use of a GAF score to describe levels of functioning for individuals with mental disorders. First, insufficient empirical evidence supports the utility of a single GAF score because the components of the GAF score may vary independently over time. Markedly different components of a single GAF score include the severity of symptoms, danger to self or others, and functional impairment. Second, proper use of the GAF requires specific training in order for the measure to have good reliability in clinical practice [33].

The GAF was eliminated from DSM-5 and was accompanied by the introduction (in the DSM) of The World Health Organization Disability Assessment Schedule (WHODAS 2.0). Based on the International Classification of Functioning, Disability, and Health (ICF), the WHODAS 2.0 was judged by the DSM-5 Disability Work Group to be the best current measure of disability for routine clinical use. The WHODAS 2.0 assesses an individual's abilities in six domains of activity: understanding and communicating; getting around; self-care; getting along with people; life activities (e.g., work/school/daily living tasks); and participation in society. The WHODAS is a self- or informant-administered instrument.

Developed in 1998, research on the use of the WHODAS provided support for its utilization as an international instrument to measure disability based on the ICF model [34]. The WHODAS 2.0 is applicable to patients with any health condition. The WHODAS 2.0 was selected to help bring DSM-5 into greater alignment with general medical disciplines by promoting the use of an assessment instrument for disability due to mental disorders that can also be used for assessing disability related to general medical conditions, thereby decreasing the separation of mental health from other health problems. The metric properties of the WHODAS-2 have been evaluated in numerous international studies, including research examining its use in samples of patients with chronic neuropsychiatric disorders such as schizophrenia, Huntington's disease, and depression [35–40]. DSM-5 field trials utilized the WHODAS 2.0 and reported its use was feasible and reliable in routine psychiatric evaluations. The WHODAS 2.0 is included in DSM5's section III as an emerging measure and model. Although its use is not required to make a DSM-5 diagnosis, its selection is consistent with WHO initiatives to move toward a clear conceptual distinction between the disorders contained in the ICD and the disabilities resulting from disorders [35].

Disability evaluations are the most common psychiatric evaluation requested for a nontreatment reason. For the forensic psychiatrist, evaluations that answer questions about disability typically provide information to an organization or a system to guide actions and aid decision-making. The American Academy of Psychiatry and the Law [AAPL] Practice Guideline for the Forensic Evaluation of Psychiatric Disability recommends that the use of rating scales may be helpful in qualifying disability. However, when these guidelines were written in 2008, they specifically noted the limitations inherent in using the GAF [41]. Gold et al. [41] noted that the GAF score blends psychological symptoms with social, academic, and occupational functioning. As a result, the relative effects of physical and mental impairment are nearly impossible to untangle from the single numerical GAF score.

The WHODAS 2.0 provides an alternative to the GAF. However, because the WHODAS 2.0 is a self-report instrument, the evaluator will need to utilize other methods to assess for malingering or feigning of reported symptoms in disability evaluations that have issues of secondary gain if they chose to use the WHODAS 2.0. Conversely, if the evaluator uses the WHODAS 2.0 in compulsory disability examinations, such as fitness for duty evaluations, the evaluator will need to evaluate for the possibility of "reverse malingering" (e.g., feigning wellness), because the evaluee may underreport their impairments in order to maintain their job [42]. The WHODAS 2.0 also has a proxy version that allows a collateral informant to rate the person being evaluated. Although this additional information may prove useful in forensic examinations, the same concerns about valid responses noted for the self-report version also apply to third parties who may have an invested interest in how impairments are rated. A thorough mental status examination and collateral information correlated with the patient's self-report, whether in clinical interview or via a rating scale such as the WHODAS, will be essential to achieve the most accurate assessment of functional impairment.

Removal of "Not Otherwise Specified"

The frequent use of the "Not Otherwise Specified" (NOS) designation was seen as a major problem to be addressed in DSM-5 [1]. The DSM-5 authors commented that clinicians over utilized the NOS designation as a "catch all" to denote clusters of symptoms that did not formally meet diagnostic criteria for any defined disorder. Variable and unreliable information about patient symptomatology resulted. DSM-5 sought to improve the psychiatric diagnostic nomenclature by replacing the NOS categories with two reportedly more precise diagnostic options: "other specified disorder" and "unspecified disorder." The "other specified disorder" designation allows the clinician to specify the reason that the criteria for a specific disorder are not met. The "unspecified disorder" designation allows the clinician to describe the clinical symptoms present but forgo specifying, or referring to, any particular mental disorder [28].

ETHICAL ISSUES AND THE USE OF DSM-5

The "imperfect fit" between a DSM diagnosis and the legal setting brings with it important ethical considerations for the psychiatrist and specifically, the forensic psychiatrist. The DSM has always been accompanied by some controversy regarding the appropriate application and meaning of diagnostic criteria, particularly in the legal setting. An ethical foundation for psychiatry in the legal system has been advanced by the seminal work of Paul Appelbaum, MD. Appelbaum [43, 44] articulated the legal principle of truth so important to courts is often at odds with the primary principle of beneficence that is required of the treating clinician towards patients. Furthermore, an individual involved in a legal matter is seeking to resolve a legal problem in contrast to a "patient" who is seeking to solve a medical problem [45]. From an ethical perspective, the forensic psychiatrist utilizing the DSM to diagnose a mental disorder in the context of answering a legal question is, in the end, assisting the court in resolving a legal matter and not a medical one. Nevertheless, the ethical use of DSM-5 in court relies on the forensic evaluator as both expert and educator in explaining the relationship (or lack thereof) of a DSM diagnosis to the relevant functional capacity and/or mental state in question. To gather and objectively present the relevant data as accurately and unbiased as possible, protecting the truth of the forensic opinion from both sides of the legal argument should be the goal of the ethical forensic psychiatrist in court [46]. The ethical guidelines of the major professional organizations for psychiatry and forensic psychiatry do not provide clear guidance on the use of the DSM in court or the ethics of testifying about some diagnoses that may have controversial reliability. For example, the American Psychiatric Association ethics procedures, Principles of Medical Ethics With Annotations Applicable Especially to Psychiatry, emphasizes the responsibility of forensic examiners to fully describe "the nature and purpose and lack of confidentiality" of forensic examinations to the examinee but does not make any explicit reference to the ethics of diagnosis or the use of the DSM in the legal setting [47].

CAUTIONARY STATEMENT FOR FORENSIC USE OF DSM-5

The use of DSM in the legal system has been an important area of concern. Courts in both civil and criminal proceedings frequently rely upon the DSM. In addition, DSM diagnostic guidelines are often utilized in state and federal statutes that define mental illness [48]. DSM-III contained the first explicit reference to concerns about the use of the DSM in legal settings. The DSM-III authors write: "... The use of this manual for non-clinical purposes, such as determinations of legal responsibility, competency or insanity, or justification for third-party payment, must be critically examined in each instance within the appropriate institutional context" [9 (p12)]. In 1987, DSM-III-R expanded the admonishment about the use of the manual in legal proceedings with the following statement:

> ... It is to be understood that inclusion here, for clinical and research purposes, of a diagnostic category such as Pathological Gambling or Pedophilia does not imply that the condition meets legal or other nonmedical criteria for what constitutes mental disease, mental disorder, or mental disability. The clinical and scientific considerations involved in categorization of these conditions as mental disorders may not be wholly relevant to legal judgments, for example, that take into account such issues as responsibility, disability determination, and competency..." [13 (pxxix)]

DSM-IV-TR authors provide an even stronger cautionary statement about the use of the DSM in the legal arena when they write: "The clinical and scientific considerations involved in the categorization of these conditions mental disorders may not be wholly relevant to legal judgments, for example, that take into account such issues as individual responsibility, disability determination, and competency" [18 (pxxxvii)].

While taking into consideration the cautionary words about the potential misuse of the DSM when applied for forensic purposes, psychiatrists and other mental health professionals testify in a wide variety of legal proceedings and routinely use the DSM to support their diagnostic conclusions. Lawyers and judges refer to the DSM to verify the foundation of expert witness testimony and may use DSM criteria to define mental disorders and identify functional impairment. The DSM has been cited in more than 5500 court opinions and over 320 times in legislation [48]. Attorneys seeking to discredit an expert witness may cite the cautionary statement regarding forensic application of the DSM and shifting medical opinion reflected in the historical changes to the diagnostic nomenclature. One reasonable answer to challenges on cross-examination of the DSM's use as a diagnostic tool is that the DSM is a living document that is continually and purposefully changing to reflect advances in medical science, and, although not perfect, the DSM is the best currently available accepted diagnostic scheme.

In the DSM-5 for the first time, the cautionary statement for the forensic use of DSM contains inclusion of language explicitly affirming the use of the DSM for courts and attorneys. Notably, the discussion of the forensic use of the manual is given its own section and an expanded discussion when compared to DSM-IV-TR. The DSM-5 cautionary statement reads: "Although the DSM-5 diagnostic criteria and text are primarily designed to assist clinicians in conducting clinical assessment, case formulation, and treatment planning, the DSM-5 is also used as a reference for the courts and attorneys in assessing the forensic consequences of mental disorders..." The authors affirm that when used appropriately, the diagnostic information can "assist legal decision makers in making their determinations..." [26 (p25)].

DSM-5 discusses the risk that diagnostic information will be misused or misunderstood and is discussed as is "imperfect fit" between the ultimate issues of the law and the information conveyed by a clinical psychiatric diagnosis. The importance of assessing an individual's functional impairments and how these impairments affect different abilities is emphasized. Last, alluding to evaluations of a person's mental state as related to their behavior, DSM-5 emphasizes "...even when diminished control over one's behavior is a feature of the disorder, having the disorder itself does not demonstrate that a particular individual is (was) unable to control his or her behavior at a particular time..." [26 (p25)].

Overall, the expanded commentary in DSM-5 regarding the forensic use of the manual offers a more balanced stance on the place of the DSM in the legal arena. The statement acknowledges both the potential helpfulness of the DSM in the courts as well as the potential limitations and risks. Forensic experts should become familiar with the new cautionary statement language because defense of one's reliance on the DSM under cross-examination may be aided by the new explicit affirmation that there is a settled and appropriate role for the DSM in legal determinations.

PSYCHIATRIC DIAGNOSIS AND LITIGATION

Legal challenges to DSM-5

The DSM has been widely accepted and relied upon in the legal system in both civil and criminal proceedings [48]. Legal challenges to the appropriate use of the DSM in court have been made based on prior DSM's cautionary statement. For example, in *Discepolo v. Gorgone* (2005), the US District Court for the District of Connecticut found that the cautionary wording in the DSM "appears to pertain to conclusions of law such as competence or criminal responsibility, and therefore is not applicable [in civil proceedings]" [49 (p130)]. Interestingly, this court distinguished between the use of the DSM in civil versus criminal proceedings and affirmed the use of DSM in civil litigation based on the lack of specific reference to civil proceedings in DSM-IV-TR's cautionary statement. As of 2012, *Discepolo v. Gorgone* had been cited in 29 other court proceedings to support the argument that the DSM is acceptable to rely upon in civil proceedings [50]. In *State v. Lockhart*, expert testimony on the subject of Dissociative Identity Disorder (DID) was excluded in criminal court based on the cautionary statement in the DSM. However, the Supreme Court of Appeals of West Virginia found that the trial court erred in excluding the testimony related to an insanity plea, finding that the inclusion of DID in the DSM reflected current consensus in the field [51]. In *State v. Galloway*, the New Jersey Supreme Court also noted the cautionary statement in the DSM, but it affirmed the use of a DSM diagnosis (in this case, borderline personality disorder) to establish diminished capacity [52].

The appropriate use of the DSM to establish the presence or absence of a diagnosis has also been litigated extensively from both sides of the argument. For example, in civil commitment proceedings, virtually all state statutes require proof of a mental disorder, disease or defect as a predicate condition for commitment. However, most states define mental illness by descriptive language and do not require a DSM diagnosis per se. In the 1965 case *Dodd v. Hughes*, a petitioner diagnosed as a "sociopath" challenged his commitment, arguing that mental illness in the Nevada legislation meant a psychotic reaction as classified in the DSM. His appeal was denied by Supreme Court of Nevada. In explaining their ruling, the court writes:

> . . . We seriously doubt that the legislature ever intended medical classifications to be the sole guide for judicial commitment. The judicial inquiry is not

to be limited so as to exclude the totality of circumstances involved in the particular case before the court... The assistance of medical examination and opinion is a necessary concomitant of the court hearing, but the court alone is invested with the power of decision. That power is to be exercised within the permissible limits of judicial discretion" [53 (p1)]

In this statement, the Nevada Supreme Court clearly articulated the importance of expert testimony to assist the trier of fact, but ultimately noted the prerogative of the court to consider all of the factors relevant to the judicial decision, above and beyond medical and/or psychiatric classification.

The case of Clark v. Arizona

In the case of *Clark v. Arizona* (2006), the United States Supreme Court issued a cautionary statement acknowledging that certain designations in the DSM may suggest "that a defendant suffering from a recognized mental disease lacks cognitive, moral, volitional, or other capacity, when that may not be a sound conclusion at all." [54 (p35)]. The Supreme Court spoke to the dangers of testimony related to diagnoses being misunderstood and/or misapplied by juries. In the wake of *Clark v. Arizona*, various courts have grappled with how mental disorders should be defined. Some state courts have struggled in how to articulate the relationship between a diagnosed mental illness and the legal standard of mental disease or defect [55]. With the controversies regarding the scientific reliability of some of the DSM-5 diagnoses, the acceptability of the DSM-5 in court may face challenges similar to those posed by previous editions.

The DSM's admissibility as evidence in court

In the 1923 case *Frye v. United States*, the D.C. Circuit Court of Appeals held that evidence could be admitted in court only if "the thing from which the deduction is made" is "sufficiently established to have gained general acceptance in the particular field in which it belongs" [56 (p1)]. Essentially, the Frye test involves a two-step analysis: (1) defining the relevant scientific community; and (2) evaluating the testimony and publications to determine the existence of a general consensus in the field. Over the years, legal scholars have argued the proper scope and application of the *Frye test*, also known as the "general acceptance" test.

Daubert v. Merrell Dow Pharmaceuticals (1993) is a United States Supreme Court case that determined the standard for admitting expert testimony and scientific reliability in federal courts [57]. In *Daubert*, the plaintiffs successfully argued that after Congress adopted the Federal Rules of Evidence in 1975, *Frye* was no longer the governing standard for admitting scientific evidence in trials held in federal courts. The Supreme Court agreed and cited Rule 702 of the Federal Rules of Evidence which reads: "If scientific, technical, or other specialized knowledge will assist the trier of fact to understand the evidence or to determine a fact in issue, a witness qualified as an expert by knowledge, skill, experience, training, or education, may testify thereto in the form of an opinion or otherwise" [58].

Experts will find it helpful to know what standard the court is using to determine the admissibility of expert testimony. If the case is in Federal Court, then the *Daubert* standard always applies. However, in state court the standard for admissibility of expert testimony varies. Since *Daubert*, some states continue to apply *Frye* and others have explicitly rejected *Frye* and adopted the *Daubert* standard or a similar test. Previous versions of the DSM have been widely accepted by the courts as satisfying both *Daubert* and *Frye* criteria. The criteria established by *Daubert* articulated four basic criteria. The four criteria are as follows: general acceptability; established standards controlling the technique's operation and accuracy; a known or potentially known rate of error; and the testability of the procedure. DSM diagnoses have been tested and reviewed based on evidence from research. In terms of general acceptability, many of the DSM-5 diagnoses have been widely peer-reviewed and articulated published literature. However, some DSM-5 diagnoses are likely more controversial than others and may not be uniformly accepted by all practitioners. In addition, whether or not proposed "conditions for further study" listed in DSM-5's Section III have met "general acceptability" in the field and meet *Daubert* and *Frye* standards has yet to be established. However, the fact that these proposed conditions were determined by the DSM-5 Task Force as not sufficiently reliable or valid to warrant inclusion as a mental disorder in Section II raises likely and justified questions about their admissibility in a legal setting.

Considering the *Daubert* criteria of known error rates, standards for quality control and accuracy and testability, the field trials established good interrater reliability for some diagnoses but yielded less sufficient interrater reliability for others, including the common diagnosis of major depressive disorder. However, because other factors in addition to interrater reliability were considered in determining those disorders to include as an official DSM-5 diagnosis, most Section II DSM-5 diagnoses will likely meet both the *Daubert* and Frye standards.

The history of legal challenges to the DSM-IV-TR may foreshadow future challenges to the DSM-5. Despite the *Clark* Court's cautionary statement about using the DSM-IV-TR, many states continued to find that the DSM-IV-TR was acceptable and admissible in civil and criminal proceedings [50]. Diagnoses in the DSM-IV-TR rarely failed to meet the threshold requirements for reliability, validity, and admissibility. The New Jersey Supreme Court, while citing the United States Supreme Court's language from *Clark v. Arizona*, noted that the DSM-IV-TR does not necessarily determine a defendant's capacity. Nevertheless, this same court ruled that the DSM-IV-TR was admissible as evidence and appropriate in reaching a final determination [59]. Similarly, the Supreme Court of Appeals of West Virginia held that regardless of the warning issued by the United States Supreme Court in *Clark*, the DSM-IV-TR meets the *Daubert* test for admissibility of expert evidence and that the inclusion of a disorder in the DSM reflects general acceptance by the psychiatric community [50].

In *Mancuso v. Consol. Edison* (1997), the DSM-IV-TR was used in a legal argument to contest the admission of mental health evidence on the grounds that the diagnosis did not rely on the DSM and therefore did not satisfy *Daubert* [60]. With the advent of DSM-5 and with the introduction of possible assessment instruments such as the WHODAS 2.0, courts and psychiatrists may face future legal challenges to test whether this most current edition meets court admissibility standards. DSM-5 may also face legal challenges in the future. It is likely that the manual's utility will ultimately weigh in favor of its continued use as a valuable resource for both experts and litigants in the courtroom.

SUMMARY

For more than 60 years, the DSM has provided the standard language used by mental health clinicians of various disciplines, public health policy makers, and mental health researchers. Like all preceding editions of the DSM, the development of the 5th Edition of the DSM attracted considerable controversy, criticism, and a robust debate about the meaning and nomenclature of the diagnosis of mental disorders. Key points regarding the development and implementation of DSM-5 highlighted in this chapter include the following:

- Overarching structural changes to psychiatric nomenclature in DSM-5 included the integration of dimensional aspects of diagnosis; the removal of the multiaxial system; the removal of the GAF; the removal of the "Not Otherwise Specified" specifier; and the addition of cross-cutting symptom measures.
- Despite legal challenges, the DSM is widely accepted and relied upon in the legal system in both civil and criminal proceedings.
- In the past, the DSM has been widely accepted by the courts to satisfy both *Daubert* and *Frye* criteria. Despite current controversies surrounding the DSM-5, this new manual will likely remain a diagnostic cornerstone in future legal arenas.

REFERENCES

1. Kupfer DJ, First MB, Regier DA. *A Research Agenda for DSM-5*. 1st ed. Arlington, VA: American Psychiatric Association, 2002: pp 31–72.
2. First MB. Paradigm shifts and the development of the diagnostic and statistical manual of mental disorders: past experiences and future aspirations. *Can J Psychiatry* 2010; 55:692–700.
3. Kupfer DJ, Regier DA. Neuroscience, clinical evidence, and the future of psychiatric classification in DSM-5. *Am J Psychiatry* 2011; 168:672–674.
4. Wanke P. American military psychiatry and its role among ground forces in World War II. *J Mil History* 1999; 63:127–146.
5. Grob GN. Origins of DSM-I: A study in appearance and reality. *Am J Psychiatry* 1991;148:421-431.
6. American Psychiatric Association. *Diagnostic and Statistical Manual, Mental Disorders*. Washington, D.C.: American Psychiatric Association; 1952.
7. Fischer BA. A review of American psychiatry through its diagnoses: the history and development of the Diagnostic and Statistical Manual of Mental Disorders. *J Nerv Ment Dis* 2012; 200:1022–1030.
8. American Psychiatric Association. *Diagnostic and Statistical Manual of Mental Disorders*. 2nd ed. Washington, D.C.: American Psychiatric Association; 1968.
9. American Psychiatric Association. *Diagnostic and Statistical Manual of Mental Disorders*. 3rd ed. Washington, D.C.: American Psychiatric Association; 1980.
10. Feighner JP, Robins E, Guze SB, et al. Diagnostic criteria for use in psychiatric research. *Arch Gen Psychiatry* 1972; 26:57–63.
11. Kendler KS, Munoz RA, Murphy G. The development of the Feighner Criteria: a historical perspective. *Am J Psychiatry* 2009; 167:134–142.
12. Williams JW, Spitzer MD. Research diagnostic criteria and DSM-III. *Arch Gen Psychiatry* 1982; 39:1283–1289.
13. American Psychiatric Association. *Diagnostic and Statistical Manual of Mental Disorders*. 3rd ed Revision. Washington, D.C.: American Psychiatric Association, 1987.
14. Zimmerman M, Spitzer RL. Classification in psychiatry. In: Sadock BJ, Sadock VA, eds. *Kaplan and Sadock's comprehensive textbook of psychiatry*. 8th ed. Philadelphia, PA: Lippencott Williams & Wilkins; 2005: pp 1003–1052.
15. Francis AJ, Widiger TA, Pincus HA. The development of DSM-IV. *Arch Gen Psychiatry* 1989; 46:373–375.
16. Widgier TA, Frances AJ, Pincus HA, et al. Toward an empirical classification for the DSM-IV. *J Abnorm Psychiatry* 1991; 100:280–288.
17. American Psychiatric Association. *Diagnostic and Statistical Manual of Mental Disorders*. 4th ed. Washington, D.C.: American Psychiatric Association, 1994.
18. American Psychiatric Association. *Diagnostic and Statistical Manual of Mental Disorders*. 4th ed Text Revision. Washington, D.C.: American Psychiatric Association, 2000.
19. DSM-5 Overview: The Future Manual. American Psychiatric Association Web site. Available at: http://www.dsm5.org/about/pages/dsmvoverview.aspx. Accessed 12 December 2013.
20. Narrow MD, First MB, Sirovatka MS, et al. *Age and Gender Considerations in Psychiatric Diagnosis*. Arlington, VA: American Psychiatric Publishing; 2007.

21. Clarke DE, Narrow WE, Regier DA, et al. Field Trials in the United States and Canada, Part I: study design, sampling strategy, implementation, and analytic approaches. *Am J Psychiatry* 2013; 170:43–58.
22. Regier DA, Narrow WE, Clarke DE, et al. DSM-5 Field Trials in the United States and Canada, Part II: test-retest reliability of selected categorical diagnoses. *Am J Psychiatry* 2013; 170:59–70.
23. Narrow WE, Clarke DE, Kuramoto SJ. DSM-5 Field Trials in the United States and Canada, Part III: development and reliability of a cross-cutting symptom assessment for DSM-5. *Am J Psychiatry* 2013; 170:71–82.
24. DSM-5 Field Trials Posted Online by AJP. Psychiatric News Alert Web site. Available at: http://alert.psychiatricnews.org/2012/10/dsm-5-fi eld-trials-posted-online-by-ajp.html. Accessed 15 December 2013.
25. Regier DA, Narrow WE, Kuhl EA. The conceptual development of DSM-V. *Am J Psychiatry* 2009; 166:6.
26. American Psychiatric Association. *Diagnostic and Statistical Manual of Mental Disorders*. Fifth Edition. Arlington, VA: American Psychiatric Association; 2013.
27. Salvador-Carulla L, Reed GN, Vaez-Azizi LM, et al. Intellectual developmental disorders: towards a new name, definition and framework for "mental retardation/intellectual disability" in ICD-11. *World Psychiatry* 2011; 10:175–180.
28. Regier DA. Dimensional approaches to psychiatric classification: refining the research agenda for DSM-V: an introduction. *Int J Methods Psychiatr Res* 2007; 16(Suppl 1):S1–S5.
29. Cloniger CR. A new conceptual paradigm from genetics and psychobiology for the science of mental health. *Aust N Z J Psychiatry* 1999; 33:174–186.
30. Löwe B, Spitzer RL, Williams JB, et al. Depression, anxiety and somatization in primary care: syndrome overlap and functional impairment. *Gen Hosp Psychiatry* 2008; 30:191–199.
31. Kendler KS. Toward a philosophical structure for psychiatry. *Am J Psychiatry* 2005; 162:433–440.
32. Mezzich JE. Multiaxial diagnosis: purposes and challenges. *Psychiatric Diagnosis* 1994; 167–174.
33. Hisenroth MJ, Ackerman SJ, Blagys MD. Reliability and validity of DSM-IV Axis V. *Am J Psychiatry* 2000; 157:1858–1863.
34. Insurance Implications of DSM-5. American Psychiatric Association Web site. Available at: http://www.psych.org/.../DSM/DSM-5/Insurance-Implications-of-DSM-5.pdf. Accessed 22 December 2013.
35. Ustun TB, Kostanjsek N, Chatterji S, Rehm J. Measuring Health and Disability Manual for WHO Disability Assessment Schedule 2.0. World Health Organization. Available at: http://whqlibdoc.who.int/publications/2010/9789241547598_eng.pdf. Accessed 28 December 2013.
36. Garin O, Ayuso-Mateos JL, Almansa J. Validation of the "World Health Organization Disability Assessment Schedule WHODAS-2 in patients with chronic diseases. *Health and Quality of Life Outcomes* 2010; 8:51.
37. Chopra PK, Couper JW, Herrman H. The assessment of patients with long-term psychotic disorders: application of the WHO Disability Assessment Schedule II. *Aust N Z J Psychiatry* 2004; 38:753–759.
38. McKibbin C, Patterson TL, Jeste DV. Assessing disability in older patients with schizophrenia: results from the WHODAS-II. *J Nerv Ment Dis* 2004; 192:405–413.

39. Chwastiak LA, Von Korff M. Disability in depression and back pain: evaluation of the World Health Organization Disability Assessment Schedule (WHO DAS II) in a primary care setting. *J Clin Epidemiol* 2003; 56:507–514.
40. Downing NR, Kim JI, Williams JK, et al. WHODAS 2.0 in prodromal Huntington disease: measures of functioning in neuropsychiatric disease. *Eur J Hum Genet* 2014; 22:958–963.
41. Gold LH, Anfang SA, Drukteinis AM, et al. AAPL Practice guideline for the forensic evaluation of psychiatric disability. *J Am Acad Psychiatry Law* 2008; 36(4 Suppl):S3–S50.
42. Lurati AR. Reverse malingering-staying on the job at any cost. *Workplace Health Saf* 2013; 61:297–298.
43. Appelbaum PS. The parable of the forensic psychiatrist: ethics and the problem of doing harm. *Int J Law Psychiatry* 1990; 13:249–249.
44. Appelbaum PS. Ethics and forensic psychiatry: translating principles into practice. *J Am Acad Psychiatry Law* 2008; 36:195–200.
45. Grubin D. Mapping a changing landscape in the ethics of forensic psychiatry. *J Am Psychiatry Law* 2008; 36:185–190.
46. Gutheil TG, Hauser M, White MS, et al. The "whole truth" vs. the "admissible truth": an ethics dilemma for expert witnesses. *J Am Acad Psychiatry Law* 2003; 31:422–427.
47. American Psychiatric Association. *Principles of Medical Ethics With Annotations Especially Applicable to Psychiatry.* Washington, D.C.: American Psychiatric Association; 2013.
48. Slovenko R. The DSM in litigation and legislation. *J Am Acad Psych Law* 2011; 39:6–11.
49. *Discepolo v Gorgone*, 399 F. Supp. 2d 123, 127 n.2 (D. Conn. 2005).
50. Bearden C. The reality of the DSM in the Legal Arena: a proposition for curtailing undesired consequences of an imperfect tool. *Hous. J Health L & Policy* 2012; 13:80–102.
51. *State v Lockhart*, 542 S.E.2d 443 (W.Va 2000)
52. *State v Galloway*, 628 A.2d 735 (N.J. 1993)
53. *Dodd v Hughes*, 398 P.2d 540 (Nev. 1965)
54. *Clark v Arizona*, 548 U.S. 735, 740 (2006)
55. Frances A, First MB. Paraphilia NOS, Nonconsent: not ready for the courtroom. *J Am Acad Psychiatry Law* 2011; 39:555–561.
56. *Frye v. United States*, 293 F. 1013 (D.C. Cir. 1923).
57. *Daubert v. Merrell Dow Pharmaceuticals, Inc.*, 509 US 579, 589 (1993).
58. Federal Rule of Evidence 702 (Apr. 22, 1993, eff. Dec. 1, 1993).
59. Shuman DW. The Diagnostic and Statistical Manual of Mental Disorders in the courts. *Bull Am Acad Psychiatry Law* 1989; 17:25–32.
60. *Mancuso v. Consolidated Edison Co. of New York*, 967 F. Supp. 1437 (S.D.N.Y. 1997).

CHAPTER 2

The DSM-5 and Major Diagnostic Changes

INTRODUCTION

This chapter is designed to introduce mental health clinicians and forensic evaluators to how diagnostic and organizational changes made from the Diagnostic and Statistical Manual of Mental Disorders, Fourth Edition, Text Revision (DSM-IV-TR) to the Diagnostic and Statistical Manual, Fifth Edition (DSM-5) will impact their work. The chapter highlights six of the 21 diagnostic categories with the most pronounced changes and summarizes important changes to the other categories. The six highlighted categories are presented in the same order used by the DSM-5, to reflect the developmental and lifespan considerations intended by the manual's authors. Figure 2.1 illustrates significant changes in chapter names and diagnostic organization.

All references in this chapter to diagnostic criteria from the DSM-IV are based on DSM-IV-TR text, unless cited otherwise [1]. Likewise, all references to diagnostic criteria from DSM-5 are based on DSM-5 text, unless cited otherwise [2]. This chapter also reviews the American Psychiatric Association's (APA) "Highlights of Changes from DSM-IV-TR to DSM-5," to ensure that the APA's reasoning for the changes is accurately reflected [3].

DEFINITION OF MENTAL DISORDERS

The definition of mental disorders changed slightly from the DSM-IV to DSM-5. DSM-IV carried the existing definition from DSM-III of a mental disorder as follows: "a clinically significant behavioral or psychological syndrome or pattern that occurs in an individual and that is associated with present distress (e.g., a painful symptom) or disability (e.g., impairment in

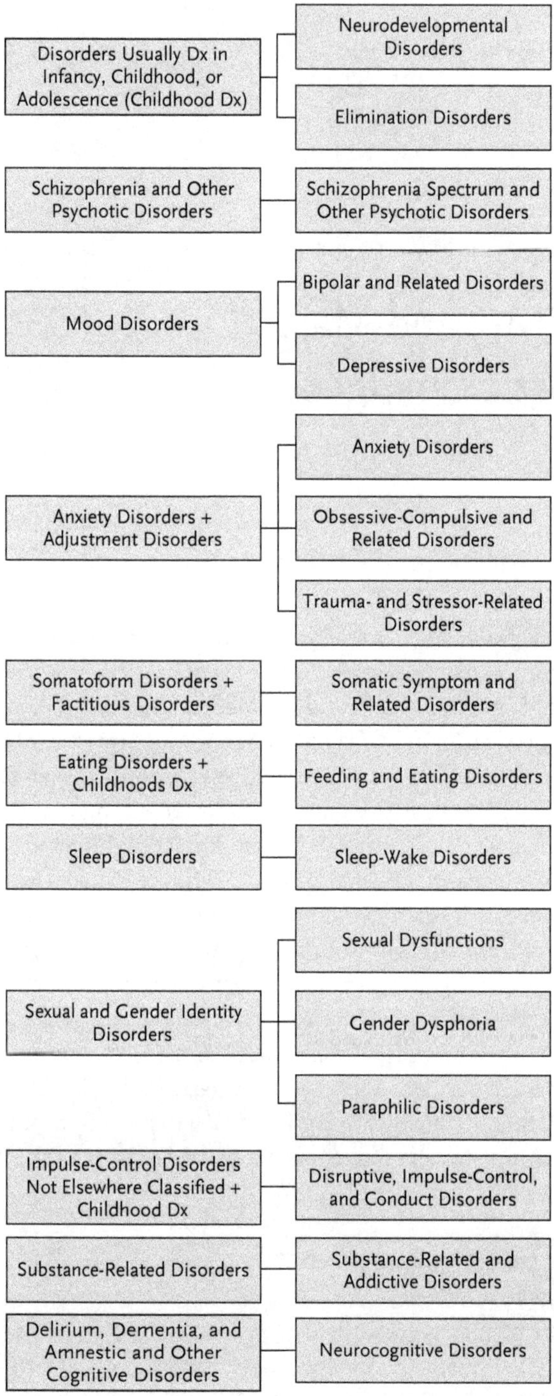

Figure 2.1:
Significant changes in chapter names and organization from DSM-IV (left) to DSM-5 (right).

one or more important areas of functioning) or with a significantly increased risk of suffering death, pain, disability, or an important loss of freedom." [1 (pxxxi)]. In contrast, DSM-5 redefined a mental disorder as follows: "a syndrome characterized by clinically significant disturbance in an individual's cognition, emotion regulation, or behavior that reflects a dysfunction in the psychological, biological, or developmental processes underlying mental functioning. Mental disorders are usually associated with significant distress or disability in social, occupational, or other important activities." [2 (p20)]. DSM-5 maintains DSM-IV's explanation that culturally appropriate responses to events and certain conflicts between individuals and the overall society (e.g., political, religious, or sexual) are not considered mental disorders [1 (pxxxi, 2 (p20)].

NEURODEVELOPMENTAL DISORDERS

The Neurodevelopmental Disorders Work Group, chaired by Dr. Susan Swedo of the National Institute of Mental Health, consisted of 13 members [4]. This work group tackled DSM-IV's broad chapter titled, Disorders Usually First Diagnosed in Infancy, Childhood, or Adolescence. The resulting chapter in DSM-5, titled "Neurodevelopmental Disorders," is the first chapter in the new edition, consistent with the newly introduced developmental and lifespan approach of the manual. This work group's implemented changes were among the most controversial.

The Neurodevelopmental Disorders Work Group both renamed and reconceptualized mental retardation from the DSM-IV. The renaming effort was largely related to a 2010 U.S. federal statute replacing the term "mental retardation" with "intellectual disability" (Rosa's law) [5]. Rosa's law was named in recognition of Rosa Marcellino, a 9-year-old girl with Down syndrome who worked with her family and state officials to have the term "mentally retarded" officially removed from the health and education code in Maryland [6]. DSM-5's reconceptualization of mental retardation into intellectual disability involved shifting from the severity of impairment being strictly based on cognitive capacity, to the severity being based primarily on adaptive functioning. Table 1 in the Neurodevelopmental Disorders chapter of DSM-5 describes the severity levels (mild, moderate, severe, profound) using three domains: conceptual, social, and practical [2 (pp34–6)]. Intelligence quotient (IQ) testing remains one acceptable aspect of determining an individual's overall cognitive functioning. However, severity ratings now require a broader determination of adaptive functioning in various contexts.

The work group also implemented significant changes to the definition of autism, which created controversy and public scrutiny. The group effectively consolidated DSM-IV's autistic disorder, Asperger's disorder, childhood disintegrative disorder, and pervasive developmental disorder not otherwise specified (PDD-NOS) into a single DSM-5 condition named autism spectrum disorder (ASD). Under the new formulation, the four previous disorders are now considered a single condition displaying varied levels of symptom severity in two core domains: "deficits in social communication and social interaction"; and "restricted, repetitive patterns of behavior, interests, or activities" (RRBs) [2 (p50)]. Frances [7] suggested that DSM-5 introduced uncertainty regarding the number of symptoms in the social-communication domain (Criterion A) required to meet criteria for ASD. He wrote that the description of Criterion A is vaguely worded and noted that the three listed criteria are described in the DSM-5 as "illustrative, not exhaustive." This degree of uncertainty could create significant challenges for both clinicians and forensic evaluators in reaching reliable ASD diagnoses.

McPartland et al. [8] presented data to show that only approximately 60% of cases they reviewed that met criteria for pervasive developmental disorders (PDD) based on DSM-IV would continue to meet criteria under DSM-5's definition of ASD. They concluded that the revised criteria might significantly alter the autistic spectrum and exclude a substantial portion of individuals diagnosed with ASDs other than autistic disorder. Another group published similar results, again with only approximately 60% of the cases reviewed meeting criteria for an ASD under DSM-5 [9]. In response, the DSM-5 Work Group on Neurodevelopmental Disorders published a commentary in which they criticized the methodologies used by McPartland's group [10]. Mandy et al. [11, 12] also published studies supporting the construct validity of the DSM-5 criteria for ASD (compared with the DSM-IV criteria) both domestically and abroad. Other authors have raised concerns regarding the potential impact of the changes on research, particularly ongoing longitudinal research [13].

With evidence of both core domains required to establish a diagnosis of ASD in the DSM-5, communication disorders would apply if individuals do not display RRBs. DSM-5 includes a newly defined disorder known as social (pragmatic) communication disorder, a condition thought to include many individuals previously diagnosed with PDD-NOS based on lack RRBs. Initial evidence regarding social communication disorder as a separate condition remains mixed, with some psychiatrists viewing the condition as well-validated while other psychiatrists are less certain about the validity [14, 15]. Other communication disorders in DSM-5 include language disorder (combining DSM-IV's expressive and mixed receptive-expressive language disorders), speech sound disorder (renaming of phonological disorder), and childhood-onset fluency disorder (renaming of stuttering) [3 (p1)].

This work group was also responsible for determining the diagnostic criteria for attention-deficit/hyperactivity disorder (ADHD). They retained the same 18 diagnostic criteria from DSM-IV to DSM-5, also retaining the two core domains, inattention and hyperactivity/impulsivity. For individuals less than age 17, at least six criteria in a domain are required to diagnose ADHD. The criteria mirror the DSM-IV. However, the work group made four important changes to the text in DSM-5. First, the necessity for cross-situational symptoms now requires several inattentive or hyperactive-impulsive symptoms in two or more settings. Second, the work group substantially eased the age requirement for symptom onset. Now an individual may qualify for ADHD if several symptoms are present prior to age 12, in contrast to DSM-IV, which required symptom onset prior to age 7. Third, three specifiers replace the DSM-IV's ADHD subtypes. The specifiers are noted as "combined presentation," "predominantly inattentive presentation," and "predominantly hyperactive/impulsive presentation" [2 (p60)]. Fourth, DSM-5 requires fewer symptoms to establish ADHD in older adolescents and adults (17 and older), for whom only five symptoms must be present in one of the two core domains.

The following vignette demonstrates a possible implication of the changes to DSM-5's Neurodevelopmental Disorders.

> Mr. A is a 31-year-old man who lives with his mother. She brings him to an outpatient psychiatric clinic for an initial evaluation after he lost his third job in a year, all due to verbal conflicts with coworkers. She reports that Mr. A "nearly ruined Christmas" because he made inappropriate and offensive comments during a large family gathering. You meet with Mr. A, who ruminates about coworkers and family members upsetting him when they force him to deviate from his usual routines, which include eating the same meals daily and watching Star Trek reruns at least three times a day during specified times, regardless of what is happening. During your evaluation, Mr. A demonstrates minimal social reciprocity, displays minimal eye contact, and misses basic non-verbal cues. You ask Mr. A for permission to meet with his mother, which he gladly grants in favor of watching Star Trek on his iPad. While gathering a developmental history from his mother, you learn that Mr. A displayed no delay in language development and has an IQ of 105. However, she notes that he was enrolled in "some special classes" in grade school while living with his father and stepmother in another state. His mother explains that when having a conversation with Mr. A when she states, "It seems like he's talking at you, not to you." She adds that he has never had friends his own age, but did not seem to mind his lack of peer relationships. She reports growing tired of having him live in the house, but worries he would struggle on his own.

According to DSM-IV, Mr. A would likely meet criteria for Asperger's disorder. For example, he had two or more of the required impairments in social interaction (failure to develop appropriate peer relationships, lack of emotional reciprocity) and at least one of the required impairments in RRBs (inflexible adherence to routines). He did not demonstrate a history of language or cognitive delays. Using DSM-5 criteria, Mr. A would not meet criteria for an ASD with only one reported or observed RRB, unless he had a "well-established DSM-IV diagnosis" [2 (p51)] of Asperger's disorder. However, he may meet criteria for a communication disorder. In Mr. A's case, the diagnostic change in DSM-5 may be less problematic, unless his insurance coverage was an issue. However, if Mr. A was instead a third grader, his lack of an ASD diagnosis may impact services available to him. How communication disorders will be addressed by the educational system remains unclear.

DEPRESSIVE DISORDERS

The Mood Disorders Work Group, chaired by Dr. Jan Fawcett of the University of New Mexico, consisted of 11 members [16]. Although the group acknowledged that symptoms of depression and anxiety commonly occur together, they decided to keep them separated in DSM-5. However, DSM-5 divided DSM-IV's Mood Disorders chapter into two separate chapters: Bipolar and Related Disorders and Depressive Disorders.

Although the core criteria and duration of symptoms for major depressive disorder remained unchanged, the group's removal of the bereavement exclusion created controversy and resulted in significant public scrutiny. The bereavement exclusion in DSM-IV involved major depressive episodes not being diagnosed within 2 months after the loss of a loved one, unless the individual experienced specified severe depressive symptoms. DSM-5 instead notes, "In distinguishing grief from a major depressive episode (MDE), it is useful to consider that in grief the predominant affect is feelings of emptiness and loss, while in an MDE, it is persistent depressed mood and the inability to anticipate happiness or pleasure" [2 (p126)]. Justifications for removing the bereavement exclusion included that depressive episodes occurring during or after bereavement share features of nonbereavement depression, tend to be chronic and/or recurrent if left untreated, and respond to treatment. Some psychiatrists have opined that the bereavement exclusion may have inappropriately implied that a person's grief should end after 2 months [17]. Another change to major depressive disorder involved adding the specifier "with mixed features" when a major depressive episode coexists with at least three manic symptoms (although does not qualify as a manic episode) [2 (p184)]. This change resulted partially from the group's decision to split DSM-IV's Mood Disorders chapter into two separate chapters and eliminate DSM-IV's mixed episodes.

The work group also modified the conceptualization of chronic depressive symptoms. Persistent depressive disorder, new to DSM-5, replaces DSM-IV's chronic major depressive disorder and dysthymia. Rhebergen and Graham [18] propose that this modification merely took a poorly validated construct and repackaged it under a new name. Of particular significance, the group also added other new Depressive Disorders, including premenstrual dysphoric disorder (PMDD) and the highly controversial disruptive mood dysregulation disorder (DMDD).

The group indicated that they added DMDD to address "potential overdiagnosis and overtreatment of bipolar disorder in children up to age 18 who display" "persistent irritability and frequent episodes of extreme behavioral dyscontrol" [3 (p4)]. Many psychiatrists have expressed concerns that the addition of DMDD merely serves to pathologize normal childhood behaviors. Published research both supports and challenges the validity of DMDD as a psychiatric diagnosis during early childhood [19, 20].

The following vignette demonstrates a possible implication of the changes to the Depressive Disorders:

> Ms. B is a 76-year-old woman who recently moved into a retirement community with her husband, soon after celebrating their fiftieth anniversary. While planning their first post-retirement trip abroad, her husband suddenly and unexpectedly died from cardiac arrest. Six weeks after her husband's death, the visits and phone calls from loved ones tapered off considerably. On the day the couple's trip was scheduled to begin, Ms. B finds herself alone in the house. Ms. B reports that she has cried so much over the last six weeks that she can no longer produce tears. She also notices that for the last several weeks she has been sleeping over 10 hours a day, has lost 15 pounds because she rarely eats or feels hungry, has minimal energy, has trouble focusing on reading or television, and feels sad and empty all day. Ms. B has not experienced improvement in the symptoms during that time. After discussing her symptoms during a phone call, Ms. B's daughter encourages her to call her primary care provider for an appointment.

According to DSM-IV, Ms. B would not meet criteria for major depressive disorder. Because her symptoms occurred entirely in the setting of the loss of her husband (less than two months ago), the bereavement exclusion would apply. In this case, there is not a clear presence of the specified severe depressive symptoms outlined in the DSM-IV, any of which would have automatically moved the diagnosis to being classified as a major depressive episode. According to the DSM-5, however, Ms. B would meet criteria for major depressive disorder.

TRAUMA- AND STRESSOR-RELATED DISORDERS

The Anxiety, Obsessive-Compulsive Spectrum, Posttraumatic, and Dissociative Disorders Work Group, chaired by Dr. Katharine A. Phillips of Brown University, consisted of 14 members [21]. The work group first met in October 2008, tasked with assessing the rather large DSM-IV chapter containing the Anxiety Disorders. Given the size of the Anxiety Disorders chapter, they elected to break into three subgroups. Ultimately, the main group decided to split the Anxiety Disorders chapter of DSM-IV into three separate chapters, each more narrowly focused [22]. The three resulting chapters in DSM-5 are titled: Anxiety Disorders; Obsessive-Compulsive and Related Disorders; and Trauma- and Stressor-Related Disorders. The most substantial changes are noted in the Trauma- and Stressor-Related Disorders section of DSM-5 and represent the focus of this section.

In addition to posttraumatic stress disorder (PTSD) and acute stress disorder, the Trauma and Stressor-Related Disorders chapter also includes adjustment disorder and reactive attachment disorder. The decision to separate PTSD away from the Anxiety Disorders was hotly debated. Opponents of this change opined that moving PTSD out of the Anxiety Disorders chapter was unsupported by existing data and that classically conditioned fear (i.e., anxiety) was central to its development [23].

PTSD and acute stress disorder also experienced significant diagnostic changes in addition to their separation from the Anxiety Disorders chapter. The stressor criterion (Criterion A) for both conditions changed. In DSM-IV, Criterion A required that both of the following were present: "the person experienced, witnessed, or was confronted with an event or events that involved actual or threatened death or serious injury, or a threat to the physical integrity of self or others;" and "the person's response involved intense fear, helplessness, or horror" [1 (p467)]. DSM-5 instead requires "exposure to actual or threatened death, serious injury, or sexual violence" [2 (p271)] in one (or more) of the following ways: directly experiencing the traumatic event; witnessing, in person, the event(s) as it occurred to others; learning that the traumatic event(s) occurred to a close family member or close friend (actual or threatened death must have been violent or accidental); or experiencing repeated or extreme exposure to aversive details of the traumatic event(s) (e.g., first responders collecting human remains, police officers repeatedly exposed to details of child abuse, etc). The work group also eliminated DSM-IV's requirement that the individual experience "intense fear, helplessness, or horror" [1 (p467)].

DSM-5 also redefined the symptom clusters that must follow a traumatic event to diagnose PTSD. In DSM-IV, the three major symptom clusters include re-experiencing, avoidance/numbing, and arousal. In DSM-5, the re-experiencing and arousal clusters remain. However, the avoidance/numbing cluster is now divided into two separate clusters, "avoidance" and persistent "negative alterations in cognitions and mood" [2 (p271)]. The newly formed persistent negative alterations cluster retained most of the numbing symptoms (with some rewording) and added additional symptoms including the following: persistent and exaggerated negative beliefs or expectations about oneself, others, or the world; persistent, distorted cognitions about the cause or consequences of the traumatic event(s) that lead the individual to blame himself/herself or others; persistent negative emotional state (e.g., fear, horror, anger, guilt, or shame); and persistent inability to experience positive emotions. The group also attempted to account for different reactions based on developmental age by providing a separate set of criteria for children age 6 or younger.

Reactive attachment disorder and adjustment disorder are the other DSM-IV conditions now included in the Trauma- and Stressor-Related Disorder chapter. In DSM-IV, reactive attachment disorder featured two subtypes, emotionally withdrawn/inhibited and indiscriminately social/disinhibited. In DSM-5, each subtype is named as a separate disorder, namely reactive attachment disorder and disinhibited social engagement disorder. In DSM-5, adjustment disorder is described as a collection of emotional or behavioral symptoms in response to an identifiable stressor occurring within 3 months of onset of the stressor(s).

The following vignette demonstrates a possible implication of the changes to the Trauma- and Stressor-Related Disorders:

> Dr. C is a 53-year-old forensic psychiatrist who has been in practice for over 20 years. His oldest daughter left home recently to enroll as a freshman at an out-of-state university. Dr. C finds that he seems to be having a harder time "letting work go" when he gets home in the evening. He feels particularly shaken by a recent case involving a freshman coed who was kidnapped, tortured, repeatedly raped, and murdered. He finds himself frequently picturing the gruesome autopsy photos, worrying about his daughter's safety, and ruminating about how the crime impacted the victim's family. Dr. C starts avoiding new cases and his production decreases considerably. He begins finding reasons to avoid the office altogether and starts calling in sick frequently. Worried about Dr. C, a colleague suggests that he make a therapy appointment. During the intake appointment, the clinician finds that Dr. C meets sufficient criteria in each of the four symptom clusters for PTSD.

According to DSM-IV, Dr. C would not meet criteria for PTSD because he was not directly exposed to a traumatic event that caused a significant negative emotional reaction at the time the event occurred. In DSM-5, he likely meets criteria for PTSD based on his experiencing work-related recurrent and significant exposure to negative traumatic situations with emotionally upsetting characteristics. His distress seems particularly related to the case involving the freshman coed, although repeated exposure to disturbing details of other cases could also be relevant.

How these changes impact the overall prevalence of PTSD in clinical samples and forensic referrals remains unclear. Some authors have suggested that the overall prevalence will change minimally, if at all [24]. Other authors have suggested that the prevalence may actually decrease due to the new requirement that at least one avoidance symptom be present [25]. Given the largely subjective nature of establishing criteria for PTSD, the risk of feigning in civil and criminal forensic cases remains a concern.

SOMATIC SYMPTOM AND RELATED DISORDERS

The Somatic Symptoms Disorders Work Group, chaired by Joel E. Dimsdale of the University of California, San Diego, consisted of 9 members [26]. The group sought to address specific concerns with DSM-IV somatoform diagnoses. First, the group eliminated somatization disorder, undifferentiated somatoform disorder, pain disorder, and hypochrondriasis, due to their often-overlapping diagnostic criteria, which reduced the diagnoses' validity and clinical utility [27]. The group eliminated many terms included in DSM-IV, such as "somatoform" and "somatization" that patients and primary care physicians often found unhelpful [28]. The group abolished DSM-IV's use of "medically unexplained" symptoms because they believed this approach perpetuated the concept of mind-body dualism and confounded diagnostic reliability and validity [29, 30]. With no distinction between medically explained and medically unexplained somatic complaints in DSM-5, an individual can meet criteria for a somatic symptom disorder despite having a clear medical explanation [31].

Although many somatoform diagnoses changed dramatically from the DSM-IV to the DSM-5, some remained largely unchanged. Previously known as factitious disorder and factitious disorder by proxy, DSM-5 includes factitious disorder "imposed on self" and "imposed on another." These diagnoses remained conceptually intact as falsified physical or psychological symptoms to assume the sick role. There are now "single episode" and "recurrent episodes" specifiers [2 (p325)]. Psychological factors affecting other medical conditions moved to this chapter from DSM-IV's chapter titled Other Conditions That May Be a Focus of Clinical Attention, with unchanged criteria but newly added severity specifiers.

DSM-5's somatic symptom disorder (SSD) is a major change from the DSM-IV. Criterion A specifies that an individual has one or more somatic symptoms that are distressing or significantly disruptive. As mentioned above, DSM-5 abolished medically unexplained symptoms (MUS) to establish this diagnosis, so an individual may be diagnosed even when medically explained diseases result in distressing somatic symptoms. Criterion B specifies behavioral and psychological features of the disorder, emphasizing the importance of how patients interpret symptoms. Individuals must demonstrate one or more of the following: "disproportionate and persistent thoughts about the seriousness of one's symptoms," "persistently high level of anxiety about health or symptoms," or "excessive time and energy devoted to these symptoms or health concerns" [2 (p311)]. The B criteria demonstrate the emphasis that the group placed on generating "positive" symptom criteria and eliminating the rule-out "after appropriate investigation" criterion necessary in DSM-IV [32]. The first two B criteria overlap, and some authors have questioned whether the presence of both supplies incremental information; the third B criterion seems valid based on studies involving increased healthcare needs in somaticizing patients, but critics have questioned whether "inappropriate excessive time" devoted to somatic symptoms would be more valid [33]. Criterion C specifies that an individual need not have the same somatic symptom present continuously, but the state of being symptomatic must be persistent "typically more than 6 months" [2 (p311)]. SSD has multiple specifiers, including: "with predominant pain," which DSM-5 notes would previously have been pain disorder; "persistent" for disorders characterized by increased severity, impairment, and duration; in addition to "mild," "moderate," and "severe."

The SSD diagnosis has come under considerable scrutiny. First, Frances [34] argued that the diagnostic criteria are overly inclusive and that 15% of patients with cancer and heart disease, plus 25% of patients with irritable bowel syndrome and widespread pain, would be diagnosed with SSD. He estimated that DSM-5's criteria would result in a 7% false-positive rate in the general population. Based on these estimates, he expressed concerns about the mislabeling of medically ill individuals as mentally ill [35].

Illness anxiety disorder is another new disorder in DSM-5. Like DSM-IV's hypochondriasis, the primary diagnostic feature is a preoccupation with having (or acquiring, in DSM-5) a serious illness. Whereas hypochondriasis required that an individual's concern arise from "misinterpretation of bodily symptoms" [1 (p507)], Criterion B of illness anxiety disorder specifies that if any somatic symptoms are present, they are mild in intensity and the preoccupation is "clearly excessive or disproportionate" [2 (p315)] to any risk of acquiring a medical condition. The criteria necessitate that an individual has a high anxiety level about their medical status. "Care-seeking type" and "care-avoidant type" specifiers indicate whether individuals obtain frequent medical attention or avoid medical attention regarding these health concerns.

Conversion disorder, known as functional neurological symptom disorder in DSM-5, remains in the chapter, but with multiple changes. Criterion A still requires one or more symptoms of altered voluntary motor or sensory function, but it no longer includes DSM-IV's requirement to "suggest a neurological or other general medical condition" [1 (p498)]. Rather, Criterion B now indicates that clinical findings suggest incompatibility between the symptom and recognized neurological or medical conditions. Eliminated are the DSM-IV's criteria that the deficit be associated with psychological factors (conflict or stress), not be intentionally produced or feigned, and that the symptom cannot be fully explained by a general medical condition, the effects of a substance, or as a cultural experience.

The final major change by this group was moving body dysmorphic disorder from the DSM-IV's Somatoform Disorders chapter to DSM-5's Obsessive-Compulsive and Related Disorders chapter. Based on studies comparing the phenomenology, epidemiology, comorbidities, neurobiology, genetics, and treatment of body dysmorphic disorder, the group considered the condition as similar to obsessive-compulsive disorder (OCD) and therefore more appropriately grouped with that disorder [36].

The following vignette demonstrates a possible implication of the changes to the Somatic Symptom and Related Disorders:

> Ms. D is a 43-year-old woman diagnosed with breast cancer two years ago. Twelve months ago she underwent radical mastectomy and adjuvant chemotherapy. Since then she has complained of excruciating, sharp chest wall pain near the surgical site. She finds herself staying home and avoiding social events with her friends because the pain is disabling. She thinks about the pain constantly and experiences considerable anxiety about recurrence of her breast cancer. She has visited her primary care physician at least monthly since the surgery and tried multiple medications for pain with limited improvement.

Based on DSM-IV, Ms. D could have received diagnoses of undifferentiated somatoform disorder or pain disorder associated with both psychological factors and a general medical condition, chronic. Using DSM-5, however, Ms. D instead meets criteria for SSD, given her distressing somatic symptom (Criterion A) and the disproportionate and persistent thoughts about her somatic symptom, her persistently high level of anxiety, and the excessive time and energy she devotes to the symptom (Criterion B). Because she meets all three B criteria, her disorder has lasted more than 6 months, and her symptom involves predominantly pain, Ms. D would be diagnosed with SSD, with predominant pain, persistent, severe.

DISRUPTIVE, IMPULSE-CONTROL, AND CONDUCT DISORDERS

The ADHD and Disruptive Behavior Disorders Work Group, chaired by David Shaffer of Columbia University and F. Xavier Castellanos of New York University, consisted of 10 members [37]. The group, charged with working on a broad set of conditions, broke into three subgroups. One subgroup focused on disorders now contained in the DSM-5 chapter entitled Disruptive,

Impulse-Control, and Conduct Disorders. First, the subgroup considered whether there was sufficient evidence to justify dividing oppositional defiant disorder (ODD) and conduct disorder (CD) into separate disorders. Second, the subgroup evaluated the diagnostic criteria of conduct disorder and antisocial personality disorder to determine whether they could be modified to achieve additional concordance. Finally, the subgroup considered whether to define a category of psychopathy, perhaps as a subcategory of CD [38].

DSM-5 brought together disorders from several DSM-IV chapters. Kleptomania and pyromania (previously in the DSM-IV chapter titled Impulse-Control Disorders Not Elsewhere Classified) remained unchanged in the DSM-5. ODD and CD remained as separate disorders because of their differential associations with other disorders. The diagnostic criteria of CD remained largely unchanged from the DSM-IV. To address the concept of psychopathy, the group added a "with limited prosocial emotions" specifier for individuals with persistent evidence for at least 12 months of two of the following: "lack of remorse or guilt," "lack of empathy," "unconcern about performance," and "shallow or deficient affect."

Of the eight diagnoses included in this chapter, the work group made the most significant changes to ODD and intermittent explosive disorder (IED). ODD's A criteria are now grouped into three categories defined as "angry/irritable mood," "argumentative/defiant behavior," and "vindictiveness" to emphasize the possible presence of both emotional and behavioral symptoms. After the A criteria, a note reads, "The persistence and frequency of these behaviors should be used to distinguish a behavior that is within normal limits from a behavior that is symptomatic" [2 (p462)]. DSM-5 no longer excludes the option to diagnosis ODD if the individual meets criteria for CD, so individuals can now be diagnosed with both concurrently. The work group also added severity specifiers (mild, moderate, severe) based on research showing that symptom pervasiveness is a useful indicator of severity [3].

DSM-5 criteria for IED are significantly expanded compared with DSM-IV. Criterion A now includes acts of verbal aggression, whereas DSM-IV only acknowledged assaultive and noninjurious physical aggression. The frequency of behavioral outbursts includes descriptors of both the number and duration of aggressive acts required to establish the diagnosis. Criterion B emphasizes that the magnitude of aggression is grossly out of proportion to the stressor and is impulsive in nature. However, the text does not provide guidance on how to objectively evaluate whether an individual's reaction is grossly out of proportion to a stressor. Furthermore, aggression is not considered impulsive if premeditated and performed to achieve some tangible objective (such as money, power, or intimidation). Individuals cannot be diagnosed with IED unless they are at least 6 years old and have impairment in functioning or negative consequences resulting from the outbursts.

A separate note in DSM-5 states that IED may be diagnosed concurrently to ADHD, CD, ODD, or ASD when the impulsive outbursts are "in excess of those usually seen in these disorders and warrant independent clinical attention" [2 (p466)]. This guideline may prove problematic because the DSM-5 does not delineate the expected number or severity of impulsive outbursts in these other conditions.

Because CD and ODD both have a high prevalence of impulsive aggressive acts, the evaluator may find it difficult to clearly determine when an individual should be additionally diagnosed with IED [39]. DSM-5 also does not specifically exclude diagnosing IED in individuals with antisocial personality disorder or borderline personality disorder and describes that the impulsive aggression in these two disorders is "lower than that in individuals with intermittent explosive disorder" [2 (p468)]. How clinicians and evaluators will determine the level of impulsive aggression that is "lower than" what is expected for IED is unclear. Based on DSM-5, a clinician could make a diagnosis of both IED and a personality disorder.

The following vignette demonstrates some of the possible implications of the changes to the Disruptive, Impulse-Control, and Conduct Disorders:

> J.E. is a 13-year-old boy whose parents bring him to the outpatient clinic for a psychiatric evaluation after his teachers reported a range of worsening behavioral problems. Over the last two years, he has repeatedly lost his temper when not getting his way, cursed out his teachers over homework assignments, blamed other children for his inability to complete tasks during class time, and gleefully thrown spitballs at his peers. Over the last few months, J.E. has been truant from class with no explanation. During his sessions with a therapist, J.E. reveals that since age 11 he has been fascinated with killing small mammals with a hatchet. He also relishes lighting fires in the woods to see how much foliage he can burn. J.E. states that he does not feel remorseful about these behaviors, despite the harm or pain they cause. He states that he gets away with it by lying to his parents, usually telling them that he is doing homework at a friend's house.

Using DSM-IV criteria, J.E. would be diagnosed with conduct disorder, adolescent-onset type, moderate. Now that ODD and CD can be diagnosed together based on DSM-5, he would receive diagnoses of oppositional defiant disorder, moderate severity, and conduct disorder, adolescent-onset type, moderate. In addition, due to his profound lack of remorse and lack of concerns about his performance in daily tasks at school and home over the last 12 months, he meets criteria for the specifier, "with limited prosocial emotions" [2 (p470)].

Because J.E. shows evidence of impulsive, aggressive behaviors such as verbal sparring with his teachers, he could also meet criteria for IED. Given DSM-5's somewhat unclear criteria about the magnitude of aggression that is out of proportion to the provocation (teachers scolding him for not completing homework) and excessiveness of impulsive, aggressive outbursts seen in his comorbid disorders (ODD and CD), the evaluator would have to subjectively determine whether J.E. meets criteria for IED in addition to his other diagnoses.

SUBSTANCE-RELATED AND ADDICTIVE DISORDERS

The Substance-Related Disorders Work Group, chaired by Charles O'Brien of the University of Pennsylvania and (until late 2011) co-chaired by Thomas Crowley of the University of Colorado, Denver, consisted of 14 members [40]. The overarching issue that the group addressed during the DSM-5's development was whether substance abuse and dependence should remain as two separate diagnoses [41]. After deciding to collapse abuse and dependence into a single substance use disorder, the group determined whether to add or withdraw diagnostic criteria. Finally, the group addressed specific disorders related to substance use.

Although the DSM-5 Substance-Related Disorders chapter differs considerably from DSM-IV, there also remains considerable overlap. The substances recognized by both texts are largely unchanged, although the group collapsed amphetamines and cocaine into a more general stimulant category and expanded hallucinogens into two categories, phencyclidine and other hallucinogens. As in DSM-IV, each substance class has diagnosable substance-induced disorders, including: intoxication and withdrawal, plus psychotic, bipolar, depressive, anxiety, obsessive-compulsive, sleep, sexual dysfunctions, delirium, and neurocognitive disorders. Caffeine remains in DSM-5 with associated substance-induced disorders but without a separate caffeine use disorder.

DSM-IV's division of abuse and dependence into separate disorders was guided by the opinion that substance use disorders consisted of a "dependence syndrome" (substance dependence) and social and interpersonal problems secondary to heavy substance use (substance abuse) [42]. The writers of DSM-IV considered substance dependence more severe than substance abuse. An individual with substance dependence could not also be diagnosed with substance abuse. The dependence diagnosis was highly reliable and validated by indicators such as substance consumption, treatment utilization, comorbidity, and impairment in functioning [43]. However, the DSM-5 work group identified many problems with the DSM-IV formulation, including reduced reliability and validity of the abuse diagnosis, the ability to diagnose individuals with substance abuse based on a single criterion, and the "diagnostic orphans," defined as cases in which two dependence criteria and one abuse criteria were met yet no diagnosis could be made [44]. The work group also cited studies showing that abuse was not simply a prodrome to dependence and that not all individuals who met criteria for dependence also met criteria for abuse, as the hierarchical organization suggested [45, 46].

Another diagnostic issue the group considered was whether to add or eliminate criteria to improve the accuracy of diagnosing substance use disorders. The group ultimately decided to eliminate legal problems as a criterion due to its low prevalence in adult samples and many adolescent samples, low discrimination, limited ability to add information to the diagnosis, and its poor fit with other criteria for substance use disorders [47, 48]. Craving is a somewhat controversial new criterion due to its limited psychometric benefit. However, due to craving's centrality to substance use disorders from behavioral, imaging, genetic studies, and the need to address craving in management of substance use disorders, the group added it as a new criterion [49]. See Table 2-1 for a summary of the changes in diagnostic criteria between DSM-IV's abuse and dependence diagnoses and DSM-5's substance use disorder.

After defining substance use disorder, the group evaluated where to set the diagnostic threshold, how to assess severity, and what changes should be made to diagnostic specifiers. Using general population data and clinical samples to compute prevalence of DSM-IV substance abuse and dependence and DSM-5 substance use disorder, the group identified two criteria as the appropriate threshold for making a diagnosis of substance use disorder. In determining how to rate severity, the group considered weighting different criteria but found that weighting had no advantage in predicting consumption, functioning, and family history. Therefore, the group adopted a strict counting approach [50]. In DSM-5, individuals must meet two or three criteria for "mild," four or five for "moderate," and six or more for "severe" [2 (p484)]. For seven of the substance use disorders (alcohol; cannabis; opioid; sedative, hypnotic, or anxiolytic; stimulant; tobacco; and other), there are 11 possible criteria. Other substance use disorders have 10 possible criteria due to the substances not causing withdrawal.

The group eliminated the "physiological" specifier (tolerance or withdrawal) [1 (p195)], citing the lack of clinical relevance to support its inclusion [41]. They eliminated the "full remission" and "partial remission" specifiers [1 (p196)] and changed the "in early remission" time course modifier to require at least 3 months of no criteria (aside from craving) being met [2 (p491)]. The "in sustained remission" specifier is unchanged and continues to require at least 12 months of no criteria being met [2 (p491)]. Likewise, the "in a controlled environment" and "on agonist therapy" ("on maintenance therapy" in DSM-5) specifiers remain essentially unchanged [2 (p541–542)].

Some substance-induced disorders were revised in DSM-5. Due to evidence that cannabis withdrawal is commonly observed in regular users, the work group formally added withdrawal as a criterion for cannabis

Table 2-1. COMPARISON OF CRITERIA FOR DSM-IV-TR SUBSTANCE ABUSE AND DEPENDENCE AND DSM-5 SUBSTANCE USE DISORDER

Criterion	DSM-IV-TR Substance Abuse (one or more criteria)	DSM-IV-TR Substance Dependence (three or more criteria)	DSM-5 Substance Use Disorder (two or more criteria)
Legal problems	X		
Social/interpersonal problems	X		X
Role obligation failure	X		X
Hazardous use	X		X
Larger amounts/longer than intended		X	X
Repeated attempts to quit/ control use		X	X
Time spent obtaining or using		X	X
Social, occupational, recreational activities given up		X	X
Continued use despite health problems related to use		X	X
Tolerance		X	X
Withdrawal		X	X
Craving			X

use disorder along with a separate diagnosis of cannabis withdrawal [51]. DSM-IV did not have established criteria for a nicotine abuse diagnosis. As a result, the group questioned whether DSM-5 criteria for tobacco use disorder should align with other substance use disorders. Research demonstrated that the proposed tobacco use disorder is strongly associated with a variety of predictors, including quantity smoked and smoking upon awakening, and therefore more accurate at identifying individuals with problematic tobacco use [52]. In addition, the DSM-5 tobacco use disorder criteria create a higher prevalence, an original criticism of the DSM-IV nicotine dependence criteria, so the group aligned the criteria with the other substance use disorders [53].

Although adding a behavioral addiction to DSM-5's chapter on substance use disorders faced some resistance, the group ultimately brought the DSM-IV diagnosis of pathological gambling into the chapter as gambling disorder due to its frequent comorbidity with substance use disorders and similarities in symptom presentation, biological dysfunction, genetic risk, and treatment [54, 55]. In keeping with eliminating legal problems from addiction criteria, the group removed illegal acts to finance gambling as a criterion. In addition, the group added time course and severity specifiers to increase the similarity to substance use disorders [2 (p586)].

The introduction of substance use disorders and their associated severity specifiers are important for both clinical and forensic assessments. Previously, an evaluator could establish a diagnosis of dependence based on the presence of three or more criteria and abuse based on the presence of one criterion (after ruling out dependence). Now, to accurately diagnose the severity of substance use disorders, evaluators would instead screen for each substance use disorder symptom for each substance in question.

The following vignette demonstrates a possible implication of the changes to the Substance-Related and Addictive Disorders:

> Mr. F is a 35-year-old man with a history of heavy drinking since his mid-teens. Over the last 10 years he has given up seeking employment due to being fired frequently for intoxication on the job. More recently he has needed to drink more to become intoxicated. If he does not drink every day, he develops shakes, sweats, and anxiety. He also finds that he frequently craves alcohol. He spends most of his day planning where to purchase cheap alcohol and consuming it. After driving while intoxicated, Mr. F is arrested and requires treatment to prevent complicated withdrawal.

Mr. F would meet DSM-IV criteria for alcohol dependence based on the fulfillment of three or more diagnostic criteria (tolerance, withdrawal, time spent to obtain and consume). Under the DSM-5, however, each criterion becomes relevant to accurately list a severity specifier. Because Mr. F meets six DSM-5 criteria (tolerance, withdrawal, craving, time spent to obtain and consume, giving up occupational activities, failure to fulfill obligations at work) for alcohol use disorder, he would be diagnosed with alcohol use disorder, severe.

OTHER DIAGNOSTIC CHANGES

In the Schizophrenia Spectrum and Other Psychotic Disorders chapter, the work group made two changes to the criteria for schizophrenia. They eliminated bizarre delusions and Schneiderian first-rank auditory hallucinations as single symptoms that could qualify for a diagnosis of schizophrenia. The decision to eliminate Schneiderian symptoms was due to their lack of specificity and clinicians' unreliable ability to distinguish nonbizarre from bizarre delusions [3 (p3)]. An individual must now demonstrate two of the five Criterion A symptoms, namely delusions, hallucinations, disorganized speech, disorganized behavior, and negative symptoms, with at least one of the first three present to establish the diagnosis [2 (p99)]. The group also eliminated the DSM-IV schizophrenia subtypes due to limited predictive value for patients' treatment response and disease progression [56]. The main change to schizoaffective disorder is required that a "major mood episode" occur for the majority of the illness after meeting Criterion A of schizophrenia [3 (p3)]. This specific time requirement was added to improve the criteria's diagnostic accuracy, validity, and stability [57]. Now that bizarre delusions alone are no longer sufficient to diagnose schizophrenia, an individual with isolated bizarre delusions may meet criteria for delusional disorder, which now has a specifier for "bizarre content" [2 (p91)]. Finally, the number of criteria required for a diagnosis of catatonia has changed, and the "catatonia" specifier can be used as a specifier across many diagnoses [2 (p119)]. DSM-IV required one cluster of symptoms to diagnose catatonia in the context of a general medical condition and two clusters of symptoms to diagnose catatonia in the context of psychosis or a mood disorder. Using DSM-5, an individual must demonstrate three of 12 criteria to establish the diagnosis [2 (p119)].

In the Bipolar and Related Disorders chapter, Criterion A for manic and hypomanic episodes now requires "abnormally and persistently increased goal-directed activity and energy" [2 (p124)] in addition to elevated, expansive, or irritable mood over a period of at least 1 week because of research indicating that subthreshold hypomanic symptoms of decreased need for sleep, unusual energy, and increased goal-directed activity predict progression to mania [58]. The seven B criteria for these episodes and the criteria for bipolar I disorder and bipolar II disorder otherwise remain unchanged. As with the Depressive Disorders, the "with mixed features" and "with anxious distress" specifiers are available to address additional symptoms present during a manic or hypomanic episode [2 (p149)].

The Anxiety Disorders chapter underwent significant revisions beyond its division into three separate chapters in DSM-5. Within the DSM-5 chapter entitled Anxiety Disorders, the diagnostic criteria of the disorders experienced minor changes. For agoraphobia, specific phobia, and social phobia, the group eliminated the requirement that individuals be over 18 years old. The 6-month duration of illness has been extended to all, not just individuals under 18. The group added separation anxiety disorder to the chapter, which can now be diagnosed in all ages as long as symptoms are present for at least 6 months. Panic disorder and agoraphobia are now distinct disorders with separate criteria, and a linkage between the two is no longer required. Finally, the group added selective mutism to the chapter.

The Obsessive-Compulsive and Related Disorders chapter, new to DSM-5, brought together many diagnoses previously located apart. The diagnoses include OCD, body dysmorphic disorder (BDD), and trichotillomania. In addition, the chapter features new diagnoses of hoarding disorder and excoriation disorder. The group eliminated DSM-IV's Criterion A for OCD that an individual must recognize the obsessional experiences as a product of his or her own mind in favor of an insight specifier (good or fair, poor, absent insight/delusional beliefs), emphasizing different degrees of insight into obsessions. An identical specifier is present for body dysmorphic disorder and hoarding disorder, recognizing the obsessive component of each disorder. When an individual's obsessional content reaches delusional levels, the relevant obsessive-compulsive and related disorder should be diagnosed over a psychotic disorder [2 (p237)]. There is now a "tic-related" specifier for OCD due to the clinical importance of identifying individuals with past or current comorbid tic disorder. For BDD, there is a "with muscle dysmorphia" specifier for individuals whose perception involves being insufficiently muscular. Hoarding disorder is new to the DSM-5, due to mounting evidence of its validity and clinical importance as a diagnosis separate from OCD. For hoarding disorder, there is a specifier for "with excessive acquisition" to distinguish traditional hoarders (those who have difficulty discarding items) from those who purposefully acquire them.

The work group made several changes to the Dissociative Disorders in DSM-5. Criterion A of dissociative identity disorder now includes possession-type experiences and indicates that transitions in identity may be either observed by others or self-reported. Criterion B highlights that dissociative experiences are inconsistent with ordinary forgetting and include recurrent gaps in recalling everyday events and/or traumatic events, important personal information, and/or traumatic events. The group also combined DSM-IV's depersonalization and derealization disorders into DSM-5's depersonalization/derealization disorder.

The DSM-IV chapter on Eating Disorders was expanded into the chapter titled Feeding and Eating Disorders in the DSM-5. The new chapter incorporates several conditions previously classified as disorders of childhood in DSM-IV. Perhaps the most significant change involved adding binge eating disorder as a separate eating disorder. Binge eating disorder is defined by recurring episodes of eating significantly more food in a short period of time than most people would eat under similar circumstances. A subjective lack of control is one characteristic of the disorder. Binge eating episodes must occur at least once a week over the last 3 months to establish the diagnosis, in line with the requirement for bulimia nervosa in DSM-5. The most significant change to anorexia nervosa is that the requirement for amenorrhea was eliminated.

The DSM-IV chapter on Sleep Disorders was renamed as Sleep-Wake Disorders in the DSM-5. The work group primarily focused on bringing together medical and mental disorders' impact on sleep, consistent with the overall philosophy in DSM-5. Primary insomnia was renamed insomnia disorder to avoid the need to differentiate primary and secondary insomnia. The group divided the breathing-related sleep disorders into three separate disorders named obstructive sleep apnea hypopnea, central sleep apnea, and sleep-related hypoventilation [3 (p13)]. The group expanded the subtypes of circadian rhythm sleep-wake disorders to include advanced sleep phase syndrome, irregular sleep-wake type, and non-24-hour sleep-wake type; they removed jet lag type [3 (p13)]. The group added rapid eye movement sleep behavior disorder and restless leg syndrome as separate diagnoses [3 (p13)]. Nonrapid eye movement sleep arousal disorders now includes sleepwalking and sleep terrors, which include the specifier "with sleep-related sexual behavior (sexsomnia)." DSM-5 notes, "In sexsomnia, varying degrees of sexual activity (e.g., masturbation, fondling, groping, sexual intercourse) occur as complex behaviors arising from sleep without conscious awareness" [2 (p400–1)].

The work group separated the DSM-IV's chapter on Sexual and Gender Identity Disorders into distinct chapters on Sexual Dysfunctions, Gender Dysphoria, and Paraphilic Disorders. The new criteria for gender dysphoria emphasize the concept of "gender incongruence" over cross-sexual identification. There are now two separate disorders, one for children and one for adolescents and adults, each requiring 6 months of incongruence between experienced or expressed gender and assigned gender. Recognizing that gender identify is unrelated to sexual orientation, the "sexually attracted to" specifiers were eliminated. There are now specifiers for "with a disorder of sexual development," such as androgen insensitivity and "posttransition," if the individual lives full-time as the desired gender and has had or plans to have a cross-sex medical treatment regimen or procedure to confirm the individual's desired gender.

In the chapter on Paraphilic Disorders, DSM-5 distinguishes between a paraphilia and disordered paraphilic behavior. The manual defines a paraphilia as "any intense and persistent sexual interest other than sexual interest in genital stimulation or preparatory fondling with phenotypically normal, physically mature, consenting human partners" [2 (p685–6)]. DSM-5 defines a paraphilic disorder as follows: "a paraphilia that is currently causing distress or impairment to the individual or a paraphilia whose satisfaction has entailed personal harm, or risk of harm, to others" [2 (pp685-686)]. Consistent with this new perspective, the term disorder was added to the names of each diagnosis in the chapter, although the diagnostic criteria remain largely unchanged. This change reflects the goal of preventing automatic labeling of nonnormative sexual behavior as psychopathological, even when it is does not result in negative consequences for the individual. The DSM-5 also includes course specifiers of "in a controlled environment" and "in remission" for individuals without opportunities to act on their urges and who no longer meet either the Criterion A or B of the disorder, respectively. Although the Highlights of Changes From DSM-IV-TR to DSM-5 document published by the APA states that these specifiers are available for all paraphilic disorders, the DSM-5 text does not include them for use with pedophilic disorder, raising the question of whether pedophilic disorder can enter remission or not.

The DSM-IV chapter titled Delirium, Dementia, and Amnestic and Other Cognitive Disorders predominantly moved into the chapter titled Neurocognitive Disorders in DSM-5. In DSM-5, dementia and amnestic disorder are combined under the condition named major neurocognitive disorder (NCD). DSM-5 also introduced a disorder called mild NCD, a less severe form of cognitive impairment. The work group's stated purpose was to recognize a less severe impairment that is itself concerning and becomes a focus of treatment [3 (p17)]. Some authors applauded the change, noting the potential benefits of diagnosing cognitive impairments earlier after onset [59]. Other authors expressed concerns about creating an unclear distinction between mild cognitive impairment and dementia [60].

The Personality and Personality Disorders Work Group considered overhauling the entire process of diagnosing personality disorders. After much debate, they decided to keep the personality disorders unchanged in DSM-5 and present the alternative formulation in Section III. The proposed system met resistance during the development, particularly based on the somewhat cumbersome diagnostic process [61].

DSM-5 introduced a new chapter titled, Medication-Induced Movement Disorders and Other Adverse Effects of Medication. Although these are included in DSM-5's Section II, DSM-5 specifically states that these diagnoses are not mental disorders [2 (p709)]. DSM-5 still contains a chapter of Other Conditions That May Be a Focus of Clinical Attention that primarily includes the v-codes.

SUMMARY

DSM-5 introduced several important diagnostic changes. Even for individuals working in systems that are slow to adopt the diagnostic changes, DSM-5 criteria can easily be presented for questioning during the course of forensic work (e.g., depositions, testimony, etc). Key points from this chapter include the following:

- The Neurodevelopmental Disorders Work Group implemented major changes, which include defining intellectual disability as a new way to diagnose cognitive impairment and redefining ASDs.
- The Mood Disorders Work Group added disruptive mood dysregulation disorder (DMDD) to address "potential overdiagnosis and overtreatment of bipolar disorder in children" up to age 18 who exhibit "persistent irritability and frequent episodes of extreme behavioral dyscontrol" [3 (p4)].
- The Anxiety, Obsessive-Compulsive Spectrum, Posttraumatic, and Dissociative Disorders Work Group separated posttraumatic stress disorder (PTSD) from the Anxiety Disorders and significantly altered the criteria.

- The Somatic Symptoms Disorders Work Group defined somatic symptom disorder (SSD), a condition which can be diagnosed even when medically explained diseases result in distressing somatic symptoms.
- The ADHD and Disruptive Behavior Disorders Work Group made significant diagnostic changes to both oppositional defiant disorder (ODD) and intermittent explosive disorder (IED). They also made it possible to concurrently diagnose children and adolescents with ODD and conduct disorder (CD).
- The Substance-Related Disorders Work Group collapsed abuse and dependence into a single substance use disorder, creating a new set of criteria.

REFERENCES

1. American Psychiatric Association: *Diagnostic and Statistical Manual of Mental Disorders*. 4th ed., Text Revision. Washington, DC: American Psychiatric Association; 2000.
2. American Psychiatric Association: *Diagnostic and Statistical Manual of Mental Disorders*. 5th ed. Arlington, Virginia: American Psychiatric Association; 2013.
3. American Psychiatric Association. "Highlights of Changes from DSM-IV-TR to DSM-5." Available at: http://www.dsm5.org/Documents/changes%20from%20dsm-iv-tr%20to%20dsm-5.pdf. Accessed 12 January 2014.
4. American Psychiatric Association. "Meet Us" page for Neurodevelopmental Disorders Work Group. Available at: http://www.dsm5.org/MeetUs/Pages/Neurodevelopmental%20Disorders.aspx. Accessed 3 January 2014.
5. Rosa's Law, Pub L No. 111-256 124 stat. 2643 (2010).
6. Office of the White House Press Secretary. Remarks by the president at the signing of the 21st century communications and video accessibility act of 2010. Available at: http://www.whitehouse.gov/the-press-office/2010/10/08/remarks-president-signing-21st-century-communications-and-video-accessib. Accessed 4 January 2014.
7. Frances A. Psychiatric Times Blog. "DSM-5 badly flunks the writing test." Available at: http://www.psychiatrictimes.com/blogs/dsm-5/dsm-5-badly-flunks-writing-test. Published November 20, 2012. Accessed 12 May 2014.
8. McPartland JC, Reichow B, Volkmar FR. Sensitivity and specificity of proposed DSM-5 diagnostic criteria for autism spectrum disorder. *J Am Acad Child Adolesc Psychiatry* 2012; 51:368–383.
9. Young RL, Rodi ML. Redefining autism spectrum disorder using DSM-5: the implications of the proposed DSM-5 criteria for autism spectrum disorders. *J Autism Dev Disord* 2014; 44:758–765.
10. Swedo SE, Baird G, Cook EH, et al. Commentary from the DSM-5 workgroup on neurodevelopmental disorders. *J Am Acad Child Adolesc Psychiatry* 2012; 51:347–349.
11. Mandy WP, Charman T, Skuse DH. Testing the construct validity of proposed criteria for DSM-5 autism spectrum disorder. *J Am Acad Child Adolesc Psychiatry* 2012; 51:41–50.
12. Mandy W, Charman T, Puura K, Skuse D. Investigating the cross-cultural validity of DSM-5 autism spectrum disorder: evidence from Finnish and UK samples. *Autism* 2014; 18:45–54.

13. Hazen EP, McDougle CJ, Volkmar FR. Changes in the diagnostic criteria for autism in DSM-5: controversies and concerns. *J Clin Psychiatry* 2013; 74:739–740.
14. Gibson J, Adams C, Lockton E, Green J. Social communication disorder outside autism? A diagnostic classification approach to delineating pragmatic language impairment, high functioning autism and specific language impairment. *J Child Psychol Psychiatry* 2013; 54:1186–1197.
15. Norbury CF. Practitioner review: social (pragmatic) communication disorder conceptualization, evidence and clinical implications. *J Child Psychol Psychiatry* 2014; 55:204–216.
16. American Psychiatric Association. "Meet Us" page for Mood Disorders Work Group. Available at: http://www.dsm5.org/MeetUs/Pages/MoodDisorders.aspx. Accessed 3 January 2014.
17. Iglewicz A, Seay K, Zetumer SD, Zisook S. The removal of the bereavement exclusion in the DSM-5: exploring the evidence. *Curr Psychiatry Rep* 2013; 15:413.
18. Rhebergen D, Graham R. The re-labeling of dysthymic disorder to persistent depressive disorder in DSM-5: old wine in new bottles? *Curr Opin Psychiatry* 2014; 27:27–31.
19. Copeland WE, Angold A, Costello EJ, Egger H. Prevalence, comorbidity, and correlates of DSM-5 proposed disruptive mood dysregulation disorder. *Am J Psychiatry* 2013; 170:173–179.
20. Axelson D, Findling RL, Fristad MA, et al. Examining the proposed disruptive mood dysregulation disorder diagnosis in children in the Longitudinal Assessment of Manic Symptoms Study. *J Clin Psychiatry* 2012; 73:1342–1350.
21. American Psychiatric Association. "Meet Us" page for Anxiety, Obsessive-Compulsive Spectrum, Posttraumatic, and Dissociative Disorders Work Group. Available at: http://www.dsm5.org/MeetUs/Pages/Anxiety.aspx. Accessed 3 January 2014.
22. Friedman M. Finalizing PTSD in DSM-5: getting here from there and where to go next. *J Trauma Stress* 2013; 26:548–556.
23. Zoellner LA, Rothbaum BO, Feeny NC. PTSD not an anxiety disorder? DSM committee proposal turns back the hands of time. *Depress Anxiety* 2011; 28:853–856.
24. Frueh BC, Elhai JD, Acierno R. The future of posttraumatic stress disorder in the DSM. *Psychol Inj Law* 2010; 3:260–270.
25. McFarlane AC. Redefining PTSD in DSM-5:conundrums and potentially unintended consequences. In: Stein DJ, Friedman MJ, Blanco C, eds. *Post-traumatic Stress Disorder.* 1st ed. West Sussex, UK: Wiley-Blackwell; 2011:42–47.
26. American Psychiatric Association. "Meet Us" page for Somatic Symptoms Disorders Work Group. Available at: http://www.dsm5.org/MeetUs/Pages/SomaticDistressDisorders.aspx. Accessed January 3, 2014.
27. Dimsdale JE, Creed F, Escobar J, et al. Somatic symptom disorder: an important change in DSM. *J Psychosom Res* 2013; 75:223–228.
28. Mayou R, Kirmayer LJ, Simon G, et al. Somatoform disorders: time for a new approach in DSM-V. *Am J Psychiatry* 2005; 162:847–855.
29. Lowe B, Mundt C, Herzog W, et al. Validity of current somatoform disorder diagnoses: perspectives for classification in DSM-V and ICD-11. *Psychopathology* 2008; 41:4–9.
30. Fink P, Toft T, Hansen MS, et al. Symptoms and syndromes of bodily distress: an exploratory study of 978 internal medical, neurological, and primary care patients. *Psychsom Med* 2007; 69:30–39.

31. Rief W, Martin A. How to use the new DSM-5 somatic symptom disorder diagnosis in research and practice: a critical evaluation and a proposal for modifications. *Annu Rev Clin Psychol* 2014; 10:339–367.
32. Dimsdale J. The proposed diagnosis of somatic symptom disorders in DSM-V to replacement somatoform disorders in DSM-IV—a preliminary report. *J Psychosom Res* 2009; 66:473–476.
33. Rief W, Mewes R, Martin A, et al. Are psychological features useful in classifying patients with somatic symptoms? *Psychosom Med* 2014; 72:648–655.
34. Frances A. DSM-5 somatic symptom disorder. *J Nerv Ment Dis* 2013; 201:530–531.
35. Frances A. The new somatic symptom disorder in DSM-5 risks mislabeling many people as mentally ill. *Br Med J* 2013; 346:f1580.
36. Hollander H, Kim S, Zohar J. OCSDs in the forthcoming DSM-V. CNS Spectrums 2007; 12:320–323
37. American Psychiatric Association. "Meet Us" page for ADHD and Disruptive Behavior Disorders Work Group. Available at: http://www.dsm5.org/MeetUs/Pages/ADHD.aspx. Accessed 3 January 2014.
38. First MB. Externalizing Disorders of Childhood (Attention-deficit/Hyperactivity Disorder, Conduct Disorder, Oppositional Defiant Disorder, Juvenile Bipolar Disorder) (February 14-16, 2007). American Psychiatric Association DSM-5 Development. Available at: http://www.dsm5.org/Research/Pages/ExternalizingDisordersofChildhood(Attention-deficitHyperactivityDisorder,ConductDisorder,Oppositional-DefiantDisorder,Juven.aspx). Accessed 11 November 2013.
39. Coccaro EF. Intermittent Explosive Disorder as a Disorder of Impulsive Aggression in DSM-5. *Am J Psychiatry* 2012; 169:577–588.
40. American Psychiatric Association. "Meet Us" page for Substance-Related Disorders Work Group. Available at: http://www.dsm5.org/MeetUs/Pages/Substance-RelatedDisorders.aspx. Accessed 3 January 2014.
41. Hasin DS, O'Brien CP, Auriacombe M, et al. DSM-5 Criteria for substance use disorders: recommendations and rationale. *Am J of Psychiatry* 2013; 170:834–851.
42. O'Brien CP. Addiction and dependence in DSM-V. *Addiction* 2011; 106:866–867.
43. Hasin DS, Hatzenbuehler ML, Keyes K, Ogburn E. Substance use disorders: Diagnostic and Statistical Manual of Mental Disorders, fourth edition (DSM-IV) and International Classification of Diseases, tenth edition (ICD-10). *Addiction* 2006; 101(Suppl):59–75.
44. Hasin D, Paykin A. Dependence symptoms but no diagnosis: diagnostic "orphans" in a community sample. *Drug Alcohol Depend* 1998; 50:19–26.
45. Pierucci-Lagha A, Gelemter J, Feinn R, et al. Diagnostic reliability of the Semi-structured Assessment for Drug Dependence and Alcoholism (SSADDA). *Drug and Alcohol Dependence* 2005; 80:303–312.
46. Hasin DS, Van Rossem R, McCloud S, Endicott J. Differentiating DSM-IV alcohol dependence and abuse by course: community heavy drinkers. *J of Subst Abuse* 1997; 9:127–135.
47. Gillespie NA, Neale MC, Prescott CA, et al. Factor and item-response analysis DSM-IV criteria for abuse of and dependence on cannabis, cocaine, hallucinogens, sedatives, stimulants and opioids. *Addiction* 2007; 102:920–930.
48. Lynskey MT, Agrawal A. Psychometric properties of DSM assessments of illicit drug abuse and dependence: results from the National Epidemiologic

Survey on Alcohol and Related Conditions (NESARC). *Psychol Med* 2007; 37:1345–1355.
49. Casey M, Adamson G, Shevlin M, McKinney A. The role of craving in AUDs: dimensionality and differential functioning in the DSM-5. *Drug Alcohol Depend* 2012; 125:75–80.
50. Dawson DA, Saha TD, Grant BF. A multidimensional assessment of the validity and utility of alcohol use disorder severity as determined by item response theory models. *Drug Alcohol Depend* 2010; 107:31–38.
51. Budney AJ, Hughes JR, Moore BA, Vandrey R. Review of the validity and significance of cannabis withdrawal syndrome. *Am J of Psychiatry* 2004; 161:1967–1977.
52. Shmulewtiz D, Wall MM, Aharonovich E, et al. Validity of proposed DSM-5 diagnostic criteria for nicotine use disorder: results from 734 Israeli lifetime smokers. *Psychol Med* 2013; 43:2179–2190.
53. Hughes JR, Helzer JE, Lindberg SA. Prevalence of DSM/ICD-defined nicotine dependence. *Drug Alcohol Depend* 2006; 85:91–102.
54. Petry NM, Stinson FS, Grant BF. Comorbidity of DSM-IV pathological gambling and other psychiatric disorders: results from the National Epidemiologic Survey on Alcohol and Related Conditions. *J Clin Psychiatry* 2004; 66:564–574.
55. Petry NM, Blanco C, Auriacombe M, et al. An overview of and rationale for changes proposed for pathological gambling in DSM5. *J Gambl Stud* 2014; 30:493–502.
56. Tandon R, Gaebel W, Barch DM, et al. Definition and description of schizophrenia in the DSM-5. *Schizophr Res* 2013; 150:3–10.
57. Malaspina D, Owen MJ, Heckers S, et al. Schizoaffective disorder in the DSM-5. *Schizophr Res* 2013; 150:21–25.
58. Fiedorowicz JG, Endicott J, Leon AC, et al. Subthreshold hypomanic symptoms in progression from unipolar major depression to bipolar depression. *Am J Psychiatry* 2011; 168:40–48.
59. Blazer D. Neurocognitive disorders in DSM-5. *Am J Psychiatry* 2013; 170:585–587.
60. Morris JC. Revised criteria for mild cognitive impairment may compromise the diagnosis of Alzheimer disease dementia. *Arch Neurol* 2012; 69:700–708.
61. Shedler J, Beack A, Fonagy P, et al. Personality disorders in DSM-5. *Am J Psychiatry* 2010; 167:1026–1028.

CHAPTER 3

DSM-5: Diagnosing and Report Writing

INTRODUCTION

DSM-5 profoundly changes how diagnoses are listed and described. With DSM-5's increasing focus on dimensional classification, decreasing emphasis on a categorical approach, and elimination of DSM-IV's multiaxial distinction, evaluators' next question very well may be, "What do we do now?" The answer: If you are going to use the DSM-5, you should have an in depth understanding of not only the manual's diagnostic changes but also the meaning of these changes. This chapter provides practical steps to help practitioners and forensic experts move forward and utilize the current manual to make DSM-5 diagnoses in both clinical and forensic contexts.

STEP 1: UNDERSTAND THE DIFFERENCE BETWEEN "DIAGNOSIS" AND "MENTAL DISORDER"

DSM-5 distinguishes the term "diagnosis" from the term "mental disorder" and evaluators should be careful to maintain this distinction. DSM-5's definition of mental disorder is described in Chapter 2. An important aspect of this definition is the need to demonstrate that the person's described dysfunction results in a "*clinically significant*" disturbance. In other words, symptoms alone do not equate with a mental disorder [1(p20)].

All of the disorders identified in Section II of the DSM-5 are "mental disorders" with two exceptions: "Medication-Induced Movement Disorders and Other Adverse Effects of Medication" and "Other Conditions That May Be a Focus of Clinical Attention." DSM-5 notes that medication-induced movement disorders are included in Section II along with mental disorders because they are frequently important in the management of medical and mental disorders and they are often important in the differential diagnosis of mental disorders.

In regard to the DSM-5 section titled "Other Conditions that May be a Focus of Clinical Attention," the DSM-5 text emphasizes that these diagnoses are included primarily to assist providers by describing common situations where individuals may seek mental health counseling but do not meet criteria for a mental disorder [1(p715)].

There are over 100 "other conditions" included in this DSM-5 section. DSM-5 "conditions" frequently seen in forensic settings include the following: malingering; academic or educational problems; other problem related to employment; homelessness; target of (perceived) adverse discrimination or persecution; victim of crime; imprisonment or other incarceration; adult antisocial behavior; child or adolescent antisocial behavior; and nonadherence to medical treatment. When writing the report or communicating findings to the legal system, the evaluator should be careful not to inadvertently label these "other conditions" as a mental disorder. For example, if an individual is assessed as malingering, the evaluator can communicate that although this person has a diagnosis of malingering, this diagnosis is *not* a DSM-5 mental disorder.

STEP 2: EVALUATE CRITERIA RELEVANT TO MAKING A DIAGNOSIS

DSM-5 provides specific diagnostic criteria and/or text descriptions for each of their diagnoses. DSM-5 notes that both clinical judgment and the clinical interview are relevant when considering diagnostic criteria [1 (p21)]. In other words, the diagnostic criteria are not the sole determinant of making a diagnosis. However, the diagnostic criteria are an important component when making a diagnosis and cannot be dismissed based solely on the evaluator's judgment or personal idiosyncratic diagnostic schema.

For some DSM-5 diagnoses, evaluators may find it difficult to understand how many criteria are necessary to establish a disorder depending on the language used to introduce the criterion set. For example, for the diagnosis of intellectual disability, when introducing Criterion A, Criterion B, and Criterion C, the DSM-5 specifically requires that all three criteria should be met [1 (p33)]. In marked contrast, the DSM-5 notes that Criterion A for autism spectrum disorder may be met when the individual has sustained deficits in the areas of social communication and interaction in a variety of contexts. DSM-5 further emphasizes that the examples provided by DSM-5 as illustrative of autism spectrum disorder are *not* all inclusive [1 (p50)]. This introduction is followed by the listing of three different types of deficits in social communication and social interaction. With this vague language, particularly compared with more specific instructions for other diagnoses, one is left to wonder: how many social deficit types are required to satisfy Criterion A? One? Two? Three? Perhaps *none* of the three provided deficit types are required as the language suggests that the evaluator may provide his or her own example of a social communication or interaction deficit. As a result, varying examiners may arise at different conclusions based on their own interpretation of this wording [2]. Evaluators may find some clarification by investigating the criteria standard used in field trials to established interrater reliability for the diagnosis in question.

There are situations in which an individual will experience symptoms that are clinically significant yet do not meet sufficient criteria for a diagnosis. Under DSM-IV, the designation "not otherwise specified" (NOS) was used in this circumstance. The NOS designation was eliminated from use under DSM-5 to reportedly enhance diagnostic specificity. DSM-5 provides two options for the evaluator to consider when the person evaluated does not meet criteria for any specific category within a diagnostic class. The two DSM-5 designations used in this circumstance are "other specified disorder" and "unspecified disorder." The designator "other specified disorder" is applied when the evaluator chooses to communicate the specific reason that an individual does not meet diagnostic criteria for any particular category. The following three steps are helpful in making a diagnosis in this circumstance:

1. Begin the diagnosis with the phrase "other specified;"
2. Use the name of the diagnostic chapter to which the diagnostic symptoms belong; and
3. State the specific reason why the diagnosis could not be made.

Consider the following situation as an example for when the "other specified" designation may be used. An individual has three clinically significant symptoms of depression lasting at least four weeks but does not meet the minimum requirement of five specified symptoms of depression for a major depressive episode or another depressive circumstance. The diagnosis in this situation would be written as follows: "other specified" + "depressive disorder" (name of diagnostic chapter) + "depressive episode with insufficient symptoms" (reason diagnosis not made) resulting in a written diagnosis that reads: Other specified depressive disorder, depressive episode with insufficient symptoms.

DSM-5 allows use of the phrase "unspecified disorder" when a person does not meet criteria for a specific disorder and the evaluator chooses not to specify the reason criteria are not met or for situations in which there is insufficient information to make a more specific diagnosis. In this situation, the diagnosis is made using the following two steps:

1. Begin the diagnosis with the word "unspecified"; and
2. Use the name of the diagnostic chapter to which the diagnostic symptoms belong.

DSM-5 notes that the use of the "unspecified" specifier may be appropriate in the emergency room setting when a person presents with a prominent symptom (e.g., delusions, hallucinations, mania, depression, or substance intoxication) but a fuller differential diagnosis is not yet possible. In the forensic context, the "other specified" designator may be preferable to "unspecified" because this allows the legal system to better understand why the individual did not meet criteria for a particular diagnosis. However, DSM-5 emphasizes that the decision to use "other specified" vs. "unspecified diagnoses" is left up entirely to the clinician's judgment.

STEP 3: EVALUATE APPLICABILITY OF DIAGNOSTIC SUBTYPES AND SPECIFIERS

After determining whether the person meets criteria for a DSM-5 diagnosis, the evaluator should evaluate if there are any diagnostic subtypes or specifiers that apply. Under DSM-5's diagnostic scheme, subtypes are mutually exclusive subgroupings within a particular diagnosis that are indicated by the manual's instruction "specify whether" included in the diagnostic criteria. Under this definition, an individual *cannot* be diagnosed with two subtypes of a disorder. Examples of mental disorders that include mutually exclusive subtypes are illness anxiety disorder, encopresis, and narcolepsy [1(p21)].

In contrast to subtypes, DSM-5 specifiers are identified in the diagnostic set by the instruction "specify" or "specify if." Specifier types include course specifiers (e.g., full or partial remission), severity specifiers, frequency specifiers, cross-cutting symptom specifiers, duration specifiers, descriptive feature specifiers (e.g., with poor insight), and environmental specifiers (e.g., in a controlled environment). Severity and course specifiers are only used to describe a person's *current* presentation and only when the person meets full criteria for a diagnosis. When a person has an "other specified/unspecified" diagnosis, severity and course specifiers cannot be used. There are a variety of specifiers and their definitions and applications are summarized below [1(p22)].

Provisional specifier

Under DSM-5, a diagnosis can also be recorded with the specifier "provisional" in two circumstances. First, when there is a "strong presumption" that full diagnostic criteria will ultimately be met but there is not enough information available to make a diagnosis at the time of the evaluation [1 (p23)]. Consider the following example where a provisional disorder may be appropriate.

VIGNETTE 1

Michael is a 39-year-old man who is taken to the emergency room after his wife found him nonresponsive in their bedroom as a result of an overdose of sleeping medication. His wife tells the emergency room psychiatrist that he has experienced severe insomnia, problems concentrating at work, and social withdrawal over the past month. However, because he is nonresponsive, the psychiatrist cannot establish that he meets full criteria for major depressive disorder. How should the psychiatrist code Michael's diagnosis?

In this situation, the psychiatrist could record Michael's diagnosis as follows: major depressive disorder (provisional). There may be presentations where the evaluator is struggling with whether to assign a "provisional" specifier diagnosis versus an "other specified/unspecified" diagnostic designation. The main point to consider in this circumstance is DSM-5's emphasis on using the provisional specifier in situations in which there is a *strong presumption* the person will meet criteria for the disorder. This contrasts with the "other specified/unspecified" designation, which can be used in circumstances where additional information does *not* (or is unlikely to) provide sufficient criteria or there remains general diagnostic uncertainty about the underlying etiology of the presenting symptoms.

Second, the provisional specifier may be used in situations in which the differential diagnosis depends exclusively on the illness duration. For example, a person who meets the duration criteria for schizophreniform disorder (i.e., symptom duration more than one month but less than six months) would be diagnosed with "schizophreniform disorder, provisional."

Severity specifiers

In DSM-5, the method of rating the severity of a mental disorder varies according to the disorder. For some disorders, the severity depends a specified number of recorded symptoms. Substance use disorders, for example, are rated as either mild, moderate, or severe based on an established number of symptoms required for each severity level. In contrast, the severity level determination of intellectual disability involves a more subjective assessment of the person's adaptive functioning in three domains, without any clear cutoff scores, specified number of symptoms, or required assessment instrument. Many disorders (e.g., depressive disorders and bipolar and related disorders) are rated as "mild, moderate, or severe" depending on how many symptoms are present, the significance of symptoms, and the degree to which the symptoms impair the individual's functioning [1 (p154, p188)]. Unlike substance use disorders, this rating method does *not* provide a specific number of required criterion symptoms but *does* require an analysis of symptom severity and degree of disability. In this context, evaluators are likely to use disparate methods to evaluate symptom severity and disability as no particular assessment tools are mandated.

Section III of DSM-5 provides examples of "emerging measures" suggested for use in further clinical evaluation and research and to assess symptom severity. "Cross-cutting symptom measures" (Level 1 and Level 2) are patient- or informant-rated measures used to assess a variety of mental health domains from a range of possible disorders. In contrast to cross-cutting symptom measures, "severity measures" are disorder-specific with criteria that generally correspond to the DSM-5 diagnostic criteria. DSM-5 discusses these severity measures, and the corresponding DSM-5 website provides specific severity disorder assessments. On the DSM-5 website, there are 10 self-report disorder-specific severity ratings for adults and 10 self-report disorder-specific severity ratings for children and adolescents. In addition, there are four clinician-rated disorder-specific severity ratings and two clinician-rated severity ratings that are not specific to any disorder (e.g., ratings of nonsuicidal behavior and psychosis). All of these rating schemes are included in Section III, "emerging measures," and therefore are not a mandatory component of assessment.

Evaluators who elect to use these assessment instruments should be familiar with the reliability and validity of these instruments and the evidence to support their use. In addition, many of these instruments have ratings that do not correspond to the DSM-5 criteria used to rate diagnosis severity. As an example, for the diagnosis of major depressive disorder, DSM-5 requires at least five depressive symptoms during the same 2-week period. According to DSM-5, the severity of depression is based on how many symptoms are present. In addition, seven of these symptoms must be present "nearly every day" over a 2-week time frame [1(p160–161)]. The suggested severity measure for depression on the DSM-5 web site is one adapted from the Patient Health Questionnaire-9 (PHQ-9). In contrast to DSM-5 depression criteria, the PHQ-9 assesses symptoms over a 1-week period and severity levels depend on the frequency of each symptom (i.e., not at all, several days, more than half the days, and nearly every day). It is very possible to receive a rating of "moderately severe depression" on the PHQ-9 but not even meet the

DSM-5 threshold to qualify for a diagnosis of depression. To prevent such conflicting and confusing results, it is recommended that the evaluator follow the DSM-5 diagnostic guidelines for rating severity included in the diagnosis criteria set.

Psychosis severity specifier

The DSM-5 section titled "Schizophrenia Spectrum and Other Psychotic Disorders" includes the following mental disorders: delusional disorder, brief psychotic disorder, schizophreniform disorder, schizophrenia, schizoaffective disorder, substance/medication-induced psychotic disorder, and psychotic disorder due to another medical condition. In each of these diagnostic criteria set, the manual instructs the evaluator to provide a "quantitative" evaluation of the following five major psychotic symptom categories: delusions, hallucinations, disorganized speech, abnormal psychomotor behavior, and negative symptoms. DSM-5 also suggests that clinicians consider rating symptom severity for the week prior to the evaluation [1 (p97)].

For all psychotic disorders listed in Section II, the DSM-5 also references an assessment instrument titled "Clinician-Rated Dimensions of Psychosis Symptom Severity" (CRDPSS). However, the actual instrument is included in Section III, a section that includes emerging measures and models that have not yet been included as part of the required DSM-5 diagnostic criteria. Because severity of psychosis may be particularly relevant in a variety of forensic and clinical contexts, an understanding of the CRDPSS is important in determining the appropriateness of its use. This instrument measures eight symptom dimensions that occur in individuals with psychotic disorders. The eight dimensions measured by this instrument include the five Criterion A symptoms of schizophrenia (hallucinations, delusions, disorganized speech, abnormal psychomotor behavior, and negative symptoms) *plus* impaired cognition, depression, and mania. The instrument's authors emphasize that symptom severity varies across individuals with psychosis thereby necessitating a dimensional assessment to measure this variability and to track the symptom course over time [3].

This CRDPSS uses a 5-point *Likert* scale to rate each of eight symptom dimensions. The five possible ratings are as follows: 0=not present; 1=equivocal; 2=present, but mild; 3=present and moderate; and 4=present and severe. Although cutoff scores are not included in the DSM-5, in a separate publication the instrument's authors note that a score of 2 or higher "should be considered sufficient severity to fulfill a Criterion A diagnostic indicator for schizophrenia" [3 (p16)]. Barsh et al. [3] provide their own definitions of how to rate each dimension. For example, the severity of hallucinations and delusions depends on the degree to which the person feels pressured to respond to the voices/delusions or is bothered by the voices/delusions. Other questions typically asked by forensic examiners to evaluate the severity of hallucinations and delusions are not included in the rating. It is unclear from the DSM-5 manual or the literature how the authors chose the final factors to determine symptom severity, the evidence base to support their inclusion or exclusion of factors, and how the validity and reliability of this instrument was established (if at all).

Because of the limited research on the use of the CRDPSS, forensic evaluators can expect a rigorous cross-examination by knowledgeable attorneys if they use this instrument to rate the severity of psychotic disorders.

The evaluator may wish to consider the following options when evaluating psychotic disorders:

Option 1: Because DSM-5 explicitly states that a severity rating is not required to make a schizophrenic spectrum disorder diagnosis, the examiner could chose to make the diagnosis without including the severity specifier. However, the severity of a person's psychosis is often very important in forensic and clinical contexts. An examiner who provides no quantitative assessment of psychosis severity may be limited on the degree of "quantitative" information they can provide relevant to key legal issues and relevant to determining the appropriate treatment and response to treatment. However, the evaluator could provide "qualitative" examples about the individual's psychotic symptoms. For example, if a woman stabs her three children to death based on command hallucinations from her deceased mother that she must do so, the examiner could appropriately communicate that this woman's psychotic symptoms are very severe when she is symptomatic.

Option 2: Because DSM-5 notes that psychosis severity is rated by a quantitative assessment of delusions, hallucinations, disorganized speech, abnormal psychomotor behavior and negative symptoms, the evaluator could rate only the first five CRDPSS items (which corresponds to these five Criterion A symptoms of schizophrenia). The caveats noted above about the known reliability and validity of this instrument and its use in a legal setting should be considered if this option is chosen.

Option 3: The evaluator could assess all eight dimensions of the CRDPSS even though not required to do so for purposes of rating severity. The caveats noted above about the known reliability and validity of this instrument and its use in a legal setting should be considered if this option is chosen.

Option 4: The evaluator could choose not to use the CRDPSS and instead administer an alternate evidence-based assessment that has demonstrated efficacy in rating the five required psychotic dimensions.

Validated measures of psychotic symptom severity are available, and two of these are briefly summarized below.

The Positive and Negative Syndrome Scale (PANNS) is a well established and valid clinician-administered instrument used to measure the severity of schizophrenia symptoms [4]. The PANSS has good interrater reliability when rated by trained and well qualified examiners [4, 5]. The PANSS has 30 items accompanied by a specific definition and detailed anchoring criteria for seven rating points (ranging from 1=absent to 7=extreme). Ratings are generally made by assessing the person's symptoms during the past week. The PANSS has three scales: the Positive Scale (P), Negative Scale (N), and General Psychopathology Scale (G). All five Criterion A symptoms that require a quantitative rating are well covered on the PANNS. In addition, the PANNS can yield a negative symptom factor score (NSFS) that includes five items from the negative scale and two items from the general psychopathology scale. This score has demonstrated good validity and test-retest reliability as a negative symptom assessment for patients with prominent negative or disorganized thought symptoms [6].

The Brief Psychiatric Rating Scale (BPRS) Expanded Version (4.0) is another commonly used instrument to assess psychiatric symptoms that include, but are not limited to, psychotic symptoms. There are 24 items on this instrument with some items rated based on the patient's self-report, some items rated based on observed behavior, and some items rated on the basis of observed behavior and speech. The items are scored on a seven-point scale, with higher ratings equating with more severe symptoms. Although there is no unique scale to measure delusions, the BPRS includes an evaluation of specific types of delusions on various scales, including the somatic concern scale, guilt scale, grandiosity scale, suspiciousness scale, and unusual thought content scale [7]. As with the PANNS, this instrument evaluates symptom severity in the five required areas.

When deciding whether or not to use one of these validated instruments, the examiner should be aware of two caveats. First, the severity ratings are for a defined period of time (e.g., typically the past week). Consider the above example of the woman who stabbed her three children to death with an obvious history of severe psychosis. If she responds to treatment, her scores on the PANSS or BPRS could indicate that her symptoms are "mild" or "absent." Although this may be useful clinical information and important to her current risk evaluation, this score alone would not accurately reflect the severity of her illness when she is not in clinical remission. In a forensic context, if an evaluator chooses to use a quantitative severity-rating instrument, it is highly recommended that they also provide a qualitative description of the person's psychosis severity when they are symptomatic. Second, retrospective ratings of a person's psychotic symptoms using the

PANNS or BPRS may be difficult and not consistent with the administration guidelines.

Although DSM-5 does not require a severity rating of cognitive impairment, depression, or mania for purposes of rating the severity of psychotic disorders, the CRDPSS includes these three dimensions. Rating the dimension of impaired cognition on this instrument may prove to be particularly difficult. The instrument instructs the evaluator to assess the degree, if any, of reduction in cognitive function below the person's expected age, socioeconomic status, and degree of standard deviation from the mean. No specific cognitive assessment instrument is cited or recommended to rate impaired cognition. The instrument's authors provide the following guidance for evaluators in rating this domain:

> We would suggest that when possible, clinicians obtain a formal clinical neuropsychological assessment in individuals with psychosis to fully understand the nature and severity of their cognitive impairments... When it is not possible to obtain a full neuropsychological evaluation, a number of studies have shown that several different brief assessment approaches provide clinically useful information concerning a patient's general level of cognitive impairment... Such measures should be administered and scored by personnel trained in the use of testing instruments and who are familiar with the expected influence of demographic factors... to ensure valid interpretation of observed scores relative to normative data... [3 (p18)]

The likelihood and availability of a formal clinical neuropsychological assessment will vary greatly depending on the treatment setting and purpose of treatment. Acute psychiatric inpatient units with short lengths of stay whose primary goal is to stabilize the patient are unlikely to have a full neuropsychological assessment immediately available or completed by the time of discharge. Likewise, many community outpatient centers and private practice clinics are unlikely to have a neuropsychologist available to help rate this domain for all of their patients with psychosis. Barsh et al. [3] acknowledge this limitation and note that if a formal assessment by trained personnel is not possible, then "the clinician should use the best available information to make a judgment about the client's function, including the clinician's interactions with the patient and/or reports of family members or clinical staff that regularly interact with the patient" [3 (p18)]. However, the instrument's authors acknowledge the limited utility of this approach as they write, "... It is likely that without objective assessments, such ratings will have poor reliability and potentially low validity" [3 (p18)]. Although DSM-5 specifically references the use of the CRDPSS to measure psychosis severity, the DSM-5 also notes that additional investigation is needed to determine whether this instrument is helpful in providing treatment [1 (p90)]. Numerous validated assessments of cognitive impairment are available and a review of these instruments is beyond the scope of this chapter.

"In remission" specifiers

DSM-5 provides the specifiers "in remission," "in full remission," or "in partial remission" for several, but not all, DSM-5 disorders. Definitions of "remission," "full remission," and "partial remission" vary depending on the specific diagnosis. One confusing application of the specifier "in full remission" is related to the Paraphilic Disorders. In the Paraphilic Disorders section, the "in full remission" specifier notes that the individual must not have engaged a "nonconsenting person" in their paraphilic interests, must not be distressed by their paraphilic interests, or must not demonstrate impairment resulting from their paraphilic interests for at least five years [1 (p687)]. This remission specifier is included in the description of every paraphilic disorder with the exception of pedophilic disorder. Therefore, an evaluator could logically conclude that the drafters of the paraphilic disorders criteria wanted to clearly communicate that a person with pedophilic disorder could never be in full remission. However, in the DSM-5 section titled "highlights of changes from DSM-IV to DSM-5," the DSM-5 text specifically notes that the "in remission" specifier applies to all paraphilic disorders [1 (p816)]. It is unclear whether the remission specifier was *mistakenly excluded* in the text description of pedophilic disorder or whether the sentence summarizing the changes from DSM-IV to DSM-5 *mistakenly included* pedophilic disorder. This confusion is extremely problematic, particularly for forensic evaluators who are asked to provide status updates of sex offenders and their treatment response.

Cross-cutting symptom specifiers

A significant focus of DSM-5 is the recognition that various psychiatric symptoms are present in a variety of mental disorders. DSM-5 provides certain *symptom* specifiers that may be used with multiple diagnoses. Two key examples of such cross-cutting symptom specifiers include "panic attack" and "catatonia."

Panic attack specifier

DSM-5 specifically notes that a panic attack is not a mental disorder and cannot be coded as such. The panic attack specifier requires the presence of four (or more) of 13 delineated symptoms that represent an abrupt surge of intense fear or discomfort from a calm or anxious state that peaks within minutes of onset. The panic attack specifier can apply to *any* DSM-5 mental disorder and some medical conditions, with the exception of panic disorder where the presence of panic attack is contained within the criteria for the disorder. DSM-5 mental disorders that have an associated panic attack specifier include bipolar disorders, depressive disorders, eating disorders, personality disorders, and psychotic disorders. Consider the following scenario as an example of how to use the panic attack specifier when making a diagnosis. Heather is a 55-year-old woman diagnosed with borderline personality disorder who describes that her heart suddenly begins to race along with trembling of her hands. She states that she also experiences dizziness and derealization when this occurs. According to DSM-5, Heather's diagnosis would be written as follows: Borderline personality disorder, with panic attack.

Catatonia specifier

DSM-5 describes that catatonia is characterized by three or more of 12 psychomotor features, such as stupor, catalepsy, waxy flexibility, mutism, and grimacing. DSM-5 does not recognize catatonia as a separate disorder but instead notes that catatonia can be associated with another mental or medical disorder. When catatonia is associated with a mental disorder, the specifier reads "catatonia *with* another mental disorder" in contrast to catatonia associated with a medical condition that reads, "catatonic disorder *due to* another medical condition" [1 (p119–120)]. In both situations, the evaluator records two separate diagnoses because the catatonia specifier is not included as part of the underlying diagnoses.

To illustrate, a 22-year-old man with schizophrenia presents with grimacing, mimicking of his peers' speech and movements, and various stereotypies. Based on this presentation, he meets criteria for catatonia associated with his diagnosis of schizophrenia. This diagnosis would read as follows: Catatonia associated with schizophrenia. The evaluator would also diagnose this man with schizophrenia and would code this disorder *first*. The final diagnoses would therefore appear as follows:

1. Schizophrenia
2. Catatonia associated with schizophrenia.

A similar diagnostic listing process occurs if the individual has catatonia associated with a medical condition.

STEP 4: APPLY THE CORRECT INTERNATIONAL CLASSIFICATION OF DISORDERS CODE (ICD) IF REQUIRED

The Mental Health Program of the World Health Organization (WHO) has developed a classification scheme for health conditions known as the International Classification of Diseases (ICD). The ICD coding system has been adopted by the United States and is used by the U.S. Centers for Medicare and Medicaid Services (CMS) and the Centers for Disease Control and Prevention's National Center for Health Statistics to ensure that physical and mental health conditions are coded consistently throughout the world. This international coding scheme allows various nations to record prevalence and mortality data for health conditions in a similar manner. In addition, clinicians use the ICD codes to identify their patient's diagnosis, which is also used by CMS to collect data on prevalence of psychiatric disorders and by insurance companies to process billing submissions [1].

The ICD has undergone numerous revisions over the years. At the time of DSM5's release in 2013, the official coding system used by the United States was the International Classification of Diseases, Ninth Revision, Clinical Modification (ICD-9-CM), even though a 10th revision of the ICD coding system, ICD-10-CM, had already been in use worldwide. Because the United States was to officially adopt the ICD-10-CM by October 2014, DSM-5 includes codes for both ICD-9-CM and ICD-10-CM to assist during this transition period. Both codes are included with the diagnostic criteria set with the ICD-9 code listed first followed by the ICD-10 code in brackets. For example, the diagnosis of schizophrenia with associated codes is identified in the following manner: 295.90 [F20.9] Schizophrenia [1]. Clinicians are generally required to include the ICD codes for billing purposes and should be aware that the coding changes and updates to the DSM-5 are posted on the DSM-5 website [8]. However, forensic evaluators are not mandated to use the associated ICD codes in their forensic reports and typically list the DSM-5 diagnoses only. [*Author's Note: For the purposes of this chapter, ICD codes are not included when diagnoses are provided.*]

When writing a DSM-5 diagnosis that includes subtypes or specifiers, the evaluator should be aware of three diagnostic coding possibilities if they choose to include the ICD codes [1]:

1. For some diagnoses, coding numbers for subtypes and specifiers are available for both ICD-9-CM and ICD-10-CM;
2. For some diagnoses, a subtype or specifier can be coded under ICD-10-CM but not under the ICD-9-CM; and
3. For some diagnoses, subtypes and specifiers cannot be coded either under the ICD-9-CM and ICD-10-CM systems.

In situations, where no ICD codes are available, the evaluator writes the name of the disorder following by the applicable subtype or specifier. For example, a 35-year-old man with obsessive-compulsive disorder who is completely convinced that his obsessional beliefs are true would qualify for the specifier, "with absent insight/delusional beliefs." However, neither ICD-9 nor ICD-10 provides a coding number for this specifier. In this situation, the evaluator would write the diagnosis as follows: 300.3 [F42] obsessive-compulsive disorder, with absent insight/delusional beliefs.

As noted above, the ICD-10 was to have been implemented starting October 2014. However on April 1, 2014, President Obama signed legislation passed by the House and Senate delaying the implementation of ICD-10. At the time of this writing, Centers for Medicare and Medicaid Services (CMS) had not announced an official 2015 compliance date; however, the ICD-10 adoption *cannot* occur prior to October 2015 [9].

STEP 5: DETERMINE WHICH DIAGNOSES ARE "CURRENT"

DSM-5 notes that a diagnosis is typically given in regard to a person's current clinical status. Many DSM-5 diagnoses, but not all, have specifiers that indicate if the diagnosis is in partial or full remission [1 (p22)]. Substance use disorders have an "early remission" and "in sustained remission" modifier. If a person has met criteria for a substance use disorder in the past but does not meet the criteria at the time of the evaluation, the substance use disorder should still be included on the list of diagnoses (with appropriate remission modifiers).

Modifiers such as "history of" or "prior history of" are not included for use in DSM-5. Evaluators should include a previous diagnosis from which the person has recovered on the DSM-5 diagnostic list when the diagnosis has the "full remission" modifier included in the criteria set. For example, if a woman being evaluated currently meets criteria for posttraumatic stress disorder but has a prior history of moderate major depressive disorder (single episode) that has completely remitted, the diagnoses would be listed as follows:

1. Posttraumatic stress disorder
2. Major depressive episode, moderate, in full remission

For situations where the individual has a prior diagnosis that has remitted but there is no DSM-5 remission modifier, the evaluator will need to determine whether the *prior* diagnosis should nevertheless remain on the *current* diagnostic list. There is no universal rule that applies to all diagnoses in regard to this issue. Consider the two following vignettes that illustrate this point.

VIGNETTE 2

Rick is a 58-year-old man convicted of 44 counts of lewd and lascivious conduct against boys and girls, all under the age of 14. After serving time in prison, he is committed as a sexually violent predator to a forensic state hospital. The state statute mandates annual progress reports to court to include current diagnoses. Rick has not had access to children in over a decade and therefore has not acted on his sexual urges nor have his continued fantasies caused him current distress. Should Rick's diagnosis of pedophilic disorder be listed as a "current" DSM-5 diagnosis?

Unlike the rest of the paraphilic disorders, pedophilia has no remission modifier in its criteria set. Therefore, his diagnosis of pedophilic disorder would remain on the current diagnostic list if the evaluator opines that individuals with pedophilic disorder generally never enter remission. [*Author's Note: recall the DSM-5 discrepancy discussed above in the application of the remission modifier to pedophilic disorder.*]

However, there are situations where previous diagnoses have completely remitted, do not have a remission modifier, and yet do not require inclusion in the current diagnostic list. The following vignette illustrates this principle.

VIGNETTE 3

Mary is a 36-year-old woman who was in a near fatal car accident when she was 16 years old. She experienced classic symptoms of posttraumatic stress disorder that resolved completely over a period of two years. Recently, her husband of 15 years goes to the hospital for a routine hernia repair. In the hospital, he is inadvertently given an incorrect dose of potassium in his intravenous fluids. As a result of this medical error, he dies instantly. Mary was not present when this occurred and learns of his death through a phone call from her daughter. Mary does not develop any symptoms of PTSD nor is there any evidence that her prior PTSD is aggravated. However, she becomes severely depressed in response to his death. She sues the hospital providers alleging that her major depressive disorder resulted from the death of her husband that was caused by the negligent hospital staff. How should the forensic evaluator code Mary's diagnoses?

Mary's current DSM-5 diagnoses would include her diagnosis of major depressive disorder (as her principal diagnosis). Her prior PTSD diagnosis is not required to be included as a current diagnosis if she has no evidence of lingering or aggravated PTSD symptoms from the accident that she experienced at age 16. However, the evaluator could discuss her prior PTSD in the diagnostic section that addresses consideration of other disorders.

STEP 6: LIST CURRENT DIAGNOSES IN ORDER OF TREATMENT PRIORITY OR FOCUS OF TREATMENT

DSM-5 abandons the recording of diagnoses in the axial format required by DSM-IV. Under DSM-IV there were five axes: Axis I included clinical disorders and other conditions that may be a focus of clinical attention; Axis II included the diagnoses of personality disorders and mental retardation; Axis III involved an enumeration of general medical conditions potentially relevant to the understanding of the person's mental disorder; Axis IV noted psychosocial and environment problems; and Axis V provided a Global Assessment of Functioning (GAF) score of the individual [10].

DSM-5 notes that under this new system, diagnoses that were previously included under Axes I, II, or III should now be enumerated as a single diagnostic list. The clinician should be aware that DSM-5 has a section titled "Other Conditions that May Be a Focus of Clinical Attention" and conditions listed in this section are also included in the single list of diagnoses. In contrast to DSM-IV, which capitalized the first letter of each word in the diagnosis, the DSM-5 does *not* capitalize diagnoses (except for the first letter when it begins a sentence or the first letter when noted on the list of diagnoses).

In regard to information previously included on the DSM-IV Axes IV and V, DSM-5 indicates that these should *not* be included in the list of diagnoses and the evaluator should note significant stressors and disability ratings separately [1 (p16)]. According to this guideline, the evaluator should document life stressors and disability independent of the list of diagnoses. There seems to be a natural overlap between what would have been listed as psychosocial stressors under Axis IV in the DSM-IV and "other conditions that may be a focus of clinical attention" in DSM-5. The DSM-5 text provides some assistance in distinguishing these two situations by emphasizing that life conditions that account for the reason for treatment or need for further evaluation can be coded as a diagnosis [1 (p16)]. In reality, many psychosocial stressors previously noted on DSM-IV Axis IV will now be recorded on the list of diagnoses (as a V or Z code) if the stressor plays a role in the need for treatment.

DSM-5 emphasizes that when a person has more than one diagnoses, diagnoses should be listed in order of the focus of attention and treatment. The first diagnosis on the list is called the "principal diagnosis." The phrase "(principal diagnosis)" or "(reason for visit)" follows the principal diagnosis in most cases. For example, an evaluator would record the diagnosis of an individual who comes for treatment because they have clinically significant distress from five symptoms of major depressive disorder for the first time in their life as follows:

1. Major depressive disorder, single episode, mild (principal diagnosis)

DSM-5 notes that when a person has a medical condition that causes a mental disorder (which is the focus of treatment), ICD coding rules require that the underlying medical condition is listed first and the resulting mental disorder is listed second. To illustrate, a person who experiences a serious head injury that causes a major neurocognitive disorder would have the following diagnostic listing:

1. Traumatic brain injury
2. Major neurocognitive disorder (principal diagnosis)

Recording diagnoses in an inpatient setting

According to DSM-5, the evaluator should identify those symptoms and behaviors that were the primary reason for the individual's admission when determining the principal diagnosis [1 (p22)]. Consider the following two inpatient scenarios where the same person may receive a different principal diagnoses in regard to two separate psychiatric hospitalizations.

Mr. Jones is a 44-year-old man with well documented schizophrenia and a comorbid alcohol use disorder. Although he has some mild residual psychotic symptoms, he has been able to function reasonably well despite his mild symptoms. However, he has trouble maintaining abstinence from alcohol and continues to drink more than eight beers a day. One day, he decides to stop "cold turkey." When he develops classic signs of alcohol withdrawal, his brother takes him to the emergency room where he is admitted to the hospital for treatment of alcohol withdrawal. Upon discharge, his diagnoses based on this presentation would be noted as follows:

1. Alcohol withdrawal (principal diagnosis)
2. Schizophrenia

In contrast, if Mr. Jones' primary reason for admission involves treatment of active psychotic symptoms rather than alcohol use, then his diagnoses would be listed as follows:

1. Schizophrenia (principal diagnosis)
2. Moderate alcohol use disorder

In situations where multiple diagnoses each contribute to the reason for admission, the evaluator may have difficulty prioritizing the diagnoses. In addition, in long-term hospital settings, such as a forensic psychiatric facility, the diagnosis that results in the hospital admission does not necessarily continue as the primary focus of treatment over the long term. The following vignette illustrates this point.

VIGNETTE 4

Richard is a 42-year-old man found not guilty by reason of insanity for the assault of his landlord while in a manic and psychotic state. Richard also has antisocial personality disorder and a methamphetamine use disorder, but neither of these diagnosis were related to his being determined criminally nonresponsible and subsequently involuntarily hospitalized. During his first year of treatment, Richard's bipolar disorder goes into complete remission. Over his subsequent 10 years of hospitalization, he is repeatedly involved in planned aggression unrelated to his bipolar disorder. In addition, his urine drug screens are repeatedly positive for methamphetamine. Should Richard's bipolar diagnosis remain the principal diagnosis because it was the condition responsible for his hospitalization?

Although bipolar disorder may have been the initial reason for Richard's hospital admission, the principal focus of his treatment centers on addressing his antisocial personality disorder actions and methamphetamine use. Therefore, the treatment team could, and should, consider changing his principle diagnosis to the one that becomes the primary focus of treatment. The treatment team can communicate this diagnostic change and reason for the change in their chart documentation and reports to court.

Recording diagnoses in outpatient setting

In the outpatient setting, where more than one diagnosis is present, the clinician notes the reason for the visit as the primary diagnosis that results in the individual seeking treatment [1 (p22)]. Because this language notes that the principal diagnosis is identified according to reason the person received services for that particular visit, a provider treating a person with multiple diagnoses could potentially change the principal diagnosis repeatedly depending on the focus and issues of a particular appointment.

Recording diagnoses in a correctional setting

DSM-5 does not provide specific guidance on how to list diagnoses in a correctional setting. In general, the evaluator should approximate the correctional setting that most closely matches an inpatient and outpatient setting. For example, for an inmate who is admitted to an acute crisis bed or correctional mental health treatment center, the rules about listing diagnoses for an inpatient setting would apply. Likewise, for inmates who are followed in other correctional settings (such as general population or enhanced treatment programs that are not acute psychiatric treatment programs), the principal diagnosis would be the primary reason they are being seen for that visit.

Recording diagnoses in forensic evaluations

DSM-5's method of listing diagnoses is not a perfect fit for recording diagnoses for many forensic evaluations. DSM-5 acknowledges the limitations of the DSM-5 for forensic use and specifically comments that the DSM-5 was developed to assist clinicians and researchers rather than courts and lawyers [1 (p25)].

Many forensic assessments address the relationship, if any, of a person's emotional or behavioral symptoms to a particular legal question. Some evaluees will have no diagnosis and for other evaluees, they may have a diagnosis in the past but none at the time of the evaluation. The following are general guidelines for listing diagnoses in forensic evaluations:

1. In criminal and civil competency evaluations, list the person's current diagnoses and record the diagnosis that most significantly impairs a person's competency as the principal diagnosis.
2. In evaluations that involve an assessment of a person's psychiatric presentation in the past (e.g., not guilty by reason of insanity evaluations), use a heading that identifies the diagnoses at that identified past point in time in addition to listing current diagnoses. To illustrate, consider the following vignette:

VIGNETTE 5

Alistair is 47-year-old man who snorts four lines of methamphetamine on March 22, 2014. He becomes extremely agitated, paranoid, and hears the voice of a "famous gospel singer" commanding him to kill his boyfriend. Moments later, Alistair brutally stabs his lover to death with an ice pick through the heart. Alistair also has moderate methamphetamine use disorder. Shortly after his arrest, all of Alistair's psychotic symptoms clear. Six months later, Alistair is referred for an evaluation of his sanity at the time of the crime. During the evaluation conducted on October 30, 2014, Alistair blatantly malingers symptoms of psychosis. Diagnostic findings could be communicated to the court as follows (using the ICD-9 format):

DSM-5 DIAGNOSES ON MARCH 22, 2014:

1. Methamphetamine-induced psychotic disorder (principal diagnosis)
2. Moderate methamphetamine use disorder

DSM-5 DIAGNOSES ON OCTOBER 30, 2014:

1. Malingering (principal diagnosis)
2. Moderate methamphetamine use disorder, in early remission, in a controlled environment.

In civil litigation, the evaluator is frequently asked to assess whether the plaintiff experienced emotional distress or a mental disorder as a result of an identified stressor *and* whether the plaintiff continues to have any current diagnoses. There are often situations in which an injured party may have had a psychiatric diagnosis that is in remission at the time of the evaluation so a list of current diagnoses will not reflect this history. One option to address this common presentation is to provide a list of current diagnoses and in the body of the report (e.g., diagnostic considerations or opinion section) discuss whether the plaintiff suffered from a diagnosis in the past that was in remission at the time of the evaluation.

STEP 7: EXPLAIN THE DSM-5 DIAGNOSES

There are some situations (e.g., outpatient clinics) in which listing DMS-5 diagnoses may be all that is required for documentation purposes. However, most forensic assessments require some explanation of the diagnoses. For clarity purposes, the evaluator may find it useful to list the current diagnoses and below this listing provide the evidence to support the diagnoses.

In situations in which there are other diagnoses that were considered but not diagnosed, the evaluator can explain in the body of the report why the diagnosis was not made. To illustrate, consider the following case.

VIGNETTE 6

Grant Wilson is a 43-year-old man diagnosed with bipolar disorder who works for a cell phone company. Over a three-week period, Grant becomes increasingly delusional and believes that all of the cell phones in the store are transmitting "super sonic saturated strychnine" to the employees. He hears the "voice of Edward Snowden" commanding him to act so he smashes all of the phones in the store. He is subsequently arrested and charged with vandalism and destruction of property. His attorney requests a competency to stand trial evaluation. The examiner determines that Grant is still psychotic during the interview, with nearly incoherent speech. He also notes that Grant clearly meets criteria for schizophrenia (with multiple previous psychotic episodes) but not bipolar disorder. Grant also has a history of mild alcohol use disorder. In jail, Grant is diagnosed with hepatitis C. When he learns this news, becomes suspicious that "liver strychnine" has been placed into his meals and stops eating. He demands that his jail physician "purify" his liver. How should the evaluator list Grant's diagnoses?

An abbreviated example of how to list Grant's diagnosis, an explanation of his diagnosis, and how other diagnoses were considered in a forensic report is provided in Table 3-1.

STEP 8: DETERMINE WHETHER AND HOW "DISABILITY" WILL BE ASSESSED

DSM-IV utilized the Global Assessment of Functioning (GAF) scale to indicate the clinician's judgment of the person's overall functioning on a scale of 0–100 (with 0 representing an extremely impaired functioning level and 100 representing an extremely high functioning level) [10 (p34)]. DSM-5 notes that the GAF was not included under this new edition because it lacked clarity in describing levels of suicide risk and disability and questionable psychometrics in clinical practice [1].

DSM-5 includes one global measure of disability, the World Health Organization Disability Schedule 2.0 (WHODAS 2.0), in Section III titled

Table 3-1. REPORT EXAMPLE FOR DSM-5 DIAGNOSES AND OTHER DIAGNOSTIC CONSIDERATIONS FOR "GRANT."

Current Diagnostic and Statistical Manual of Mental Disorders (DSM-5) Diagnoses:

1. Schizophrenia, multiple episodes, currently in acute episode (principal diagnosis)
2. Hepatitis C
3. Mild alcohol use disorder

Mr. Wilson meets criteria for schizophrenia. In particular, he has experienced delusional beliefs, such as thinking that the cell phones in his work place are beaming poisonous strychnine to employees putting them at risk to die. He also has auditory hallucinations of Edward Snowden commanding him to destroy cell phones. During my interview, Mr. Wilson was incoherent and he exhibited markedly disorganized speech. For example, when asked the role of his attorney, he responded, "Like order of the trees, to judge not lest ye be judged for all mankind is to do better or not do at all." My review of Mr. Wilson's jail records indicates that his symptoms have been present most of the time during his three months of incarceration. His outpatient records substantiate that he has had similar symptoms with multiple psychiatric hospitalizations over a 15-year period.

Mr. Wilson also been recently diagnosed with hepatitis C. This medical condition is included on the diagnostic list because he has developed delusional beliefs about the impact of his hepatitis and is requiring additional mental health treatment to address his concerns about his hepatitis.

In addition, I diagnosed Mr. Wilson with mild alcohol use disorder because he reported that often drank more beer than he intended and he had repeated, but failed, efforts to cut down on his alcohol use.

Consideration of other diagnoses:

I carefully considered the possibility that Mr. Wilson met criteria for bipolar disorder because this is the diagnosis noted in his outpatient treatment records. However, a review of his records indicates that he has never had a manic episode that has occurred concurrently with his active symptoms of hallucinations and delusions. His marked agitation when symptomatic is consistent with the paranoia he experiences when psychotic during the active phase of schizophrenia as opposed to increased energy due to mania.

I also considered the possibility that Mr. Wilson could be malingering, particularly as he is facing criminal charges. It is my opinion that Mr. Wilson is not malingering his symptoms. His mental disorder is well established over a 15-year period and multiple observers have documented that his symptoms continue in jail when he is unaware that he is being observed. I administered three tests to assess possible malingering and none of these indicated he was malingering any symptoms. Finally, Mr. Wilson repeatedly demands to be "declared competent" so that he can "fight the beams," indicating that he is not trying to avoid his trial.

"Emerging Measures and Models." DSM-5 does not require the use of the WHODAS 2.0 as a replacement for the GAF score and clearly differentiates measures included in Section III from the diagnostic criteria outlined in Section II. In particular, the DSM-5 manual emphasizes that unlike diagnoses listed in Section II, the WHODAS 2.0 and other scales included in Section III have not undergone sufficient rigorous research to support their routine use in clinical settings [1 (p23)].

Might the WHODAS 2.0 nevertheless be useful in forensic evaluations and reports? As an overview, the WHODAS 2.0 measures the impact of both physical and mental disorders on functioning and disability in the following six life domains:

1. Cognition (understanding and communication);
2. Mobility (ability to move and get around);
3. Self-care (ability to attend to personal hygiene, dress and eat, and live alone);
4. Getting along (ability to interact with other people);
5. Life activities (ability to carry out responsibilities at home, work and school); and
6. Participation in society (ability to engage in community, civil and recreational activities) [1 (p745)].

There are limitations in using the WHODAS 2.0 as a measure of disability in forensic psychiatric evaluations. For example, the WHODAS 2.0 includes several questions that address areas of functioning with limited applicability to correctional settings and patients involuntarily committed to psychiatric hospitals. To illustrate, consider how inmates or involuntarily detained psychiatric patients would respond to questions asking about their difficulty "moving around inside your home," "taking care of your household responsibilities," "or "joining in community activities in the same way as anyone else can." Evaluators should not manipulate the language of the WHODAS 2.0 questions in an attempt to force this instrument to apply to any unique setting. In fact, the manual specifically states that users of WHODAS 2.0 have no authority to make substantive changes to the assessment instrument unless given explicit permission to do so [11 (p37)]. Furthermore, the WHODAS 2.0 scoring restrictions limit how many items can be missing yet still allow the instrument to be scored. There are limited, if any, studies that involve the use of the WHODAS 2.0 in criminal evaluations, correctional settings, forensic psychiatric hospitals, or civil litigation samples. Finally, the WHODAS 2.0 is a self-report instrument. It is obvious when completing the form that higher scores equate with more disability. Unfortunately, the WHODAS 2.0 has no measure to assess malingering or over-reporting of one's limitations due to disability. For these reasons, the WHODAS 2.0 is not recommended for use in either criminal or civil forensic evaluations [12].

If the WHODAS 2.0 is not recommended for use, what should an evaluator use? There are several important issues to address to help answer this question. First, a quantitative disability measure is not required for all evaluations. For example, competency to stand trial evaluations focus on the impairment, if any, that results from a defendant's mental condition on his or her ability to assist the attorney or understand the legal process. A reasonable argument could be made that more detailed assessments of the defendant's disability in various life circumstances (e.g., home, work, school) is not necessary to render a forensic opinion on trial competency. Likewise, criminal responsibility evaluations focus on the individual's mindset at the time of the crime. The level of their current disability would have minimal, if any, relevance to that specific legal question. Second, disability assessments in civil cases (e.g., workers' compensation, private disability, and social security disability insurance) may mandate the use of a specified disability assessment instrument/s, independent of DSM-5's recommendations. The evaluator will need to comply with their state's requirement in regard to how disability is assessed. [See Chapter 9 for further discussion of this issue.] Third, evaluators could continue to use the GAF despite its known limitations. In her excellent review of the use of the WHODAS 2.0 and the GAF, Gold [12 (p180)] concludes,

> Psychiatric evaluations of impairment and disability have generally benefitted from the standardization of practice provided by the multiaxial assessment methodology that included routine assessment of functioning and use of the GAF. Given the problems associated with forensic use of WHODAS 2.0 and the possibility of the proliferation of idiosyncratic methods for evaluations of psychiatric impairment and disability, psychiatric residency programs and forensic fellowships are well advised to continue training young clinicians in the use of the GAF despite its exclusion from DSM-5.

Finally, the evaluator could provide a qualitative (i.e., nonquantitative) description of how the person's mental health impairment limits their ability in various areas of their life, such as working, going to school, interacting with others, or performing activities of daily living. Because disability ratings are not included in the DSM-5 diagnostic list, a separate heading titled "disability" assessment could be included in the report after the list of diagnoses with their accompanying explanations.

SUMMARY

DSM-5 brings many changes in how diagnoses are made and coded. Although this diagnostic overhaul may seem daunting, evaluators can utilize the basic steps outlined in this chapter as a practical guide to accurately record and describe DSM-5 diagnoses in clinical records and forensic reports. Key summary points from this chapter include the following:

- DSM-5 no longer uses the multiaxial approach to listing diagnoses. Diagnoses that would have been listed on Axis I, II, and III under the DSM-IV system are now provided on one list.
- Diagnoses should be listed in order of treatment priority or reason for the visit.
- DSM-5 has removed the GAF scoring system with no required alternative disability assessment offered. Evaluators have a range of options to now consider when a disability assessment is required.
- Although DSM-5 recommends the WHODAS 2.0 as a possible disability assessment measure, there are serious concerns about the use of this instrument in forensic evaluations.

REFERENCES

1. *American Psychiatric Association. Diagnostic and Statistical Manual of Mental Disorders.* Fifth Edition. Arlington, VA: American Psychiatric Association; 2013.
2. Frances A. DSM-5 badly flunks the writing test. *Psychiatric Times.* Available at: http://www.psychiatrictimes.com/ dsm-5-badly-flunks-writing-test. Published June 11, 2013. Accessed 9 January 2014.
3. Barch DM, Bustillo J, Gaebel W, et al. Logic and justification for dimensional assessment of symptoms and related clinical phenomena in psychosis: relevance to DSM-5. *Schizophr Res* 2013; 150:15–20.
4. Kay SR, Opler LA, Lindenmayer JP. Reliability and validity of the positive and negative syndrome scale for schizophrenics. *Psychiat Res* 1988; 23:99–110.
5. Muller MJ, Wetzel H. Improvement of inter-rater reliability of PANSS items and subscales by a standardized rater training. *Acta Psychiatr Scand* 1998; 98:135–139.
6. Edgar CJ, Blaettler T, Bugarski-Kirola D, et al. Reliability, validity and ability to detect change of the PANSS negative symptom factor score in outpatients with schizophrenia on select antipsychotics and with prominent negative or disorganized thought symptoms. *Psychiat Res* 2014; 218(1–2):219–224.
7. Overall JE, Gorham DR. The brief psychiatric rating scale. *Psychol Rep* 1962; 10:799–812.
8. American Psychiatric Association. DSM-5 coding update: supplement to Diagnostic and Statistical Manual of Mental Disorders, Fifth Edition. Available at: http://dsm.psychiatryonline.org/DocumentLibrary/DSM-5%20Coding%20Update_Final.pdf. Effective March 2014. Accessed 2 June 2014.
9. Dimick C. Senate passes ICD-10 delay bill. Journal of AHIMA. March 31, 2014. Available at: http://journal.ahima.org/2014/03/31/senate-votes-on-icd-10-delay-bill/. Accessed 2 June 2014.

10. *American Psychiatric Association. Diagnostic and Statistical Manual of Mental Disorders*, Fourth Edition, Text Revision. Arlington, VA: American Psychiatric Association; 2000.
11. Ustun TB, Kostanjsek N, Chatterji S, Rehm J. *Measuring Health and Disability. Manual for the WHO Disability Schedule.* Geneva, Switzerland: World Health Organization; 2010.
12. Gold L. DSM-5 and the assessment of functioning. The World Health Organization Disability Assessment Schedule 2.0 (WHODAS 2.0). *J Am Acad Psychiatry Law* 2014; 42(2):173–181.

CHAPTER 4

DSM-5 and Psychiatric Evaluations of Individuals in the Criminal Justice System

INTRODUCTION

Criminal defendants present with a wide variety of psychiatric disorders and many psychiatric diagnoses are overrepresented in forensic populations. A report from the Bureau of Justice Statistics indicates that half of all inmates—over 1 million persons—have at least one mental health condition [1]. In addition, epidemiologic studies have shown a prevalence of severe mental illness (psychotic or major mood disorder) in 15% to 24% of incarcerated individuals in the United States [2, 3]. Therefore, clinicians and forensic evaluators should be aware of DSM-5 diagnostic changes for these diagnoses, which are highlighted in Chapter 2.

In addition to a significant prevalence of psychotic and mood disorders, approximately 70%–90% of offenders are estimated to have an alcohol or substance use problem and up to 68% meet diagnostic criteria for substance abuse or dependence when they enter the criminal justice system [4]. In DSM-5, the distinction between abuse and dependence has been eliminated. Essentially the abuse and dependence criteria were combined from DSM-IV. The criterion *recurrent legal problem(s)* has been eliminated from the criteria, and a new criterion, *craving or a strong desire or urge to use a substance*, has been added. DSM-5 has also added a new diagnosis of cannabis withdrawal characterized by three of the following: irritability, nervousness, trouble sleeping, diminished appetite, restlessness, depressed mood, and one physical symptom (such as abdominal pain, chills, or fever) [5 (p518)]. For opioid use disorder, a new specifier, *on maintenance therapy* (rather than *on agonist therapy*), has been added to indicate individuals who are taking methadone or buprenorphine but who do not meet other criteria for opioid use disorder other than potential tolerance to or withdrawal from the agonist. Finally, gambling disorder has been added to the section on Substance-Related and Addictive Disorders because DSM-5 notes that the same brain reward areas are involved in this condition [5].

Persons with posttraumatic stress disorder (PTSD) are more likely to be encountered in a criminal forensic setting because they may be at increased risk for criminal domestic violence and other crimes [6, 7]. Therefore, evaluators need to be aware of the diagnostic criteria changes for PTSD in DSM-5. In DSM-IV, a diagnosis of PTSD required that an individual had experienced or witnessed a traumatic incident [8]. This definition of trauma contained in DSM-IV was fairly restrictive. However, DSM-5 broadens the description of the traumatic to now include learning about a nonaccidental death to a close friend or family member or being exposed to shocking and upsetting details about trauma as part of one's employment [5 ([271)].

Although this widening of the traumatic event definition may allow more individuals to be diagnosed and treated outside of the forensic setting, this change could also provide the basis for either a mental defense (in the case of a dissociative flashback) or a request for leniency or diversion to mental health court in the criminal setting [9].

In addition to major mental illness, substance use disorders and PTSD, there are several psychiatric disorders that are more commonly seen in the forensic setting compared with a general psychiatric setting and include the following: antisocial personality disorder, paraphilic disorders, intermittent explosive disorder, pyromania, and kleptomania.

The diagnostic criteria for antisocial personality disorder are unchanged, although Section III of DSM-5 contains an alternative model for personality disorder diagnosis that emphasizes deficits in personality functioning along four domains that are abnormal and ubiquitous to all personality disorders: identity, self-direction, empathy, and intimacy. In addition, this model describes specific pathological personality traits specific to antisocial personality disorder. DSM-5 does not require the use of this model. However, if the evaluator uses this proposed approach to make a diagnosis, the forensic clinician may face specific challenges in explaining the new diagnostic model in a legal setting.

In DSM-5, the paraphilias are now referred to as paraphilic *disorders* (to emphasize distress or impairment to an individual or risk of harm to others), but the diagnostic criteria for the disorders themselves have only undergone minor changes. Of note, the proposed Paraphilic Coercive Disorder—a recommendation of a DSM-5 sub-workgroup that defined coercive sexual behavior that was not sadistic as a disorder—did not make it into DSM-5 [10]. However, evaluators in sexual violent predator proceedings may potentially diagnose these individuals as having "other specified paraphilic disorder." In addition, the disorder of hebephilia—the recurrent sexual attraction to persons in early puberty (in general 11 to 14 years of age)—likewise did not make it into the DSM-5 despite early proposals [11]. These proposals as well as a failed proposal to include hypersexuality as a disorder underwent sharp criticism during DSM-5 development [12].

There have been minor changes to a few specific DSM-5 Paraphilic Disorders. Voyeuristic disorder (formerly Voyeurism in the DSM-IV-TR) now has age exclusion for persons under the age of 18. This particular exclusion was implemented to prevent pathologizing normative sexual interest and behavior during pubertal adolescence. Therefore, an individual arrested as a "peeping tom" who is under the age of 18 would no longer qualify for this disorder. This age exclusion distinguishes voyeuristic disorder from the other Paraphilic Disorders in DSM-5 in that voyeuristic behaviors in adolescents are viewed as a nonpathological stage, whereas other paraphilic behaviors among adolescents may qualify for a paraphilic disorder diagnosis. Exhibitionistic disorder (formerly Exhibitionism in DSM-IV) has also had a minor change in the definition of the paraphilic requirement. In DSM-IV, the victim had to be an "unsuspecting stranger" [8 (p569)], but this has been changed in DSM-5 to "unsuspecting person" [5 (p689)]. Therefore, an individual may expose themselves recurrently to persons they know but who are unsuspecting and still meet the diagnostic criteria for exhibitionistic disorder. This has implications for persons who expose themselves to coworkers, in educational settings, or individuals (inmates) who expose themselves to correctional officers within correctional settings. Transvestic disorder (formerly Transvestic Fetishism in DSM-IV-TR) has dropped the requirement that the individual engaging in these behaviors must be a heterosexual male. Instead, DSM-5 recognizes two specific subtypes of the disorder: *with fetishism* if aroused by fabrics, materials, or garments, and *with autogynephilia* (in males) if aroused by thoughts or images of self as female [5 (p702)].

DSM-5 significantly expands the definition of intermittent explosive disorder to eliminate the requirement for serious assaultive acts or destruction of property. In DSM-5, verbal aggression (e.g., such as temper tantrums or arguments) is sufficient for the diagnosis, as long as the acts of verbal aggression occur at least twice a week for three months, are in marked excess to the level of provocation, are not planned, and cause impairment (e.g., interpersonal, occupational, financial, or legal) [5 (p466)]. This expansion has been met with some criticism that relational anger is much different from impulsive anger and that the disorder may pathologize any person with frequent angry outbursts [13]. Intermittent explosive disorder retains an alternative criterion: three behavioral outbursts in a 12-month period that results in serious damage or destruction of property. Basically, DSM-5 recognizes two types of intermittent explosive disorder: one characterized by high frequency/low intensity outbursts and one characterized by low frequency/high intensity outbursts [14]. In addition, the person must be at least six years of age and there is an exhaustive list of diagnoses that must be excluded before a diagnosis of intermittent explosive disorder can be assigned. Given this broadening of the diagnostic criteria, there may be an increase in the prevalence of this redefined disorder.

Individuals with intellectual impairments are frequently encountered in forensic populations. The diagnosis of Mental Retardation has been changed to intellectual disability in DSM-5 and has undergone significant revisions, with an emphasis on the need to assess both cognitive capacity *and* adaptive functioning. The different severities (mild, moderate, severe, and profound) are no longer related to actual IQ score ranges, but they are based solely on an individual's adaptive functioning in three domains (conceptual, social, practical). Notably, the actual diagnostic criteria for intellectual disability do not even mention a standardized IQ measurement approximately 70 or below, but rather require "deficits in intellectual functioning" confirmed by clinical assessment and "individualized, standardized intelligence testing" [5 (p33)]. IQ scores that would meet the definition of "deficits in intellectual functioning" are suggested to be those that fall approximately two standard deviations below the mean. On IQ tests with a standard deviation of 15 and a mean of 100, this involves an IQ score of 65–75 (70 ± 5). DSM-5 places an emphasis on the importance of using clinical judgment in interpreting scores and taking into consideration the margin of error in measurement and factors that may lower or raise IQ scores. More importantly, DSM-5 clearly indicates that a diagnosis of intellectual disability might be appropriate in persons with a measured IQ greater than 70 if the adaptive functioning of the individual is comparable to that of individuals with a much lower IQ score [5 (p37)].

Finally, malingering is frequently encountered in forensic populations, and estimates among pretrial detainees referred for either competency or criminal responsibility evaluations range from as low as 8% to as high as 21% [15, 16]. Among jail inmates referred for psychiatric assessment and treatment, rates of malingering have been reported as high as 45% to 56% [17]. In a study of jail inmates that used a structured psychological instrument to detect malingering, this prevalence was even higher (66%) [18]. Among prison inmates claiming psychiatric symptoms, one study found a malingering rate of 46% [19]. DSM-5 includes malingering under the section "Other Conditions That May Be a Focus of Clinical Attention." The description of malingering remains essentially unchanged from DSM-IV-TR and retains the emphasis on motive, with the desire to assume a sick role being characteristic of factitious disorder and other secondary gain to be characteristic of malingering.

DSM-5 DIAGNOSTIC CHANGES AND DRUG COURT AND MENTAL HEALTH COURT DIVERSION PROGRAMS

Drug and Mental Health Courts have been described as "problem solving courts" and have been called the most significant criminal justice initiative of the 20th century [20]. Their basic philosophy is based on the premise that substance abuse problems or mental illness may predispose persons to criminal behavior. These courts target the defendant's underlying substance use or mental illness through the provision of treatment services in conjunction with judicial supervision. As a result, individuals are diverted from the criminal justice system to a treatment program with the goal of assisting the individual in recovery and preventing the occurrence of future criminal acts that are grounds for re-arrest.

Eligibility criteria for drug court treatment generally require that the individual is over the age of 18, has a drug charge that does not involve manufacturing or distribution, has no history of violent felony convictions, and has a demonstrated need for substance misuse treatment. The elimination of recurrent substance-related legal problems from the diagnostic criteria for a substance use disorder may prevent persons who were formerly diagnosed with substance abuse from meeting diagnostic criteria for a substance use disorder. This change could potentially impact their eligibility for drug court diversion. The following vignette illustrates how this DSM-5 diagnostic change might affect drug court eligibility for some defendants.

VIGNETTE 1

A 55-year-old married male accountant is referred for possible drug court diversion after being charged with Driving Under the Influence (DUI) with an elevated blood alcohol level. According to the accountant and his spouse, he rarely drinks alcohol and does not normally drink excessively. He had been at a Super Bowl party and states he did not realize he was impaired. He has not used more than intended and has not made attempts to cut down. He denies craving, and his overall functioning at home and at work is not impaired. He has not had social or interpersonal problems due to drinking. Other than his current charge, there is no evidence of recurrent use in situations that are physically hazardous. He has not displayed tolerance or withdrawal. Under the new DSM-5 diagnostic criteria, the man would have no substance use disorder diagnosis.

Under the DSM-IV-TR, legal difficulty related to the use of alcohol (such as the current DUI) would qualify for a diagnosis of Alcohol Abuse.

Because this legal difficulty criterion has been eliminated, this accountant would not qualify for a diagnosis of Alcohol Use Disorder. Therefore, if a substance use disorder is a requirement for drug court diversion, this individual would not qualify.

Some drug courts exclude those with significant mental health issues. Mental health evaluators are frequently requested to assist the court in identifying treatment needs. With the elimination of the distinction between Substance Abuse and Substance Dependence in DSM-5, the evaluating clinician will be called upon to provide the court with recommendations as to whether an individual needs medical detoxification from alcohol or illicit substances prior to entering a recovery program or participating in drug court supervision. The requirement for detoxification is not readily apparent from the generic diagnosis of substance use disorder, so the clinician will need to inform the court about the specific symptoms of physiological tolerance or history of withdrawal symptoms (two of the eleven diagnostic criteria). The specifiers of *mild, moderate*, or *severe* can be used to guide recommendations to the court about the needed frequency of random drug screens. The recognition of persons *on maintenance therapy* for opioid use disorder is potentially important for clinicians working with drug courts. Clinicians should be prepared to educate drug court judges and personnel about the use of methadone and buprenorphine as agonist therapy and their medically recognized role in the treatment of opioid use disorder. Finally, the recognition of cannabis withdrawal in DSM-5 may have implications for drug courts as this disorder, although not medically dangerous or requiring treatment, may lead to functional impairment [21]. Evaluators may need to educate courts about this newly recognized phenomenon.

Because most jails and detention centers do not allow many controlled substances on formulary, drug court judges should be aware that if someone is removed from drug court while on agonist therapy, they are likely to undergo significant withdrawal if agonists are not continued. In DSM-5, Amphetamine Abuse and Dependence and Cocaine Abuse and Dependence have been combined under the category of stimulant use disorder. However, these substances have widely different pharmacokinetics and half-lives. This has particular relevance to drug testing and the ability to detect illicit drug use. Therefore, it would be important for the clinician to inform the judge about which specific substance has typically been used so that appropriate monitoring may be implemented.

Mental Health Courts seek to divert an increasingly large number of mentally ill individuals into court mandated treatment programs instead of the prison system. Advantages of these courts include linking persons to mental health treatment, reducing recidivism, reducing jail time, saving costs, and decriminalizing the mentally ill [22]. Disadvantages include the perceived coercion of the participants, the usual requirement of entering a guilty plea, and potential race and gender bias [23]. Since the Broward County Mental Health Court accepted its first defendant 15 years ago, over 280 mental health courts have been developed in the United States [24]. Historically, mental health courts have targeted nonviolent misdemeanor offenders. However, new mental health courts have been accepting more serious prison-bound offenders [25].

Clinicians and forensic evaluators will play an important role in assisting the mental health court in the transition to DSM-5, especially in the explanation of issues that have been created by the removal of the multiaxial system of diagnoses. For example, the removal of the multiaxial system will require clinicians to explain the difference between highly treatable conditions (most but not all conditions formerly on Axis I) and those conditions, which appear to be chronic and less resistant to change (intellectual disability and personality disorders). Experts will have to explain to jurors, lawyers, and judges how behaviors related to an acute psychiatric illness are both the same as and different from behaviors stemming from a chronic personality disorder [26]. If medical issues are relevant in the defendant's mental health court participation, those issues will need to be presented separately as well.

In addition, the removal of Axis IV (psychosocial stressors) and the Axis V Global Assessment of Functioning (GAF) scale may eliminate one way a clinician might explain a particular patient's unique stressors and their overall functioning to the court. The usefulness of the GAF in tracking court participants' functional improvement as they progress through the mental health court program is lost if no alternate measure of disability and impaired functioning is used. The examiner must determine how to best communicate initial impairment and subsequent progress to the court, either through the forensic report or court testimony. DSM-5 proposes numerous rating scales that may be considered in evaluating illness severity and functional impairment, including an alternative to the GAF scale. These scales are described under Section III "Emerging Measures and Models" and therefore are not currently mandated for use.

One alternative offered by DSM-5 for measuring symptom severity in individuals with psychosis is the Clinician-Rated Dimensions of Psychosis Symptom Severity Scale, which is discussed in detail in Chapter 3. In section III, DSM-5 includes the World Health Organization Disability Assessment Schedule 2.0 (WHODAS 2.0), which assesses functional impairment in six domains and is discussed in Chapters 1 and 3. The WHODAS 2.0 includes many items that are not directly applicable to incarcerated individuals; therefore, its use in a correctional environment has significant limitations.

Some mental health courts exclude mentally ill individuals who have concomitant intellectual disability because of concerns that they are less likely to be able to comply with the requirements imposed by the court, although research has not concluded that those with intellectual disability are less successful in completing a mental health court program [27]. If persons with intellectual disability are excluded, that determination will rely on the revised diagnostic criteria for intellectual disability as outlined in DSM-5. Therefore, the mental health practitioner will likely have to place greater emphasis on adaptive functioning as outlined in the new criteria when assisting the court with this determination.

DSM-5 CHANGES AND IMPLICATIONS FOR VIOLENCE RISK ASSESSMENT AND SEX OFFENDER RISK ASSESSMENT

Violence risk assessment

Violence risk assessment has evolved over the last two decades from an attempt to predict violent behavior to the identification of static and dynamic risk factors that demonstrate an association with violent behavior. After these factors are identified, treatment strategies and interventions are targeted to manage and minimize the dynamic risk factors [28]. Because violent acts are rare events, prior misguided attempts to predict violent behavior were usually associated with a very high number of false positive predictions. The presence of a major mental illness (psychotic or major mood disorder) does not necessarily predispose a person to behaving violently. In fact, persons with mental illness are much more likely to be the victim of a violent act than a perpetrator. However, public perception may be shaped by high profile events involving violent acts among persons with mental illness that have garnered media coverage. In the medical literature, certain symptoms of psychosis have been linked to violence risk; however, replication of these findings has not always shown consistency [29]. Results from the MacArthur study have linked the presence of threat/control override delusions to assaultive behavior. Specifically, certain delusions that were accompanied by anger were linked to violent acts: being spied upon, being followed, being under control of a person/force, and thought insertion [30]. Even though DSM-5 has eliminated the special attribution of some of these bizarre delusions and Schneiderian first-rank auditory hallucinations for the diagnosis of schizophrenia, if threat/control override delusions are present, they should be carefully documented in a violence risk assessment. In contrast, negative symptoms of schizophrenia (diminished emotional expression, social withdrawal, avolition) have been shown to reduce the rate of serious violence among individuals with schizophrenia [31]. Although negative symptoms are one of the five DSM-5 A criteria for schizophrenia, their presence is not required to make the diagnosis. Therefore, when conducting violence risk assessments, the presence of negative symptoms should be specifically noted as a potential protective factor.

Substance use has repeatedly demonstrated an increased likelihood of violent behavior and mental illness combined with a substance use disorder appears to impose an added risk than substance use alone [32]. Because DSM-5 eliminates the distinction between abuse and dependence, the severity of the alcohol and drug use disorder (as determined by the number of present symptoms) will guide recommendations towards managing this dynamic risk factor. Therefore, utilizing DSM-5 specifiers is important. The addition of craving adds a subjective diagnostic criterion that may be quantified with rating scales, including the Obsessive Compulsive Drinking Scale (OCDS) [33].

Other potential diagnoses that increase violence risk include PTSD, intermittent explosive disorder, and antisocial personality disorder. The diagnostic changes in DSM-5 have made many diagnoses that have been associated with violent behavior easier to diagnosis. The two prime examples of these are PTSD (traumatic event now includes hearing about death or serious injury of a loved one) and intermittent explosive disorder (repeated frequent outbursts of verbal aggression or physical aggression without injury or property damage occurring on average twice weekly for three months). Because courts may be willing to provide treatment for persons with intermittent explosive disorder (IED) but not persons with antisocial personality disorder (ASPD), distinguishing these disorders is important. The DSM-5 states that the level of impulsive aggression in individuals with ASPD is less than in IED. In addition, IED is not characterized by planned or premeditated violence and does not involve other features of ASPD (other unlawful behaviors, lying, irresponsibility, lack of remorse).

In addition to clinical assessment, violence risk assessments can be supplemented with actuarial instruments designed to categorize risk based on historical and clinical data. Although a complete review of this topic is beyond the scope of this chapter, it is important to note that scores on these actuarial instruments may change with the new diagnostic criteria contained in DSM-5. For example, the Violence Risk Appraisal Guide (VRAG) [34] contains 12 items that are scored based on research demonstrating that these items have an actuarial association with increasing or decreasing violence risk. One item notes that a DSM-III diagnosis of schizophrenia lessens the overall score (and violence risk). Because delusional disorder now includes bizarre delusions, some persons formerly diagnosed with schizophrenia under DSM-III and DSM-IV-TR may now be classified as having delusional disorder, thereby raising the overall VRAG score by four points if the examiner was to utilize DSM-5 diagnostic criteria. Because the research was validated under criteria that prohibited a diagnosis of delusional disorder if bizarre delusions were present, VRAG scoring using the original VRAG must follow the former DSM-III and DSM-IV-TR diagnostic guidelines. The VRAG was revised in 2013 (VRAG-R), and the presence of schizophrenia was removed as an item. Therefore, evaluators must be aware of implications of DSM-5 on both versions of this instrument. Actuarial instruments are also used in presentencing evaluations of sex offenders, so changes in actuarial instrument scores as a result of DSM-5 diagnostic changes may have sentencing implications.

Sex offender assessment

Some forensic clinicians are also involved with the evaluation of convicted sex offenders at the end of their prison sentence to assess whether they would meet civil commitment criteria as a sexually violent predator (SVP) or sexually violent offender (SVO). SVP programs have been enacted in 20 states and the District of Columbia [35]. In addition, the Adam Walsh Child Protection and Safety Act of 2006 authorized the federal government to institute a civil commitment program for federal sex offenders [36]. These laws were enacted to address the high recidivism rates reported among offenders who have been convicted of violent sexual assaults [37]. Most SVP statutes require four general conditions for civil commitment: (1) one or more charges (if found Not Guilty By Reason of Insanity or Incompetent to Stand Trial) or convictions for a sexually violent offense, (2) a qualifying "mental abnormality," (3) a likelihood of engaging in further acts of predatory sexual violence, and (4) a causal link, at least in part, between the mental abnormality and the risk of sexual recidivism [38]. These laws have been the source of controversy but have been upheld by the United States Supreme Court as constitutional and not in violation of substantial due process or double jeopardy and ex post facto prohibitions [39]. Furthermore, the U.S. Supreme Court has held that to satisfy due process, there must be some proof of an inmate's lack of control of their sexual behaviors but not a showing of a *total* lack of control [40]. The commitment of a person as a SVP is a momentous decision because once committed the individual could be detained for life.

Prior to DSM-5's release, DSM-IV-TR paraphilias were some of the most common mental disorders noted to impair an individual's ability to control their sexual behavior. DSM-5 contains diagnostic changes in the chapter on Paraphilic Disorders that may impact SVP determinations. Many of these changes have been highly criticized [41]. First and foremost, DSM-5 defines a paraphilia (a prerequisite for a Paraphilic Disorder) not by what it is, but by what it is not. A paraphilia is defined as "any intense and persistent sexual interest *other than* sexual interest in genital stimulation or preparatory fondling with phenotypically normal, physically mature, consenting human partners" [5 (p 685)]. Given this definition, a wide variety of sexual interests would qualify as a paraphilia. To now meet criteria for a "paraphilic disorder," the person must have a paraphilia that is upsetting to the individual or results in harm to themselves or others [5 (p 685-6)]. The following vignette illustrates how the distinction between paraphilic interest and paraphilic disorder may impact diagnostic considerations in the forensic evaluation of a sex offender.

VIGNETTE 2

A 24-year-old male is referred for a sex offender evaluation after pleading guilty to five counts of indecent exposure. He exposed himself to several women at a local mall over six months, and this is his first arrest. During the evaluation he admits to exhibitionistic fantasies. In addition, he reports fantasies involving sexual encounters with prepubescent girls, but he has never acted on them. He reports he has never possessed child pornography, would never engage in a pedophilic act, and reports he is not troubled by his sexual interest in young girls. A penile plethysmography (PPG), visual reaction time screening and detailed self-reported sexual history reveal a primary interest in girls between ages eight and 10, adult women, and fantasies involving exposure of genitals to unsuspecting women. His most likely DSM-5 diagnosis is Exhibitionistic Disorder, sexually aroused by exposing genitals to physically mature individuals because he has acted on exhibitionistic fantasies. Although he has another paraphilia (pedophilia), he has not acted on these urges, and they have not caused him marked distress or interpersonal difficulty. Therefore, he does not meet diagnostic criteria for pedophilic disorder.

Because paraphilias increase the risk of a paraphilic disorder, conceptualizing a paraphilia as normal (i.e., not a mental illness) has been criticized as arbitrary [42]. However, this delineation between paraphilias and paraphilic disorders represents an effort to not pathologize unconventional sexual interests, such as sadomasochistic sexual behavior between consenting adults. As an example, if a person experiences recurrent and intense sexual urges involving prepubescent children, engages in masturbation while fantasizing about prepubescent children, but has not acted on the urges with a child or the urges/fantasies have not caused marked distress or interpersonal difficulty, then he or she would not be considered to have a mental disorder (i.e., pedophilic disorder). The courts may have difficulty with this new definition and may be reluctant to consider such a paraphilic individual as not mentally disordered (i.e., receiving a label of having pedophilia rather than pedophilic disorder may be equally damaging to an individual's reputation, social relationships, and occupational opportunities). Possessing child pornography involves victimization (children were exploited in its production); therefore, forensic evaluators may choose to opine that possession of child pornography as evidence of "acting on these sexual urges," a requirement for pedophilic disorder. DSM-5 notes that "the extensive use of pornography depicting prepubescent children is a useful diagnostic indicator of pedophilic disorder" [5 (p689)].

The paraphilic disorders require that the paraphilic interest has been present for six months. This was a steadfast rule in DSM-IV for the paraphilias, but it appears that language has been added to the DSM-5 description of the disorders that make this requirement less strict. DSM-5 states that the six month requirement for paraphilic urges is not an absolute requirement but rather a generally recommended time course to emphasize that the individual's sexual interest is not brief and fleeting [5 (p 685)]. In general, the duration of paraphilic interests has been derived from self-report, collateral records (such as witness statements), and legal convictions. Under the new DSM-5 language, if the individual meets criteria for a paraphilic disorder for five rather than six months, the attorney seeking commitment (normally the attorney general) may argue that the person has a paraphilia sufficient to qualify for a diagnosis of paraphilic disorder. This relaxation of a strict time limit may become a flashpoint of contention in SVP proceedings. Pedophilic disorder continues to exclude an individual who is in late adolescence and is involved in an ongoing sexual relationship with a 12- or 13-year-old child. However, what constitutes an "ongoing sexual relationship" is left undefined. Unlike other Paraphilic Disorders, pedophilic disorder is the only disorder that does not have the "in full remission" specifier, implying that it is a life-long disorder. However, in the section titled "Highlights of Changes from DSM-IV to DSM-5," the text notes that the "in remission specifier" applies to all paraphilias [5 (p816)]. This statement suggests that the "in full remission" specifier does apply to pedophilic disorder in direct contrast to diagnostic criteria listed in Section II.

For the first time, DSM-5 mentions physiological measures of sexual interest as providing evidence of paraphilic interests, especially in determining the strength of paraphilic interests in comparison to normophilic sexual interests. In particular, the DSM-5 mentions penile plethysmography (PPG) in males and viewing time in males and females. Historically, penile plethysmography has been used and accepted by courts in the treatment and supervision of convicted sex offenders [43]. Penile plethysmography has survived human rights challenges in Europe, but has not gained a wide admissibility in U.S. courts [44-45]. Its lack of admissibility in U.S. Courts has generally involved its potential use in the guilt and innocence phase of child sexual assault trials. In SVP proceedings, the goal of commitment is treatment, not punishment. This treatment focus may provide courts with an excuse to be more lenient in the acceptance of PPG testimony, and PPG testimony has survived admissibility challenges in SVP commitment hearings in several jurisdictions. The fact that penile plethysmography has been mentioned in the manual [5 (p 699)] may give ammunition to those seeking to have this evidence admitted and could be used to argue that plethysmography is now admissible when facing *Daubert* challenges [46]. Visual reaction time has been compared favorably to penile plethysmography in its ability to detect areas of sexual interest [47]. However, the reliability, validity, and statistical analysis of data supporting its use have been debated [48, 49]. These tests generally involve an unobtrusive measure of a subject's visual reaction time to a series of images depicting clothed children, teens and adults. Meanwhile, the subject is asked to rate his or her degree of sexual arousal to the visual stimuli. Like penile plethysmography, the admissibility of these instruments in court remains unclear [50]. Of note, under the *gender-related diagnostic issues* section of pedophilic disorder, there is a statement that psychophysiological laboratory measures of sexual interest are not necessarily useful in diagnosing pedophilic disorder in females.

DSM-5 CHANGES AS THEY APPLY TO DEATH PENALTY LITIGATION

In the 1972 case of *Furman v. Georgia*, the U.S. Supreme Court declared the death penalty as unconstitutional because it violated the 8th Amendment's ban on cruel and unusual punishment [51]. The reasoning behind the decision was that the death penalty was arbitrarily imposed, and there were little differences between those who received the death penalty and those who did not. Since the *Furman* decision, 34 of the 50 United States have enacted statutes that define criteria to be used in determining whether someone is eligible for the death penalty. These statutes were found constitutional by the U.S. Supreme Court because they created statutory sentencing guidelines written to prevent the death penalty from being arbitrarily and capriciously applied [52]. In general, these statutes define a set of aggravating circumstances, one of which is necessary in order to sentence a defendant to death. Examples of aggravating circumstances include, but are not limited to, killing of a law enforcement officer, torture, murder during commission of a violent crime, murder for hire, etc [53]. In some jurisdictions (e.g., Idaho, Oklahoma, Oregon, Texas, Virginia, Washington, and Wyoming), the future dangerousness of the defendant is also considered a potentially aggravating factor. Forensic psychiatrists and other forensic mental health professionals are involved in many stages of capital litigation: competency to stand trial evaluation, criminal responsibility evaluation, evaluation of mitigating factors, evaluation of future dangerousness, competency to be executed evaluation, and evaluation of intellectual disability for the purpose of avoiding the death penalty. The important role that a defense retained psychiatrist may have in capital cases has been described by the U.S. Supreme Court as "pivotal," and failure by the State to provide an indigent capital defendant with the use of a psychiatric expert has also been found to deny due process [54].

The standards governing competency to stand trial and criminal responsibility evaluations are the same in capital cases and noncapital cases, and these evaluations are addressed in Chapter 5 and Chapter 6. In most jurisdictions, the evaluation of potential mitigating factors includes consideration of how a mental disorder (to include substance use) may have impacted the defendant's behavior. As noted above, DSM-5 has combined the DSM-IV diagnoses of Substance Abuse and Dependence into one diagnostic category labeled "substance use disorder." The clinician should carefully review each criterion for every substance the defendant has used in order to rate the severity of substance use and how such use may have impacted the defendant's behavior. In addition, the clinician must be prepared to describe how various substances may impact a person's behavior during periods of intoxication or withdrawal. The DSM-5 has added two new withdrawal syndromes, caffeine withdrawal and cannabis withdrawal. Although caffeine withdrawal does include "dysphoric mood, depressed mood, or irritability" as one symptom [5 (p506)], caffeine withdrawal is unlikely to play a prominent mitigating role for criminal behavior. In contrast, cannabis withdrawal includes multiple symptoms, such as irritability, anger, or aggression, nervousness or anxiety, restlessness, and depressed mood, all of which may be considered as influencing a defendant's thinking and behavior.

Although many states mandate that juries consider a defendant's risk of future dangerousness when considering the death penalty, the assessment of future dangerousness has been challenged for lacking scientific validity. As outlined above, the evaluator should be familiar with those factors that have been described to increase a person's risk of future violence as well as the limitations of research in this area.

At the end of 2013, there were 3108 inmates on death row in the United States [55]. Many of these inmates will likely undergo a competency to be executed evaluation as the date of their execution approaches. In *Ford v. Wainwright*, the U.S. Supreme Court decided that the execution of an incompetent inmate constitutes cruel and unusual punishment because such an execution has questionable retributive value, presents no example to others and therefore has no deterrence value, and simply offends humanity. In addition, the Court stated that certain due process requirements were relevant and that the condemned prisoner was entitled to a hearing on the competency issue where he could present evidence from his own experts and cross-examine the state's experts [56]. However, the Court did not specify what standard should be used to determine whether a death row inmate is competent. In a concurring opinion, one Justice suggested that a narrow cognitive test would suffice—that an inmate was competent to be executed if they were aware of their pending execution and the reason for it. As a consequence, it has been left to the individual states to decide what standard should be applied in competency to be executed evaluations. Some states have expanded the narrow cognitive standard to include the ability to rationally consult with legal counsel.

The most common DSM-5 psychiatric disorders that would potentially impair an inmate's ability to be aware of their pending execution would include major mental illnesses (schizophrenia, schizoaffective disorder, and possibly bipolar I disorder), delirium, or a major neurocognitive disorder (formerly Dementia in DSM-IV). The most common psychiatric symptom that would impair a death row inmate's ability to understand the reason for their punishment is a delusion. In the case of Texas death row inmate Scott Louis Panetti, the presence of a delusion became a central issue in the questioning of his competency to be executed. Mr. Panetti believed that although the state said it wanted to execute him for a murder, the state's stated reason was a sham and the state was actually trying to execute him to prevent him from preaching. Although the lower courts found Mr. Panetti competent to be executed, the U.S. Supreme Court held that gross delusions stemming from a severe mental disorder may put the awareness of the reason for execution in a context so far removed from reality that the punishment could serve no purpose. The court added that an inmate's awareness of a state's rationale for execution is not the same as having a rational understanding of it [57]. Therefore, in assessing an inmate's competency to be executed, particular attention should be paid to delusional statements.

In general, grandiose delusions may be the type of delusion most likely to negatively impact competency to be executed. For example, a delusion that one has been anointed with special powers and will survive the lethal injection (or electrocution) may impair the ability to appreciate the permanent nature of the punishment. Paranoid delusions concerning alternative government interests (i.e., interests other than punishment) in performing the execution may also impair an appreciation of the reason for the punishment. These types of delusions could be seen in a variety of DSM-5 diagnoses that can include psychotic symptoms. In DSM-5, delusional disorder requires that apart from the delusion or its resulting consequences, the individual may otherwise appear and behave relatively normal [5 (p90)]. There is a potential for tremendous secondary gain that could be obtained from the intentional false production of a "delusional" thought that is directly related to a pending execution. Because inmates with delusional disorder generally lack the negative symptoms (blunted or flat affect, social isolation, amotivation) that are generally seen in other types of psychosis, distinguishing true delusions from malingered delusions may prove somewhat difficult.

In states that have adopted an assistance prong in their competency to be executed standards, illnesses that disrupt thought processes may be associated with impaired ability to communicate with an attorney. Psychotic disorders have the ability to disrupt thought process through the production of loose associations, tangentiality, circumstantiality, and thought blocking. Any one of these symptoms, if sufficiently severe, can also impair attorney-client communication and thereby impact competency. The average prisoner on death row has been there 13 years. Because the appeals process is very long, an inmate may spend as much as 36 years from incarceration to execution [58, 59]. As a result, death row inmates, by virtue of their lengthy incarceration, may be at risk of developing major or mild neurocognitive disorder, which could impact their competency to be executed.

In 2002, the U.S. Supreme Court, citing evolving standards of decency, ruled that the execution of those with mental retardation constituted cruel and unusual punishment under the 8th Amendment [60]. The Court concluded that such punishment was excessive and therefore prohibited by prevailing standards, and that the death penalty for persons with mental retardation did not measurably advance the deterrent retributive purposes of the death penalty. Persons with mental retardation may unwittingly confess to crimes they did not commit, have poor ability to assist counsel at trial, and may appear to lack remorse due to an impression created by their demeanor in court. Because of the *Atkins* decision, numerous individuals on death row who were convicted prior to 2002 have been or will have to be evaluated for the presence of mental retardation. Evaluators should be aware of the specific definition of mental retardation used in their jurisdiction. Most of these definitions parallel the DSM-IV and the American Association on Intellectual and Developmental Disabilities (AAIDD) definition.

As described above, DSM-5 replaces the DSM-IV diagnosis of Mental Retardation with "intellectual disability," which requires deficits in intellectual and adaptive functioning. Research on murder defendants referred for pretrial evaluation has indicated that although 15.5% presented with a valid, measured IQ score at or below 70, only 6% received an actual diagnosis of mental retardation (Intellectual Disability) [61]. Therefore, adaptive functioning did not correlate with the low IQ score or low IQ was not seen until after the developmental period, so a DSM-IV-TR diagnosis of mental retardation was not made.

Unfortunately, the assessment of adaptive functioning is very difficult when an individual is incarcerated. For clinical assessment, evaluators may need to think "outside the box." Assessment of adaptive behavior may be strengthened by the use of multiple informants. It still must be assessed in three domains: conceptual, social, and practical. The *conceptual* domain involves abstract thinking, executive functioning, memory and functional use of academic skills. Assessing this domain on death row would involve examining tasks that require these skills such as reading ability, ability to work with an appellate attorney and understand legal principles, ability to manage his/her canteen fund, and ability to problem solve. Examining letters that the inmate writes to home or to others would be useful in assessing vocabulary and basic conceptual abilities. The *social* domain involves the ability to interact socially and perceive social cues, communication and conversational skills, and social judgment. Assessing this domain would involve examining how the inmate interacts with other inmates and correctional officers. Given the environment of death row, persons with intellectual disability, due to their naiveté or gullibility, may be easily victimized or taken advantage of by other inmates. Deficits in the social domain would be manifest by other inmates easily taking advantage of the inmate or feeling a need to protect him/her because of a perceived social vulnerability. Information about relationships with others is crucial and may involve talking to numerous prison officials who are familiar with the daily activities on death row. Therefore, talking to several correctional officers and administrators may help paint a more complete picture. Evaluators will also need to consider the relationship of the informant to the individual being assessed and the potential gains for the informant. The *practical* domain involves an ability to function in age-appropriate personal care. This is the hardest domain to assess among incarcerated individuals. On death row, other inmates prepare meals and complete laundry and most inmates do not routinely participate in work assignments. To assess this domain, medical records may reveal evidence of the inmate's functioning when making medical decisions and whether they can maintain compliance with treatment. An inmate who requires assistance to complete medical requests or to fill out canteen orders may have deficits in the practical domain.

Information about an individual's level of adaptive functioning prior to incarceration may be more revealing than trying to assess adaptive functioning in prison. Therefore, school academic records, psychoeducational reports, employment records and a history from collateral sources (family members, teachers) are crucial. In addition to establishing concomitant low adaptive functioning, the onset of intellectual and adaptive deficits must begin during the developmental period (i.e., prior to adulthood). Assessments of adaptive behavior can be accomplished through the use of standardized instruments, but these have limitations in the forensic setting as well. Most of these instruments rely on information gathered from a third party familiar with the individual who is being assessed. Finding such a reliable third party on death row may prove difficult. There are a few measures, such as the Street Survival Skills Questionnaire (SSSQ) and the Adaptive Behavior Assessment System (ABAS), which may be useful for this population [62]. In addition, the American Association on Intellectual and Developmental Disabilities (AAIDD) is planning a release of a Diagnostic Adaptive Behavior Scale (DABS), which may be used in forensic populations [63].

The DSM-5's shift in focus to adaptive functioning (as opposed to a specific I.Q. score when defining intellectual disability) has heightened importance considering the U.S. Supreme Court's decision in *Hall v. Florida* [65]. Freddie Lee Hall was convicted and sentenced to death in 1978 for his part in the abduction and murder of a 21-year-old pregnant woman. During one resentencing trial, the court found that Mr. Hall was mentally retarded. Florida's statutory scheme for identifying defendants with mental retardation in capital cases categorically barred defendants who do not have an I.Q. test score of 70 or below. In subsequent hearings, evaluators testified that Hall's I.Q. scores on the Wechsler Adult Intelligence Scale were 71, 73, and 80. Because his scores were above the mandatory cut off score of 70, the court denied a motion to vacate his death sentence, and this decision was upheld by the Florida Supreme Court. Hall appealed the case to the U.S. Supreme Court, which held that Florida's statutory scheme for identifying individuals with mental retardation violated the 8th Amendment prohibition on the execution of persons with mental retardation as articulated in *Atkins v. Virginia*. The primary issue in this case involved Florida's rigid adherence to a cut off score of 70 or below without consideration of the standard error of measurement for IQ tests and without consideration of adaptive functioning. Because DSM-5's criteria for intellectual disability no longer uses IQ scores to determine the presence or severity of intellectual disability, this diagnostic change is extremely relevant to both past and future evaluations of death row inmates as well as the constitutionality of the death penalty for this population [64].

DSM 5 CHANGES AND TREATMENT REQUIREMENTS IN A CORRECTIONAL ENVIRONMENT

The U.S. Supreme Court has held that deliberate indifference to the serious medical needs of prisoners constitutes the "unnecessary and wanton infliction of pain" proscribed by the 8th Amendment [65]. Although the Supreme Court has not specifically ruled on whether the serious medical needs of prisoners includes mental health treatment, two separate U.S. Courts of Appeal have held that a lack of psychiatric care was a critical deficiency and that there is no underlying distinction between the right to medical care and its psychological counterpart [66, 67]. The definition of *serious medical needs* as it relates to mental disorders remains unclear. The Society of Correctional Physicians has defined *serious mental disorder* for the purpose of limiting administrative segregation as one of the following: (1) a psychotic disorder or major mood disorder; (2) a diagnosed mental disorder that includes being actively suicidal; (3) a diagnosis of a mental disorder that is frequently characterized by breaks with reality, or perceptions of reality that leads to significant functional impairment; (4) a cognitive disorder (delirium or dementia) that leads to functional impairment; (5) a personality disorder with frequent episodes of psychosis or depression; and (6) mental retardation [68]. Two diagnostic criteria changes to relatively common mental disorders, major depressive disorder and PTSD, are likely to increase the incidence of these disorders in correctional populations. The removal of the bereavement exclusion criterion for major depressive disorder may lead to an increase in the incidence of this disorder among incarcerated inmates who have recently lost a family member. Likewise, being informed of a traumatic but unexpected death of a family member will now qualify for the traumatic criterion in PTSD. The expansion of intermittent explosive disorder diagnostic criteria to include verbal aggression and repeated acts of anger or aggression that do not result in serious injury to persons or property may lead to this disorder being used by inmates as an excuse when facing certain disciplinary infractions in prison.

DSM-5 contains several new diagnoses that may or may not be grounds for litigation if correctional systems fail to provide treatment. These include social (pragmatic) communication disorder, premenstrual dysphoric disorder, hoarding disorder, excoriation disorder (skin picking), and mild neurocognitive disorder. It is foreseeable that prison inmates may attempt to use hoarding disorder as a defense against prison rules violation for failure to maintain an orderly cell. The expansion of the diagnosis of intermittent explosive disorder to include frequent acts of verbal or physical aggression that do not result in serious injury or damage to property likewise has potential for abuse by inmates when facing disciplinary actions by prison officials. There may be claims by inmates that they are being punished for their disorder. Likewise, the relaxation of the trauma exposure requirement of PTSD to include learning that a traumatic event occurred to a close family member or close friend has potential to both increase the prevalence of PTSD in correctional settings and the abuse of this diagnosis by inmates to avoid segregation or other disciplinary actions as well. The diagnosis of gender dysphoria (gender identity disorder in DSM-IV-TR) will continue to present unique challenges for prison administrations and the courts. Courts have arrived at different conclusions as to whether correctional systems must provide treatment for this disorder including, in some cases, gender reassignment surgery. A federal court in Massachusetts has decided in one case that failure to provide gender reassignment constituted cruel and unusual punishment. That case is currently under appeal [69].

SUMMARY

DSM-5 has significant implications for forensic evaluations and delivery of care related to the criminal justice system. The following are key points to consider when practicing in this arena:

1. Forensic clinicians should be familiar with DSM-5 diagnostic changes for illness commonly encountered in forensic setting. Relaxation of the diagnostic criteria for intermittent explosive disorder and posttraumatic stress disorder will likely result in an increase in their prevalence among forensic populations.
2. The lack of a multiaxial system of diagnosis will require additional education for courts as to which illnesses may be treatable and which are lifelong and more resistant to interventions.
3. In alcohol and drug courts, the severity of the substance use disorder will guide the needed treatment approach because the distinction between abuse and dependence has been eliminated.
4. In violence risk assessments, actuarial instruments may need to be re-normed when the presence of a newly defined mental disorder alters the score.
5. In capital litigation, intellectual disability and its severity will be determined by adaptive functioning. Clinicians should be aware of the challenges of assessing adaptive functioning in a correctional setting.
6. The existence of new DSM-5 disorders and diagnostic criteria will produce challenges for correctional administrators. Failure to provide treatment for these disorders may also become a source of future litigation against correctional facilities.

REFERENCES

1. James DJ, Glaze LE. Mental health problems of prison and jail inmates. Bureau of Justice Statistics special report, NCJ 213600. Washington, DC: US Department of Justice. Available at: http://www.ojp.usdoj.gov/bjs/pub/pdf/mhppji.pdf. Published September 2006. Accessed 27 April 2014.
2. Baillargeon J, Binswater IA, Penn J, et al. Psychiatric disorders and repeat incarcerations: the revolving prison door. *Am J Psychiatry* 2009; 166:103–109.
3. Diamond PM, Wang EW, Holzer CE III, et al. The prevalence of mental illness in prison. *Adm Policy Ment Health* 2001; 29:21–40.
4. Karberg JC, James DJ. Substance dependence, abuse, and treatment of jail inmates, 2002. Bureau of Justice Statistics special report, NCJ 209588. Washington, DC: US Department of Justice. Available at: http://www.bjs.gov/content/pub/pdf/sdatji02.pdf. Published July 2005. Accessed 27 April 2014.

5. *American Psychiatric Association: Diagnostic and Statistical Manual of Mental Disorders,* Fifth Edition. Arlington, VA: American Psychiatric Association; 2013.
6. Van Winkle EP, Safer MA. Killing versus witnessing in combat trauma and reports of PTSD symptoms in domestic violence. *J Trauma Stress* 2011; 24:107–110.
7. Teten AL, Schumaker JA, Taft CT, et al. Intimate partner aggression perpetrated and sustained by male Afghanistan, Iraq, and Vietnam veterans with and without posttraumatic stress disorder. *J Interpers Violence* 2010; 25:1612–1630.
8. *American Psychiatric Association: Diagnostic and Statistical Manual of Mental Disorders,* Fourth Edition, Text Revision. Washington, DC: American Psychiatric Association; 2000: 467.
9. Frierson RL. Combat-related posttraumatic stress disorder and criminal responsibility determinations in the post-Iraq era: a review and case report. *J Am Acad Psychiatry Law* 2013; 41:79–84.
10. Stern P. Paraphilic coercive disorder in the DSM: the right diagnosis for the right reason. *Arch Sex Behav* 2010; 39:1443–1447.
11. Wakefield JC. The DSM-5's proposed new categories of sexual disorder: the problem of false positives in sexual diagnosis. *Clin Soc Work J* 2012; 40:213–223.
12. Frances A. The risk that DSM-5 will exacerbate the SVP mess in forensic psychiatry. *Curr Psychiatry Rev* 2012; 8:264–267.
13. Anand S. Intermittent explosive disorder and DSM-5: a flawed conceptualization of pathological anger. *Aust N Z J Psychiatry* 2013; 47:578–579.
14. Coccaro EF, Lee R, McCloskey MS. Validity of the new a1 and 12 criteria for dsm-5 intermittent explosive disorder. *Compr Psychiatry* 2013; 55:260–267.
15. Cornell DG, Hawk GL. Clinical presentation of malingerers diagnosed by experienced forensic psychologists. *Law Hum Behav* 1989; 13:375–383.
16. Rogers R, Seman W, Clark CR. Assessment of criminal responsibility: initial validation of the R-CRAS with the M'Naghten and GBMI standards. *Int J Law Psychiatry* 1989; 9:67–75.
17. Norris MP, May MC. Screening for malingering in a correctional setting. *Law Hum Behav* 1998; 22:315–323.
18. McDermott BE, Sokolov G. Malingering in a correctional setting: the use of the Structured Interview of Reported Symptoms in a jail sample. *Behav Sci Law* 2009; 27:753–765.
19. Walters GD, White TW, Greene RL. Use of the MMPI to identify malingering and exaggeration of psychiatric symptomatology in male prison inmates. *J Consult Clin Psychol* 1988; 56:111–117.
20. Huddleston CW III, Marlowe D, Casebolt R. Painting the current picture: a national report card on drug courts and other problem-solving court programs in the United States. Alexandria, VA: National Drug Court Institute. Available at: http://ndci.org/publications/painting-current-picture. Published May 2008. Accessed 27 April 2014.
21. Allsop DJ, Copeland J, Norberg MM, et al.Quantifying the clinical significance of cannabis withdrawal. *PLoS One* 2000; 7:1–11.
22. Sarteschi CM, Vaughn MG, Kim K. Assessing the effectiveness of mental health courts: a quantitative review. *J Crim Just* 2011; 39:12–20.

23. Naples M, Morris LS, Steadman HJ. Factors in disproportionate representation among persons recommended by programs and accepted by courts for jail diversion. *Psychiatric Ser* 2007; 58:1095–1101.
24. Steadman HJ, Redlich A, et al. Effect of mental health courts on arrests and jail days: a Multisite study. *Arch of Gen Psychiatry* 2011; 68:167–172.
25. Redlich A, Steadman HJ, Monahan J, et al. The second generation of mental health courts. *Psychol Public Policy Law* 2005; 11:527–538.
26. Wortzel, Hal S. The DSM-5 and forensic psychiatry. *J Psychiatr Pract* 2013; 19:238–241.
27. Burke MM, Griggs M, Dykens EM, Hodapp RM. Defendants with intellectual disabilities and mental illness diagnoses: faring in a mental health court. *J Intellect Disabil Res* 2012; 56:305–316.
28. Douglas KS, Skeem, JL. Violence risk assessment: getting specific about being dynamic. *Psychol Public Policy Law* 2005; 11:347–383.
29. Appelbaum PS, Robbins PC, Monahan J. Violence and delusions: data from the MacArthur Violence Risk Assessment Study. *Am J Psychiatry* 2000; 157:566–572.
30. Ulrich S, Keers R, Cold JW. Delusions, anger, and serious violence: new finding from the MacArthur Violence Risk Assessment Study. *Schizophr Bull* 2014;40:1174–1181.
31. Swanson JW, Swartz MS, Van Dorn RA, et al. A national study of violent behavior in persons with schizophrenia. *Arch Gen Psychiatry* 2006; 63:490–499.
32. Steadman HJ, Mulvey EP, Monahan J, et al. Violence by people discharged from acute psychiatric inpatient facilities and by others in the same neighborhoods. *Arch Gen Psychiatry* 1998; 55:393–401.
33. Anton RF, Moak DH, Latham PK. The obsessive compulsive drinking scale: a new method of assessing outcome in alcohol treatment studies. *Arch Gen Psychiatry* 1996; 53:225–231.
34. Rice ME, Harris GT, Lang C. Validation of and revision to the VRAG and SORAG: the violence risk appraisal guide-revised (VRAG-R) *Psychol Assess* 2013; 25:951–965.
35. Civil commitment of sexually violent predators. Association for the Treatment of Sexual Abusers. Available at: http://www.atsa.com/civil-commitment-sexually-violent-predators Accessed 3 January 2014.
36. The Adam Walsh Child Protection and Safety Act, 42 USC §16911 (2006).
37. Snyder HN. Sexual Assault of Young Children as Reported to Law: Victim, Incident, and Offender Characteristics. Bureau of Justice Statistics. A NIRB special report. NCJ 182990. Washington, DC: U.S. Department of Justice. Available at: http://www.bjs.gov/content/pub/pdf/saycrle.pdf. Published July 2000. Accessed 27 April 2014.
38. Rucket DE, Brakel SJ. Sexually violent predator laws. In: Rosner R, ed. *Principles and Practice of Forensic Psychiatry,* 2nd ed., London: Arnold Publishers, 2003: p 717.
39. *Kansas v Hendricks*, 521 U.S. 346, 117 S.Ct. 2072 (1997).
40. *Kansas v Crane*, 534 U.S. 407, 122 S.Ct. 867 (2002).
41. Fedoroff JP, Di Gioacchino L, Murphy L. Problems with paraphilias in the DSM-5. *Curr Psychiatry Rep* 2013; 15:363–368.
42. Moser C, Kleinplatz PJ. DSM-IV-TR and the paraphilias: an argument for removal. *J Psychol Hum Sex* 2005; 17:91–109.

43. Sachsenmaier SJ, Peters JM. Sexual offender risk assessment methods and admissibility as expert witness evidence. In: Peters JM, ed. *Assessment and management of sex offenders: What prosecutors need to know*. Washington, DC: United States Department of Justice, Child Exploitation and Obscenity Section; 2002.
44. Gazan F. Penile plethysmography before the European court of human rights. *Sex Abuse* 2002; 14:89–93.
45. *North Carolina. Spencer*, 459 S.E.2d 812, 815 (N.C. Ct. App. 1995).
46. *Daubert v Merrell Dow Pharmaceuticals Inc.*, 61 U.S.L.W. 4805, 113 S.Ct. 2786 (1993).
47. Abel GG, Huffman J, Warberg B, Holland CL. Visual reaction time and plethysmography as measures of sexual interest in child molesters. *Sex Abuse* 1998; 10:81–95.
48. Smith G, Fischer L. Assessment of juvenile sexual offenders: reliability and validity of the Abel Assessment for interest in paraphilias. *Sex Abuse* 1999; 11:207–216.
49. Abel G. The importance of meeting research standards: a reply to Fischer and Smith's articles on the Abel Assessment for Sexual Interest. *Sex Abuse* 2000; 12:155–161.
50. Coric V, Feuerstein S, Fortunati F, et al. Assessing sex offenders. *Psychiatry (Edgmont)* 2005; 2:26–29.
51. *Furman v. Georgia*, 408 U.S.238, 92 S. Ct. 2726 (1972).
52. *Gregg v. Georgia*, 442 U.S.95, 99 S. Ct. 2909 (1976).
53. Aggravating factors for capital punishment by state. Death Penalty Information Center. Available at: http://deathpenaltyinfo.org/aggravating-factors-capital-punishment-state. Accessed 6 January 2014.
54. *Ake v Oklahoma*, 470 U.S. 68, 105 S.Ct. 1087 (1985).
55. The death penalty in 2013: Year-end report. Death Penalty Information Center. Available at: http://deathpenaltyinfo.org/YearEnd 2013. Accessed 30 December 2013.
56. *Ford v Wainwright*, 477 U.S. 399, 106 S.Ct. 2595 (1986).
57. *Panetti v Quarterman*, 551 U.S. 930, 127 S. Ct. 2842 (2007).
58. Liptak A. Lifelong death sentences. New York Times, October 31, 2011.
59. Time on death row. Death Penalty information Center. Available at: http://www.deathpenaltyinfo.org/time-death-row. Accessed 10 January 2014.
60. *Atkins v Virginia*, 536 U.S. 304, 122 S.Ct. 2242 (2002).
61. Dwyer RG, Frierson RL. The presence of low IQ and mental retardation among murder defendants referred for pretrial evaluation. *J Forensic Sci* 2006; 51:678–682.
62. Seay OJ. Evaluating mental retardation for forensic purposes. *Appl Psychol Crim Justice* 2006; 2:52–81.
63. Diagnostic Adaptive Behavior Scale (DABS). American Association on Intellectual and Developmental Disabilities. Available at: http://aaidd.org/intellectual-disability/diagnostic-adaptive-behavior-scale. Accessed 10 January 2014.
64. *Hall v. Florida*, Slip opinion No. 12–10882, U.S. Supreme Court (2014).
65. *Estelle v. Gamble*, 429 US 97, 97 S. Ct. 285 (1976).
66. *Newman v. Alabama*, 503 F. 2d 1320 (5th Cir. 1974).
67. *Bowring v. Goodman*, 551 F. 2d 44 (4th Cir. 1977).

68. Position Statement: Restricted housing of Mentally Ill Inmates. Society of Correctional Physicians. Available at: http://societyofcorrectional-physicians.org/resources/position-statements/restricted-housing-of-mentally-ill-inmates. Accessed 11 January 2014.
69. Naughton M, Michelle Kosilek. Appeals court to hear transgender inmate case. Available at: http://www.metro.us/newyork/news/2013/04/01/michelle-kosilek-appeals-court-to-hear-transgender-inmate-case/. Accessed 11 January 2014.

CHAPTER 5

DSM-5: Competencies and the Criminal Justice System

INTRODUCTION

Mental health professionals are frequently called upon to evaluate a criminal defendant's ability to competently participate in one or more phases of the process of a criminal investigation, trial, sentencing and/or appeal. In this chapter, the evaluation of various criminal competencies are reviewed, including competence to stand trial; to confess to a crime; to plead guilty; to waive counsel; to waive a jury trial; to testify; to waive extradition; to be sentenced; to waive appeals; and, in capital cases, to be executed.

COMPETENCE AS A CONCEPT

Competence is a general term meaning the ability or capacity to understand a concept and rationally proceed through a decision-making process. Competence refers to one's mental state at a given point in time. Because mental states and the degree of mental illness can fluctuate over time, one's competence may also vary over time. Assessing a subject's competence may be a present-state evaluation, such as in competence to make a medical decision, or a retrospective evaluation, such as whether an individual had been competent to execute a will at a prior point in time. Rarely, an evaluator is asked to opine about a future competence, such as in certain guardianship assessments. In assessing many of the criminal competencies, such as competence to stand trial, the evaluation is a present-state evaluation. However, a defendant's competence to confess to a crime or to plead guilty may be the basis of an appeal following a conviction. In those circumstances, the evaluator may be tasked with retrospectively assessing the defendant's competence in those areas.

The presence of a mental disorder does not automatically equate with incompetence. Even a severely mentally ill individual may be competent; in so far as the symptoms of their illness do not impact the areas of mental functioning required to be competent. In contrast, a single delusional belief may render an otherwise well-functioning individual incompetent. For example, a person suffering from severe major depressive disorder may be competent to make a will, manage their own affairs, and consent to treatment if their depressive symptoms do not impact their ability to carry out these activities. In contrast, an otherwise well-functioning person with the single delusional belief that their child is demonic may be incompetent to make a will because their delusional belief may cause them to irrationally disinherit their child.

Prior to the 1960s, the concept of global incompetence was embraced: a person adjudicated incompetent in one area of mental functioning was deemed incompetent in all areas. For example, many state laws at that time indicated that civilly committed patients, based on their status as an involuntarily hospitalized patient, were not competent to make decisions about their financial affairs, vote, marry, make a will, and make decisions about their treatment. Beginning in the 1950s and 1960s, courts, mental health professionals, and state legislatures realized that mental disorders may *selectively* impair functioning, and therefore the principle arose that competence is decision-specific. With that realization, the concept of specific competencies was developed, and more than 30 types of competencies have now been defined in the law. In addition, an adjudication of incompetence in one area no longer equates with incompetence in other areas. Competencies specific to the criminal justice system are listed in Table 5-1.

Table 5-1. SPECIFIC CRIMINAL COMPETENCIES

- To be a witness
- To be executed
- To confess to a crime
- To sign a waiver/waive counsel
- To waive rights
- To be transferred from juvenile to adult court
- To waive criminal appeals
- To waive mitigation
- To be sentenced
- To plead guilty
- To refuse the insanity defense
- To stand trial

COMPETENCE TO STAND TRIAL

Criminal defendants facing trial have a right to be tried only if competent to stand trial. This principle flows from the guarantees afforded in the United States Constitution, including the 6th Amendment's right to the assistance of counsel and the right to confront witnesses, and the 14th Amendment's rights to substantive and procedural due process of law. With respect to the 6th Amendment, a mentally ill defendant may be unable to cooperate with his attorney and, due to mental illness, effectively be denied assistance of counsel. Likewise, a mentally ill defendant may be unable to confront witnesses against him at trial. Regarding the substantive due process clause of the 14th Amendment, trying an incompetent defendant is fundamentally unfair. Finally, with respect to the procedural due process clause of the 14th Amendment, a mentally ill defendant may not be able to understand and exercise his procedural due process rights—such as understanding the notice of the charges, participate in a hearing, and take advantage of other procedural safeguards designed to ensure that the defendant receives a fair trial.

Trying an incompetent defendant risks the possibility of an erroneous conviction because the mentally ill incompetent defendant who cannot understand the proceedings against him and/or assist in his defense may be wrongly convicted. For that reason, defense attorneys often request an evaluation of their client's competence to stand trial. Prosecutors and judges also have an interest in evaluating a mentally ill defendant's competence to stand trial because trying and convicting an incompetent defendant will likely lead to an overturn of the conviction on appeal. It simply does not serve justice to try an incompetent defendant.

In this chapter, the legal standards for competence to stand trial, the DSM-5 diagnostic changes most relevant to trial competency evaluations, and trial competency restoration programs are reviewed.

VIGNETTE 1

Joseph, a middle-aged man with schizophrenia, has been charged with felonious assault. Joseph refused to cooperate with his defense attorney, believing that his attorney is secretly working for the FBI. Joseph's defense attorney requested that the court order a competence to stand trial evaluation.

In this example, Joseph was adjudicated incompetent to stand trial because his delusions interfered with his working relationship with his defense attorney. He was committed to a psychiatric hospital for treatment to restore his competency to stand trial.

History of competence to stand trial

The origins of competence to stand trial can be traced to 13th century trials before the king's court in England. Criminal defendants who failed to enter a plea of guilty or not guilty were given three warnings by the court, and then either confined and starved (*prison forte et dure*) or gradually crushed under increasing weights (*peine forte et dure*) until they entered a plea or died [1, 2]. The phrase "to press someone for an answer" originates from this practice. Before engaging such methods, the king's court first needed to determine whether the defendant was intentionally withholding a plea (mute by malice), or whether, due to a mental defect, the defendant was unable to understand that a plea was required of them (mute by visitation of God—having a God-given mental defect). Those mute by visitation of God were spared the extreme methods described above, and a not guilty plea was entered for them. In 1353, the first criminal defendant was formally adjudicated Incompetent to Stand Trial. Legal standards for trial competence developed over the course of several subsequent centuries, although the United States legal standard was not articulated until 1960.

Competence to stand trial legal standards

Modern American competence to stand trial standards stem from the U.S. Supreme Court ruling in *Dusky v. United States* (1960) [3]. The *Dusky* standard inquires "whether the defendant has sufficient present ability to consult with his lawyer with a reasonable degree of rational understanding—and whether he has a rational as well as factual understanding of the proceedings against him." Although the *Dusky* standard did not require that a mental illness be the cause of the defendant's incompetence, the subsequently adopted Federal Insanity Defense Reform Act of 1984 [4] required a present mental disease or defect as the cause of the defendant's incompetence to stand trial.

In response to *Dusky v. United States*, every American jurisdiction adopted a competence to stand trial standard based on the *Dusky* standard. In general, state and federal standards indicate that defendants may be incompetent to stand trial if their mental illness makes them (1) unable to understand the nature and objectives of the court proceedings and/or (2) unable to assist in their defense.

VIGNETTE 2

George, an 18-year-old man, is charged with murder for the death of his mother. George has a severe psychotic disorder, which is now in remission, except for his belief that a government official authorized George to kill his mother. George plans on subpoenaing government telephone records and government officials to testify at trial as part of his defense plan. Otherwise, George does not appear psychotic. Is he competent?

In this example, George would likely be incompetent to stand trial, given that his delusions cause him to make an irrational decision about his defense, severely hampering his ability to assist in his defense.

VIGNETTE 3

Anna, a 38-year-old woman with a severe depressive disorder, is charged with murder regarding the death of her child. Presently, in the midst of a depressive episode, Anna has no interest in an acquittal, and in fact she is hoping to be convicted and subject to the death penalty so that she can be reunited with her child in heaven. Is Anna competent to stand trial?

In this scenario, Anna is likely incompetent to stand trial based on her irrational wish to be convicted, which is the result of her depressive symptomatology.

Evaluating competence to stand trial

Defense attorneys question their client's trial competency in 8%–15% of felony prosecutions [5, 6]. Typically, a defense attorney may question his client's competency due to the defendant's past history of a mental health diagnosis or treatment, behavior suggesting the presence of a mental disorder (either currently or during the offense), and/or an uncooperative or irrational client. The defense attorney formally enters a motion for a competence to stand trial evaluation, triggering the court to order a competence evaluation.

Competence to stand trial evaluations are one of the most commonly ordered forensic mental health evaluations: approximately 60,000 are performed annually in the United States [7]. Most competence evaluations are performed on an outpatient basis, although provisions for an inpatient evaluation can be made for the defendant who is uncooperative or suspected of malingering [8]. On average, 30% of defendants evaluated for trial competency are found to be incompetent to stand trial.

The clinician performing the competency to stand trial examination should:

1. Be familiar with the competence to stand trial standard in the jurisdiction;
2. Review the defendant's relevant medical records;
3. Review relevant collateral sources of information (jail medical records, interview of family members, etc);
4. Conduct a personal interview of the defendant, consisting of:
    - A standard psychiatric diagnostic interview and mental status examination. The defendant's orientation, memory, concentration, mood, affect, and the presence of delusions, hallucinations, and loose associations are especially relevant.
    - An inquiry into the specific areas of competency to stand trial (see below); and
5. Provide a written report with a well-reasoned opinion on the competence to stand trial issue by applying the facts of the case to the legal competency standard.

Most states have statutes prohibiting data obtained from a competency to stand trial evaluation from being used to prove a defendant's guilt. For example, if a defendant confesses guilt to a clinician during a competency evaluation, the confession would be inadmissible at trial in most jurisdictions. A number of specific inquiries must be made when performing a competence to stand trial evaluation. Using the two-part legal standard for competency to stand trial described above, the following areas should to be examined:

1. *Ability to Understand Nature and Objectives of the Court Proceedings*:
    a. Charges—The defendant must be able to understand the nature of the criminal charges. Knowledge of the official name of the charge is useful, but it is more important that the defendant understand the nature of the specific act that he is accused of committing. For example, it is insufficient that a defendant knows that he is charged with Aggravated Robbery. A defendant should understand that they are charged with robbing a specific victim on a specific date.
    b. Appreciate their situation as a criminal defendant—A defendant should be able to understand that they are charged with a crime and are facing prosecution [9]. A defendant who delusionally believes that he or

she is immune from criminal prosecution is likely to be incompetent to stand trial.

c. Severity of charge—A defendant should be able to understand the severity of the charge (misdemeanor or felony) and the possible range of sentences they face if convicted.
d. Pleas—A defendant should be able to understand the various pleas available, including Guilty, Not Guilty, No Contest, and Not Guilty by Reason of Insanity (and Alford Pleas and Guilty but Mentally Ill, in some jurisdictions).
e. Courtroom personnel roles—A defendant should be able to understand the roles of the defendant, defense attorney, judge, prosecutor, jury, witness, and victim.
f. Adversarial nature of trial—A defendant must be able to understand which court personnel are acting adversely to their interests and demonstrate self-protective behavior. A defendant who, due to a mental disorder, seeks to confess to the prosecutor while waiting for the trial to begin may well be incompetent to stand trial.

2. *Ability to Assist in Defense*:
   a. Cooperate with defense attorney—A defendant must be able to have logical and coherent discussions with their attorney and be free of paranoid thinking about their attorney. A defendant should also be able to communicate relevant information to their defense counsel. An incoherent or mute defendant is likely to be incompetent [9].
   b. Understand plea-bargaining—Approximately 85% of criminal defendants plea bargain, by agreeing to plead guilty in exchange for a reduced charge and/or sentence. Therefore, it is important that a defendant understands the concept of plea-bargaining and have the capacity to rationally make decisions about plea-bargaining in their own case.
   c. Willingness to consider a mental illness defense—A defendant must possess sufficient insight into their mental illness to consider pleading Not Guilty by Reason of Insanity, Guilty but Mentally Ill, or seeking mitigation due to mental illness, if relevant. Defendants who are otherwise competent to stand trial but irrationally refuse a mental illness defense may have such a defense imposed on them by the court and still proceed to trial [10].
   d. Appraisal of evidence, estimate of likely outcome of trial—A defendant must be able to evaluate evidence, determine which evidence is helpful or harmful to their case, and estimate their chances of conviction. The defendant must also be able to apply this data in deciding whether to enter a plea.

e. Sufficient memory and concentration to understand the events at trial—A defendant must be able to pay attention during trial and have sufficient memory to retain and apply the information during trial.
f. Understand appropriate courtroom behavior—A defendant must be able to understand appropriate courtroom behavior and possess sufficient impulse control to exercise appropriate courtroom demeanor. It is important to differentiate between a defendant who (due to a mental disorder) is not capable of acting appropriately from a defendant who elects to act inappropriately to make a political statement or other reasons.
g. Give a rational, consistent, and coherent account of the offense—A defendant must be able to give a consistent and organized account of the offense. Such an account may help to achieve alibi, acquittal, insanity or mitigation. However, a defendant with permanent amnesia for the offense is not categorically incompetent to stand trial [11].
h. Formulate a basic plan of defense—A defendant should be able to work with their attorney to develop a basic plan of defense, working toward the goal of acquittal or mitigation.
i. Make reasonable defense decisions—Using their knowledge of the information listed above, a defendant must be able to rationally apply their knowledge to their defense and make reasonable, logic-driven decisions.
j. Freedom from self-defeating behavior—A defendant must be motivated to seek the best possible outcome for their criminal trial. Defendants who consciously seek an unfavorable outcome, due to mental illness, may be incompetent to stand trial. For example, a depressed, suicidal defendant who is seeking capital punishment is likely incompetent to stand trial.
k. Testify at trial—A defendant must be able to give rational, organized, and logical trial testimony that may assist in their defense. A defendant must also be able to withstand the stress of testifying and being subject to cross-examination.

Competence to stand trial structured assessment instruments

Many structured instruments have been developed to assess competence to stand trial, including the Competency Screening Test [12], Competency to Stand Trial Assessment Instrument [13], Interdisciplinary Fitness Interview [14], Competence Assessment for Standing Trial for Defendants with Mental Retardation (CAST*MR) [15], and Georgia Court Competency Test [16]. Many of these instruments are of only limited utility because they only assess a defendant's factual understanding, not reasoning ability [17]. Canadian researchers have developed the Fitness Interview Test, specifically designed to address the Canadian competency to stand trial standard [18].

The MacArthur Competence Assessment Tool-Criminal Adjudication (Mac-CAT-CA) is an instrument that assesses "adjudicative competence," which includes competence to enter a plea, stand trial, and participate in pretrial proceedings [17]. It is a standardized instrument that assesses both factual knowledge and decisional competence. In recent years, additional competence assessment tools have been introduced, including the Computer-Assisted Determination of Competency to Stand Trial (CADCOMP) [19], Evaluation of Competency to Stand Trial-Revised (ECST-R) [20], and the Inventory of Legal Knowledge (ILK).

The designers of structured competency assessment instruments do not intend that the instruments be used as diagnostic tests that decide whether an individual is capable of proceeding with adjudication. Rather, the instruments' designers recommend that forensic mental health professionals treat test results as one source of information, interpreting those results in light of the full clinical interview and other available data [7].

Outcome of competency to stand trial evaluations

Once raised as a legal issue, a defendant's competency to stand trial is usually addressed by the court in a competency hearing [21]. The competency issue is ultimately a legal question to be adjudicated by a judge. Clinical opinions on the issue of competence are admitted into evidence at a competency hearing. Courts usually (up to 90% of the time) base the adjudication of competence on the clinical opinion by the court-appointed forensic mental health professional [22, 23].

The majority of defendants clinically examined for competency to stand trial are found to be competent. The presence of a mental disorder is insufficient to conclude that a criminal defendant is incompetent to stand trial. In one study, almost one-third of defendants referred for competency evaluations and found competent to stand trial were diagnosed with a psychotic disorder [24]. Although a mental disorder is necessary to conclude that a defendant is incompetent to stand trial, incompetency also requires that the mental disorder impair the defendant's performance on the specific functional areas relevant to the competency standard.

On average, 30% of defendants evaluated for competence to stand trial are adjudicated incompetent [25], although there is a wide range (4%–77%) of incompetency rates in different jurisdictions [26]. From 37% to 50% of geriatric defendants are found to be incompetent [27–29]. Males and females are equally likely to be found incompetent to stand trial [29]. Younger adults are more likely to be incompetent due to a psychotic or mood disorder or

Table 5-2. COMMON REASONS FOR INCOMPETENCE TO STAND TRIAL FINDINGS

1. Low intelligence or dementia that impairs the defendant's understanding of the trial process.
2. Depression and self-defeating behavior that limit the defendant's motivation for the best outcome at trial.
3. Mania that impairs the defendant's ability to act appropriately in the courtroom.
4. Paranoid delusions that impair the defendant's ability to work with their defense counsel.
5. Disorganized thinking that impairs the defendant's concentration and attention.
6. Irrational decision-making about their defense as the result of delusions, disorganized thinking, low intellect or dementia.
7. Hallucinations that distract the defendant from attending to the trial.

mental retardation, whereas older defendants are more likely to be incompetent due to dementia [27]. Preteens and young adolescents are frequently incompetent due to numerous deficiencies, including inability to disclose relevant data to defense counsel, susceptibility to outside influence, inability to appraise the quality of their legal representation, and difficulty making decisions about their defense [30, 31]. Table 5-2 lists common reasons for a finding of incompetence to stand trial.

Defendants adjudicated incompetent to stand trial are usually committed to a hospital for treatment in order to restore them to competency. Approximately 7000 defendants are involuntarily committed to public hospitals annually for restoration to competence [32]. Restoration to competence is accomplished by treating the defendant's underlying mental illness and providing education about the trial process [33]. Incompetent defendants who incompetently refuse antipsychotic medication may receive involuntary treatment to restore their trial competency, if the trial court so authorizes. However, a criminal defendant adjudicated as incompetent to stand trial who nevertheless competently refuses antipsychotic medications may still receive involuntary treatment, if the prosecution can prove that there is a compelling governmental interest at stake, such as bringing the defendant to trial on major charges [34]. Approximately 80%–90% of defendants found incompetent to stand trial will eventually be restored to competence. However, this rate varies, depending on the severity of the defendant's illness and the statutory time allowed for restoration to competency.

Some defendants, due to the nature of their mental disorder, will not be restored to competency to stand trial. Common reasons for unrestorability include treatment-resistant psychosis, dementia, and moderate to severe intellectual disability. Defendants who are incompetent to stand trial may not be committed for restoration to competency unless there is a substantial likelihood that they can be restored [35]. Therefore, a clinician who opines that a defendant is incompetent to stand trial should offer an opinion about whether the defendant is likely to be restored to competency. Charges are dismissed or held in abeyance for defendants adjudicated incompetent to stand trial and not restorable. Incompetent, unrestorable defendants may remain hospitalized only if they are civilly committed.

DSM-5'S IMPACT ON COMPETENCE TO STAND TRIAL

As mentioned above, no particular diagnoses equates with incompetence to stand trial. Defendants who are adjudicated as incompetent to stand trial have diagnoses of mental disorders or defects, but a relatively low percentage of persons with mental disorders or defects that are evaluated for trial competence are ultimately adjudicated as incompetent. The most common conditions associated with trial incompetence include psychotic illnesses, brain disorders, and intellectual disability [36].

The Diagnostic and Statistical Manual (DSM) is the standard diagnostic manual used by mental health professionals in the United States. Evaluators of competence to stand trial most commonly rely on the DSM to convey diagnostic material. Discussed here are those DSM-5 [37] diagnoses most frequently represented in trial competence assessments and DSM-5 changes that impact these evaluations.

Intellectual disability

Nicholson and Kugler [25] described a small negative correlation between incompetence and intelligence scores. However, others have found the opposite. Cochrane et al. [26] for example, reported a rate of 12%–36% from literature review of adjudicative incompetence among evaluees with diagnoses of mental retardation. In looking at a sample of evaluees from a federal evaluation center, the same authors reported that 30% of defendants with diagnoses of mental retardation were assessed as incompetent by forensic evaluators. Because persons with the most severe forms of intellectual disability are more often under constant supervision, these individuals are less likely to commit criminal acts [38]. Persons with milder intellectual disabilities are, then, more likely to be evaluated for competence to stand trial. Past studies have reported that persons with mental retardation commonly report understanding of terms when, in fact, they did not understand them [39]. What was formerly called Mental Retardation is now termed intellectual disability in DSM-5. In contrast to DSM-IV, DSM-5 emphasizes both cognitive capacity and also adaptive functioning. Severity of disability is determined by adaptive functioning in three areas: conceptual, social, and practical. Accordingly, this DSM-5 diagnosis requires the forensic evaluator to conduct a more thorough assessment of functional skills rather than relying solely on IQ testing scores.

Social (pragmatic) communication disorder

DSM-5 adds a new diagnosis titled social (pragmatic) communication disorder (SPCD) to its list of mental disorders. SPCD involves persistent difficulties in the social use of verbal and nonverbal communication. To qualify for this new diagnosis, DSM-5 requires that the person demonstrates deficits in four areas: (1) problems in social communication, (2) difficulties in altering how one communicates with another individual based on the unique aspects of that individual, (3) impairments in adhering to basic conversational principles, such as telling a story, and, (4) problems understanding the more subtle aspects of verbal communication (such as humor or metaphors) [37 (p47–48)]. However, SPCD is distinguished from the DSM-5 diagnosis of autism spectrum disorder because it does *not* require the presence of "restricted, repetitive patterns of behavior, interests, or activities" to make the diagnosis [37 [p49)]. Because the ability to communicate with one's attorney is generally an important component of trial competency, might a defendant diagnosed with SPCD claim that they are incompetent due to their associated communication deficits? For example, consider a defendant who is socially rude, refuses to greet others, easily misunderstands what others say and angrily responds, and does not change the way he speaks to match the decorum of the courtroom. This presentation could describe many criminal defendants.

However, the application of SPCD diagnosis should not be taken out of context and applied inappropriately to persons who have difficulty communicating primarily due to their maladaptive personality style. In reality, SPCD would be a difficult diagnosis for most defendants to claim if the criteria are applied correctly. In particular, the defendant needs to substantiate three important elements to qualify for this diagnosis: (1) The onset of communication problems must begin in the early developmental period; (2) The communication difficulties must encompass all communication domains described by the DSM-5; and (3) The deficits must "result in functional limitations in effective communication, social participation, social relationships, academic achievement, or occupational performance, individually or in combination" [37 (p48)]. Clinicians and evaluators should carefully apply DSM-5 criteria to avoid a misdiagnosis that incorrectly labels antisocial communications as SPCD.

Schizophrenia spectrum and other psychotic disorders

DSM-5 psychotic disorders are "defined by abnormalities in one or more of the following five domains: delusions, hallucinations, disorganized thinking (speech), grossly disorganized or abnormal motor behavior (including catatonia), and negative symptoms" [37 (p87)]. These symptoms are those most commonly associated with trial incompetence. Nicholson and Kugler's [25] meta-analysis of 30 studies revealed that defendants diagnosed with a psychotic disorder had a significant correlation with incompetence. Likewise, Pirelli et al. [41] demonstrated that defendants with psychotic diagnoses had more had an 8-fold increased likelihood of being adjudicated incompetent as defendants without a psychotic diagnosis. Schizophrenia and other psychotic disorders may affect individuals in several ways that impact trial competence. For example, defendants with delusional beliefs may misattribute motives of their attorney or the prosecution against them (see Vignettes 1 and 2). Hallucinations may distract and impair a person's ability to focus and understand the course of the proceeding. Psychotic symptoms may limit reasoning abilities.

Changes in DSM-5 from DSM-IV are likely to have little overall impact on trial competency assessments for persons with psychotic disorders in terms of making diagnoses and assessing the relationship between diagnosis and the legal abilities required for trial competence. DSM-5 eliminates the subcategories of schizophrenia. The A criterion of delusional disorder no longer requires that the delusions be nonbizarre. The most significant change to impact competency to stand trial assessments is DSM-5's emphasis on severity of psychotic symptoms. New to DSM-5, the manual introduces a framework for assessing the severity of key symptoms. For all of the psychotic disorders, DSM-5 notes that the severity of psychotic symptoms is should be determined by a "quantitative assessment" of delusions, hallucinations, disorganized speech, abnormal psychomotor behavior, and negative symptoms [37 (p91)]. DSM-5 references an assessment instrument included in Section III (Emerging Measures and Models) titled the "Clinician-Rated Dimensions of Psychosis Symptom Severity Scale," and this instrument provides a dimensional rating scale for the primary symptoms of psychosis. Although use of this or another rating instrument is not required for diagnostic purposes, the forensic evaluator should be mindful of the emphasis on symptom severity and be prepared to comment on psychosis severity if needed.

Bipolar and related disorders and depressive disorders

Several studies have reported that defendants with diagnoses of mood disorders are more likely to be adjudicated incompetent to stand trial compared with the general population of trial competence evaluees [42, 43]. Defendants with bipolar mania, for example, may lack the ability to adequately control their behavior in the courtroom or in their interactions with their attorney. Depressive symptoms, such as severe emotional blunting, can impair trial competence when the defendants do not care about what happens to them, including the outcome of their legal case (see Vignette 3). DSM-5 changes in the category of Bipolar and Related Disorders are few and are unlikely to change competency assessments from DSM-IV in any meaningful way. For Depressive Disorders, the DSM-5 includes two new diagnoses that merit special attention in evaluating possible claims of trial incompetency.

Disruptive mood dysregulation disorder

The DSM-5 text notes that the essential feature of disruptive mood dysregulation disorder (DMDR) is "chronic, severe persistent irritability" [37 (p156)]. The diagnostic criteria for DMDR includes the presence of significant and repeated temper problems (either verbally or physically) that typically occur three or more times a week and are a mismatch with the youth's level of development. In addition, the symptoms must be present for at least 12 months without any symptom free period lasting three or more months. DSM-5 notes that this disorder was added to help differentiate *non*-episodic irritability from a pattern of episodic-irritability, which is more consistent with bipolar disorder in children. DSM-5 particularly emphasizes that bipolar disorder is specifically designated for psychiatric presentations that include discrete periods of bipolar symptoms [37 (p157)].

Many adult defendants facing trial may have recurrent temper outbursts; however, they will not meet criteria for DMDD, even if they have verbal or behavioral problems that interfere with their ability to cooperate with counsel. The text criteria states that the diagnosis should not be made for the *first* time in those older than 18. Could an adult defendant continue to retain this diagnosis into adulthood if he or she was diagnosed with DMDD at age 18 or less? The DSM-5 text suggests not. In particular, the DSM-5 notes, "...use of the diagnosis should be restricted to age groups similar to those in which validity has been established (7–18 years) [37 (p157)]. Based on this statement, the diagnosis of DMDD appears strictly limited to those less than age 19.

The real issue is the how the diagnosis of DMDD may be used as the predicate diagnosis to establish trial incompetency for juveniles (i.e., age 18 or less). Because youth often present with difficulties controlling their temper and behavior, the evaluator will need to carefully apply DMDD criteria to distinguish this diagnosis from other common mental health presentations found in juvenile delinquent populations (e.g., oppositional defiant disorder or conduct disorder). The following guidelines may assist the evaluator in making these distinctions:

1. The diagnosis of DMDD cannot be made prior to age 6 in contrast to oppositional defiant disorder and conduct disorder.
2. The diagnosis of DMDD must begin prior to age 10. Therefore, juveniles who first present with symptoms characteristic of DMDD at age 10 or older cannot be diagnosed with DMDD.
3. The diagnosis of DMDD cannot be made alongside the diagnosis of oppositional defiant disorder (ODD). In distinguishing DMDD from ODD, the DSM-5 comments that mood symptoms are rare in children with ODD, that children with DMDD have a persistent disruption in mood between temper outbursts (unlike momentary mood disruptions with ODD), and that children with DMDD must have "severe impairment in at least one setting…and mild to moderate impairment in a second setting" [37 (p159)]. If the youth meets criteria for both disorders, DMDD is the only diagnosis that should be made.
4. The diagnosis of DMDD cannot be made alongside the diagnosis of bipolar disorder. If the juvenile independently meets criteria for bipolar disorder in addition to DMDD, only the diagnosis of bipolar disorder should be made.

Premenstrual dysphoric disorder

This is a completely new DSM-5 diagnosis. For a woman to meet criteria for premenstrual dysphoric disorder (PMDD), she must have at least five symptoms that occur during the week prior to menstruation, an improvement of symptoms within a few days after her menses begin, and minimal if any symptoms in the week after menstruation has stopped (Criterion A) [37 (p171)]. A female defendant could possibly claim she cannot cooperate with counsel during periods when she is experiencing PMDD due to her marked irritability, feelings of hopelessness, high anxiety, mood swings, and difficulty concentrating. However, it is important for the examiner to note that the DSM-5 criteria for this disorder must be met for most menstrual cycles that occurred during the prior year. In addition, Criterion A should be verified by "prospective daily ratings during at least two symptomatic cycles," the symptoms must cause "clinically significant distress," and the symptoms are not related to another mental disorder [37 (p172)]. PMDD would only apply to a small minority of woman and unlikely to have a significant impact on the number of women claiming trial incompetence. If this issue is raised, careful evaluation of PMDD diagnostic criteria, potential personality traits or disorders, and malingering will be especially relevant.

Posttraumatic stress disorder

The diagnostic changes for posttraumatic stress disorder (PTSD) have been covered extensively in other chapters of this book (see Chapters 2, 8, and 11). The most relevant issue for potential concerns related to trial competency includes the new DSM-5 specifier "with dissociative symptoms" [37 (p274)]. This specifier includes the possibility that the individual could experience either depersonalization (feeling separated from one's own body) or derealization (a sustained sense that one's environment is not real). A defendant might claim that his or her PTSD results in dissociation thereby preventing them from being able to assist counsel in real time during the trial or trial preparations. PTSD, as described by DSM-IV, was not a common diagnosis resulting in a finding of trial incompetency. It is unclear what, if any, impact this new specifier might have in future claims of trial competency related to a PTSD diagnosis claim.

Dissociative identity disorder

The diagnosis of dissociative identity disorder (DID) has been typically used to question trial competency in two situations: (1) The defendant cannot control his or her personalities, and therefore their behavior is unpredictable and impairs their ability to attend to the trial process or testify; and/or (2) The defendant's personality who was involved in the alleged crime is not consistently present, or he/she does not remember the crime thereby, impairing their ability to assist in their own defense [44]. Although DID was included in DSM-IV, DSM-5 has made some changes to the diagnostic language which may raise new issues in the legal setting. First, both DSM-IV and DSM-5 describe that the individual has two or more distinct personality states. However, in Criterion A, DSM-5 adds that distinct personality states "may be described in some cultures as an experience of possession" [37 (p292)]. DSM-5 describes these "possession-form identities" as those that commonly present as if a spirit or supernatural force has taken over the individual and as a result the individual talks or behaves in an obviously different manner than usual. DSM-5 asserts that these possessions may present as a ghost of a girl, a demon, or a deity [37 (p293)].

With this new language, will malingerers try to present that they are "possessed" and therefore cannot assist counsel, testify, or behave in court? DSM-5 cautions that few possession states will represent genuine cases of DID. The relevant text emphasizes that most possession states are considered normal and are often part of a religious or spiritual ceremony [37 (p293)]. Second, DSM-IV Criterion C noted that DID memory gaps were characterized by failing to remember personal information in excess of simple forgetting [40 (p529)]. In contrast, the DSM-5 significantly broadens this criteria and notes that a person will meet this criterion if he or she has repeated memory lapses for everyday incidents in addition to impairment in remembering personal information [37 (p292)]. One can imagine situations where a defendant claiming DID might now allege that they cannot remember basic everyday events, such as information that was presented to them about the legal process or when to appear for a court hearing. However, DSM-5 adds one criterion that likely narrows who can be diagnosed with DID when compared with the DSM-IV diagnostic criteria. In particular, DSM-5 now requires that the reported symptoms must cause "clinically significant distress or impairment in social, occupational, or other important areas of functioning" [37 (p292)], a requirement not included in the DSM-IV. Therefore, if DID claims are raised, the forensic examiner should carefully review not only the claim, but evidence that that the symptoms causes clinically significant distress or impairment. The assessment of malingering will be particularly relevant for this diagnosis and is discussed in more detail in Chapter 11.

Intermittent explosive disorder

The intermittent explosive disorder (IED) criteria have greatly expanded under DSM-5. Under DSM-IV, the person had to demonstrate physical aggression to qualify for this diagnosis. Under the new DSM-5 criteria, the individual only need recurrent behavioral outbursts characterized by (1) verbal aggression or (2) damage or destruction to property and/or physical assault [37 (p466)]. Consider the situation of a criminal defendant who frequently yells out in court and has a verbal tirade. His attorney states that it is impossible to work with him because when he tries to meet with him, he gets in repeated verbal arguments at least twice a week, and this pattern has been present during the entire three months that he has been working with him. The defendant's behavior has resulted in the judge holding him in contempt of court and having him physically removed from the courtroom.

Could this attorney raise a doubt of trial competency based on a diagnosis of IED? Should this diagnosis be raised for consideration, the examiner should carefully document the frequency and duration criteria as required by DSM-5. More importantly, a distinction between impulsivity and aggression characteristic of ASPD and Borderline Personality Disorder is highly relevant. In making this distinction, the evaluator will need to determine the degree, if any, that the behavior is planned and whether the degree of aggression is greater than expected based on the triggering incident. DSM-5 does not provide clear guidance on how to distinguish between IED and ASPD, only that "the level of impulsive aggression in individuals with antisocial personality disorder is lower than that in individuals with intermittent explosive disorder" [37 (p468)].

Neurocognitive disorders

Using the MacArthur Competence Assessment Tool-Criminal Adjudication (McCAT-CA) [17], Ryba and Zapf [45] sampled male forensic patients and found a positive association between cognitive function and competency. The DSM-IV diagnosis of Dementia is now classified as major neurocognitive disorder under DSM-5, and DSM-5 now recognizes less severe cognitive dysfunction with the diagnosis of mild neurocognitive disorder. With formal inclusion of the milder diagnosis, more individuals are likely to be diagnosed with cognitive dysfunction. Nevertheless, this change should not meaningfully impact adjudicative competence because the evaluator must assess how any cognitive impairment ties to the capacity requirements. The mild neurocognitive disorder criteria dictate that the disorder does not interfere with a person's independence or activities of daily living. This exemplifies the point that this diagnosis alone is likely insufficient to cause such significant cognitive impairment that the defendant would be incompetent to stand trial.

DSM-5 AND OTHER TRIAL COMPETENCIES

Although discussed in the context of trial competence, the DSM-5 diagnoses reviewed above are likely to be those most applicable in other areas of criminal competencies. A discussion of several additional types of criminal competencies is summarized below.

COMPETENCE TO CONFESS TO A CRIME

The 5th Amendment indicates that a criminal defendant cannot be compelled to be a witness against him/herself, also known as the privilege against self-incrimination. In 1966, the U.S. Supreme Court ruled in *Miranda v. Arizona* [46] that the 5th Amendment requires that the police inform a defendant in custody that they have the right to remain silent; the right to counsel; and that any statements the defendant makes can be used against them. A defendant may choose to waive his 5th Amendment (*Miranda*) rights and provide investigators with a confession that may later be introduced at trial by the prosecution as evidence of guilt. The standard for waiving one's *Miranda* rights (or any Constitutional right) is whether the defendant knowingly, intelligently [47] and voluntarily waived that right.

Forensic mental health professionals may be asked to evaluate whether a defendant competently or incompetently waived his or her *Miranda* rights. Mental disorders such as intellectual disability, schizophrenia spectrum and other psychotic disorders, bipolar disorder, or severe depression may impair a defendant's ability to competently make a decision whether to invoke or waive their *Miranda* rights, or to be susceptible to making a false confession. However, in 1986 the U.S. Supreme Court ruled in *Colorado v. Connelly* [48] that *police coercion* is a necessary predicate to a court finding that a defendant's confession was incompetently made, and that police officers and courts are not required to make inquiries into a defendant's reasons (rational or otherwise) for waiving their *Miranda* rights. Therefore, the forensic mental health professional's evaluation may be limited to retrospectively evaluating the defendant's mental state at the time of the confession and their susceptibility to potentially coercive police behavior.

COMPETENCE TO PLEAD GUILTY

Many criminal defendants agree to plead guilty to their charges in exchange for a reduced sentence or the dismissal of a portion of the indictment in the process known as plea bargaining. Pleading guilty involves waiving specific rights, including the right to freedom from self-incrimination, the right to a jury trial, and the right to confront witnesses. Mental health professionals may be requested to contemporaneously evaluate a defendant's competence who wishes to plead guilty, or (more frequently) retrospectively evaluate a defendant's competence to plead guilty as the basis of an appeal. At issue is whether the defendant had a mental disorder at the time that the decision to plead guilty was made, and whether the symptoms of the defendant's mental disorder impaired their ability to intelligently, knowingly and voluntarily waive those rights.

COMPETENCE TO WAIVE COUNSEL

An early decision a criminal defendant faces is whether to obtain legal representation. The 6th Amendment affords criminal defendants the right to counsel. The purpose of counsel includes assisting the defendant through the adjudicative process as well as ensuring the validity of the plea and court process [49]. However, a defendant may want to waive counsel for a variety of reasons, including mistrust of the legal system, financial reasons, a belief that they do not need representation because they are "innocent," a belief that they could better represent their situation than an attorney, a belief that they will earn sympathy by proceeding *pro se* against the government, or any number of psychotic or self-defeating beliefs.

In *Faretta v California* (1975) [49], the U.S. Supreme Court held that a criminal defendant has a Constitutional right (via the 6th Amendment) to knowingly and intelligently refuse legal representation. Although a related concept (and both may be subjects of forensic assessment), it is important to point out that refusing counsel is not the same thing as representing oneself (proceeding *pro se*). The *Faretta* court added that a defendant's ability to represent himself has no bearing on his competence to elect to represent himself. In *Indiana v. Edwards* (2008) [50], the Court ruled that courts may require a higher standard of competence for self-representation than that necessary for trial competence. The right to represent oneself is not absolute; courts have discretion in maintaining the validity of the court process.

Forensic evaluators in the position to evaluate defendants for competence to waive counsel should familiarize themselves with jurisdictional law. Under *Faretta*, the mental health professional evaluating competence to waive counsel must assess whether the defendant understands that he or she is abandoning the right to representation by legal counsel and that there may be disadvantages as a result of the waiver of counsel. Although the evaluator may not agree with the defendant's rationale, the evaluator must be careful not to equate poor judgment with incompetence. The focus should be on whether the defendant has symptoms of a mental disorder or defect that impair the defendant's ability to make the decision to waive counsel.

COMPETENCE TO WAIVE A JURY TRIAL

There is a constitutional right to be tried by an impartial jury of one's peers. There is no constitutionally guaranteed right to waive a jury trial. However, defendants may seek to waive a jury trial and be tried by the trial judge if they perceive that a bench trial is in their legal interests, which is frequently the case in contested insanity trials. There is not a specific legal standard with respect to waiving the right to trial by jury; however, one may extrapolate from other legal standards that in order for a defendant to competently waive trial by jury, the waiver must be made intelligently, knowingly, and voluntarily. Therefore, the mental health professional evaluating whether a defendant can competently waive trial by jury and proceed to a bench trial must evaluate whether the defendant has a mental disorder that impairs any ability to understand the right to be impartially tried by a jury of peers, and investigate the rationality of the decision to waive trial by jury.

COMPETENCE TO TESTIFY

Competence to testify as a defendant in a criminal trial is traditionally encompassed in the evaluation of competence to stand trial, as addressed above. In contrast, competency to testify as a fact witness (also known as testimonial competency) in a civil or criminal proceeding is a separate determination, and may be questioned if the witness is a child or mentally ill.

In general, testimonial competency requires that the witness be able to offer reliable and credible testimony. Common reasons for the finding that a witness is incompetent to testify include cognitive deficits, confabulation, disorganized thinking, and/or mania. Therefore, the evaluating mental health professional should assess whether the witness has a present mental disorder that impairs their ability give reliable and credible testimony.

COMPETENCE TO WAIVE EXTRADITION

Criminal defendants may be arrested in a jurisdiction different from where their charges originated and where they will be tried. Defendants can challenge extradition (their transfer) to a requesting state. Only a handful of states have explicitly considered the issue of a defendant's right to be competent to proceed with an extradition hearing. In some states, competence to participate in an extradition hearing is similar to competence to stand trial, in that the defendant must understand factual material related to extradition under the Uniform Criminal Extradition Act and be able to assist their defense counsel at the extradition hearing. Some states apply a more limited competency standard related solely to particular requirements of extradition (as to identity and fugitive status). Finally, a limited number of states have found that a fugitive has no right to be competent to proceed in an extradition hearing.

COMPETENCE TO BE SENTENCED

A mentally ill defendant who is competent to stand trial or to plead guilty may nevertheless experience an exacerbation of his/her illness during the period of time between trial and sentencing and potentially become incompetent to be sentenced. Competence to be sentenced deals with evaluating the defendant's understanding that they have been convicted of a crime; the reason for the conviction; and the reasons that sentencing will be imposed. Competence to be sentenced also requires that the defendant be able to rationally participate in a presentence investigation; to assist their defense attorney in minimizing the negative impact of their conviction; and to assist their attorney in offering mitigating factors that may cause the court to reduce their sentence.

COMPETENCE TO WAIVE APPEALS

Defendants who have been convicted may appeal their conviction, and, in fact, defendants who are convicted and sentenced to death have numerous appeals filed automatically on their behalf. A mentally ill defendant may irrationally instruct his attorney to not file appeals on his behalf, or he/she may refuse to cooperate with his attorney in preparing appeals. In contrast, a defendant may rationally waive his appeals in the belief that pursuing further appeals is not likely to be fruitful or not in his/her best interests. Evaluating competence to waive appeals involves assessing the defendant's current mental state and understanding whether current symptoms impair the defendant's ability to rationally make a decision of whether to pursue appeals and to assist his/her defense counsel in that pursuit. A depressed defendant who, as a result of their depression, lacks energy/motivation to pursue appeals may be incompetent to waive appeals. A suicidal defendant seeking capital punishment may be incompetent to waive appeals, as is a defendant with paranoid delusions about his/her attorney or the court. In contrast, a defendant who prefers capital punishment compared with a life of imprisonment may be competent to waive appeals if his/her decision is rational and not the product of his/her mental disorder.

COMPETENCE TO BE EXECUTED

Presently, 34 states and the federal jurisdiction have the ability to sentence a defendant to death. On average, in American jurisdictions, 15 years pass between when the defendant is sentenced to death and when the sentence is carried out. Defendants on death row may develop a mental disorder during those 15 years that may impair their competence to be executed.

The U.S. Supreme Court has ruled that executing a mentally retarded defendant is unconstitutional [51] as is executing a defendant who was under the age of eighteen years at the time of the commission of the offense [52]. In *Ford v. Wainwright* [53], the U.S. Supreme Court ruled that it is cruel and unusual punishment, in violation of the 8th Amendment, to execute an incompetent defendant, and that states must have sufficient procedures in place to allow a defendant to challenge their competence to be executed. The *Ford* court held that the trial court should determine the defendant's competence to be executed by evaluating the defendant's understanding of the nature of the death penalty and the reason that the death penalty is being imposed.

In *Panetti v. Quarterman* [54], the U.S. Supreme Court broadly interpreted their ruling in *Ford v. Wainwright*, indicating that a defendant's simple awareness of the state's rationale for their execution was insufficient to prove that the defendant is competent to be executed. Instead, a defendant must have a more substantive understanding of the nature of the death penalty and the reason for its imposition. Although not giving a bright-line definition of what a more substantive understanding of the death penalty constitutes, the Court held that simple "yes" or "no" responses by the defendant to a series of questions about the death penalty do not constitute a substantive understanding of the death penalty.

Forensic evaluators may be called upon to evaluate a defendant's competence to be executed. Such an evaluation must assess the defendant's mental state and the presence/absence of a mental disorder that may impact the defendant's understanding of:

1. The general concept of punishment;
2. The nature of the death penalty;
3. The nature of death row;
4. The personnel present at the execution;
5. The role of the defense attorney;
6. What will happen when their execution is carried out;
7. The reason that the death sentence has been imposed; and
8. Symptoms that may impact their perception of reality.

SUMMARY

Competence to stand trial is a necessary predicate to criminal adjudication. Trial competence is the most frequently performed criminal capacity assessment. The forensic evaluator has a role to assess a defendant's mental condition and determine whether any mental disorder impacts the defendant's trial competence or adjudicative capacities. The presence of a mental disorder does not equate with trial incompetence nor other criminal competencies. The DSM-5 brings several diagnostic changes, and the most significant of these have been reviewed in regard to trial competency.

Key points to consider when evaluating competencies in the criminal justice system include the following:

- When asked to perform a forensic assessment of a criminal defendant, the evaluator should determine the specific question or type of legal competency to be evaluated.
- Competence to stand trial evaluations focus on the defendant's present mental state.
- Legal standards for competence to stand trial uniformly assess for the presence of a mental disorder that impairs the defendant's ability to either (1) understand the nature and objectives of the court proceedings and/or (2) assist in their defense.
- Defendants adjudicated as incompetent to stand trial are referred for competency restoration treatment if there is a probability that they can be restored to competence.
- Restoration of trial competence does not require remission of psychiatric symptoms.
- For any criminal competency, mental health evaluators should focus on the relationship between symptoms and the specific legal abilities required for the competence.
- Forensic evaluators need to be aware of their jurisdiction's specific requirements for any criminal competence.

REFERENCES

1. Statute of Westminster of 1275 (3 Edw. I).
2. Grubin D. *Fitness to Plead in England and Wales*. East Sussex, England: Psychology Press; 1996.
3. Dusky v United States, 362 US 402 (1960).
4. Insanity Defense Reform Act, 18 USC § 4241 (1984).
5. Hoge SK, Bonnie R, Poythress N, Monahan J. Attorney-client decision-making in criminal cases: client competence and participation as perceived by their attorneys. *Behav Sci Law* 1992; 10:385–394.
6. Poythress N, Bonnie R, Hoge S, et al. Client abilities to assist counsel and make decisions in criminal-cases: findings from 3 studies. *Law Human Behav* 1994; 8:437–452.
7. Mossman D, Noffsinger SG, Ash P, et al. Practice guideline: forensic psychiatric evaluation of competence to stand trial. *J Am Acad Psychiatry Law* 2007; 35:S3–S72.
8. Grisso T, Cocozza J, Steadman HJ, et al. The organization of pretrial forensic evaluation services: a national profile. *Law Human Behav* 1994; 18: 377–394.
9. Bonnie R, SK Hoge, Monahan J, et al. The MacArthur adjudicative competence study: a comparison of criteria for assessing the competence of criminal defendants. *J Am Acad Psychiatry Law* 1997; 25:249–259.
10. *Frendak v United States*, 408 A.2d 364 (DC Cir 1979).
11. *Wilson v United States*, 391 F.2d 460 (DC Cir 1968).
12. Lipsitt L, Lelos D, McGarry AL. Competency for trial: a screening instrument. *Am J Psychiatry* 1971; 128:105–109.

13. *Laboratory of Community Psychiatry, Harvard Medical School: Competency to Stand Trial and Mental Illness* (DHEW Pub. No. ADM-77-103). Rockville, MD: US Department of Health Education and Welfare; 1973.
14. Golding SL, Roesch R, Schreiber J, et al. Assessment and conceptualization of competency to stand trial: preliminary data on the Interdisciplinary Fitness Interview. *Law Human Behav* 1984; 9:321–334.
15. Everington C: The Competence Assessment for Standing Trial for Defendants with Mental Retardation (CAST-MR): a validation study. *Crim Just Beh* 1990; 17:147–168.
16. Nicholson RA, Briggs SR, Robertson H. Instruments for assessing competency to stand trial: how do they work? *Prof Psychol* 1988; 19:383–394.
17. Hoge SK, Bonnie RJ, Poythress N, et al. The MacArthur adjudicative competence study: development and validation of a research instrument. *Law Human Behav* 1997; 21: 141–179.
18. Zapf PA, Roesch R, Viljoen JL. Assessing fitness to stand trial: the utility of the fitness interview test (revised edition). *Can J Psychiatry* 2001; 46:426–432.
19. Barnard GW, Thompson JW Jr, Freeman WC, et al. Competency to stand trial: description and initial evaluation of a new computer-assisted assessment tool CADCOMP. *Bull Am Acad Psychiatry Law* 1991; 19:367–381.
20. Rogers R, Tillbrook CE, Sewell KW. *Evaluation of Competency to Stand Trial-Revised (ECST-R) and Professional Manual.* Odessa, FL: Psychological Assessment Resources; 2004.
21. *Pate v Robinson*, 383 US 375 (1966).
22. Freckelton I. Rationality and flexibility in assessment of fitness to stand trial. *Int J Law Psychiatry* 1996; 19:39–59.
23. Reich J, Tookey L. Disagreements between court and psychiatrist on competency to stand trial. *J Clin Psychiatry* 1986; 47:29–30.
24. Roesch RD, Eaves D, Sollner R, et al. Evaluating fitness to stand trial: a comparative analysis of fit and unfit defendants. *Int J Law Psychiatry* 1981; 4:145–157.
25. Nicholson R, Kugler K. Competent and incompetent criminal defendants: a quantitative review of comparative research. *Psychol Bull* 1991; 109:355–70.
26. Cochrane RE, Grisso T, Fredrick RI. The relationship between criminal charges, diagnoses, and psycholegal opinions among federal pretrial defendants. *Behav Sci Law* 2001; 19:565–582.
27. Frierson RL, Shea SJ, Shea ME. Competence-to-stand-trial evaluations of geriatric defendants. *J Am Acad Psychiatry Law* 2002; 30: 252–256.
28. Heinik J, Kimhi R, Hes K. Dementia and crime: a forensic psychiatry unit study in Israel. *Int J Geriatr Psychiatry* 1994; 9:491–494.
29. Riley SE. Competency to stand trial adjudication: a comparison of female and male defendants. *J Am Acad Psychiatry Law* 1998; 26:223–240.
30. McKee GR. Competency to stand trial in preadjudicatory juveniles and adults. *J Am Acad Psychiatry Law* 1998; 26:89–99.
31. Slovenko R. The prosecution of Nathaniel Abraham: a minor. *J Am Acad Psychiatry Law* 2000; 28:89–101.
32. Steadman H, Hartstone E. Defendants found incompetent to stand trial. In: Monahan J, Steadman H, eds. In: *Mentally Disordered Offenders.* New York, NY: Plenumn 1983: pp 39–64.
33. Noffsinger SG. Restoration to competency practice guidelines. *Int J Off Therapy Comp Criminology* 2001; 45:356–362.

34. *Sell v United States*, 539 US 166 (2003).
35. *Jackson v Indiana*, 92 Supreme Court Reporter 1845 (1972).
36. Hubbard KL, Zapf PA, Ronan KA. Competency restoration: an examination of the differences between defendants predicted restorable and not restorable to competency. *Law Human Behav 2003*; 27:127–139.
37. American Psychiatric Association. *Diagnostic and Statistical Manual of Mental Disorders, Fifth Edition (DSM-5).* Arlington, VA: American Psychiatric Association, 2013.
38. Wall BW, Christopher PP. A training program for defendant's with intellectual disability who are found incompetent to stand trial. *J Am Acad Psychiatry Law* 2012; 40:366–373.
39. Ericson K, Perlman N. Knowledge of legal terminology and court proceedings in adults with developmental disabilities. *Law Human Behav* 2001; 25:529–545.
40. American Psychiatric Association. *Diagnostic and Statistical Manual of Mental Disorders, Fourth Edition, Text Revision*. Arlington, VA: American Psychiatric Association; 2000.
41. Pirelli G, Gottdiener WH, Zapf PA. A meta-analytic review of competency to stand trial research. *Psychol Public Pol L*, 2011; 17:1–53.
42. Rogers R, Gillis JR, McMain S, Dickens SE. Fitness evaluations: a retrospective study of clinical, criminal and sociodemographic characteristics. *Can J Behav Sci* 1998; 20:192–200.
43. Warren JI, Rosenfeld B, Fitch WL, Hawk G. Forensic mental health clinical evaluation: an analysis of interstate and intersystemic differences. *Law Human Behav* 1997; 21: 372–390.
44. Lewis D, Bard J. Multiple personality disorder and forensic issues. *Psychiatr Clin North Am* 1991; 14:741–746.
45. Ryba NL, Zapf PA. The influence of psychiatric symptoms and cognitive abilities on competence-related abilities. *Int J Forensic Ment Health* 2011; 10:29–40.
46. *Miranda v Arizona* 384, US 436 (1966).
47. *Johnson v Zerbst*, 304, US 458 (1938).
48. *Colorado v Connelly*, 479 US 157 (1986).
49. *Faretta v California*, 422 US 806 (1975).
50. *Indiana v Edwards*, 554 US 164 (2008).
51. *Atkins v Virginia*, 536 US 304 (2002).
52. *Roper v Simmons*, 543 US 551 (2005).
53. *Ford v Wainwright*, 477 US 399 (1986).
54. *Panetti v Quarterman*, 551 US 930 (2007).

CHAPTER 6

DSM-5 and Not Guilty by Reason of Insanity and Diminished Mens Rea Defenses

INTRODUCTION

Courts, defense attorneys, and prosecutors often request assistance from mental health professionals when a criminal defendant's mental state at the time of the offense is at issue and the defendant enters a mental health defense. Mental health defenses are frequently raised when a defendant has a history of a preexisting mental disorder; behaved bizarrely during the offense; or evidenced other signs of a mental disorder after being arrested. The defense of Not Guilty by Reason of Insanity (NGRI) is the most widely discussed concept related to criminal responsibility, and it provides a total defense for the defendant who is adjudicated legally insane. Diminished Capacity and Guilty but Mentally Ill are additional mental health defenses that exist in some jurisdictions and may provide a partial defense that mitigates the defendant's criminal responsibility for the offense. Because the topic of mental health defenses is expansive, this chapter focuses on basic principles of criminal responsibility with particular attention to the elements of a crime and defenses that relate to criminal defendant's mental state. The Diagnostic and Statistical Manual of Mental Disorders, Fifth Edition (DSM-5) made several changes and additions to how mental disorders are defined and the potential impact of these changes on the concepts of insanity and other mental health defenses are discussed.

ELEMENTS OF A CRIME: CONCEPTS OF MENS REA AND ACTUS REUS

Criminal law and societal standards strive to establish a consistent and practical method to describe behaviors for which society may punish. Accordingly, federal, state, and municipal jurisdictions establish sources of criminal law—most commonly through statute—which outline the elements necessary for a defendant to be found guilty of a crime. Criminal guilt is established only if the prosecution can demonstrate and prove all of the required elements of the crime charged. The prosecution must prove each required element of the crime to the standard of beyond a reasonable doubt in a criminal trial. A defendant is to be found *not guilty* of a crime if the prosecution fails to prove all of the required elements of the crime or if the defendant establishes an affirmative defense to the crime.

In general, for a defendant to be guilty of a crime, two elements must be established and proven by the prosecution: the actus reus (Latin: "prohibited act") and the mens rea (*guilty mind*—the intent to commit the actus reus). The actus reus is further defined as either a voluntary physical act committed by the defendant or the defendant's failure to act when there was a legal duty to act. The law is usually concerned with preventing individuals from committing a harmful act to another. However, there are some obligations imposed by the law, such as a parent must provide food and shelter to a child, and failure to do so would constitute an actus reus. Both the actus reus and the mens rea must occur together in order to constitute a criminal act.

For example, person A is angry and intentionally strikes person B. A is charged with Battery. The actus reus is A striking B. The mens rea is A's purposeful intent to strike B, motivated by A's anger at B. In this example, A could be convicted of Battery. In a contrasting example, A strikes B as the result of an unintentional bump. A has struck B, therefore a forbidden act has occurred. But because the striking was accidental, no mens rea is present and no criminal liability exists (although civil liability may result). For nearly all crimes, the prosecution must prove the requisite mental state (mens rea). An exception is strict liability offenses, such as Statutory Rape or Driving Under the Influence, which require only an actus reus to result in a criminal conviction.

The concept of mens rea is important because the criminal law recognizes that a person who intends to harm another is more blameworthy than the person who accidentally harms another [1]. It is important to note that a defendant with a major mental illness may still be able to form the requisite level of mens rea for a given crime. Mentally ill defendants may intentionally commit criminal acts that occur for reasons and motives independent of their mental illness. For example, a psychotic individual may still purposely assault another for reasons unrelated to his psychosis, such as anger, revenge, financial gain, etc.

Even if the prosecution establishes all of the criminal elements (actus reus and mens rea) beyond a reasonable doubt, the defendant my nevertheless avoid criminal responsibility by raising an affirmative defense. An affirmative defense is a legal defense in which the defendant affirms that he indeed

Table 6-1. EXAMPLES OF AFFIRMATIVE DEFENSES
• Automatism (unconsciousness) • Duress (compulsion) • Entrapment (inducement by law enforcement) • Necessity (justification due to emergency) • Not guilty by reason of insanity • Self-defense (danger of imminent bodily harm) • Statute of limitations (expiration of time to pursue prosecution)

committed the actus reus, but, due to the special conditions alleged via the affirmative defense, seeks an acquittal. An affirmative defense justifies or excuses a criminal defendant of legal responsibility even though the elements of the crime have been proved. A state may, at its discretion, place the burden of proof for establishing an affirmative defense on either the prosecution or defense. Some affirmative defenses are legal justifications for the criminal act, such as in self-defense. The law recognizes that harm to another may be justified when a person is defending against imminent physical harm. Another category of affirmative defenses are legal excuses. The defense of NGRI falls into this category. For these, society has determined that the defendant is not blameworthy of the criminal act, usually based on a moral ground. Table 6-1 lists common affirmative defenses.

VIGNETTE 1

Frank has been diagnosed with Schizophrenia. He experiences intermittent auditory hallucinations and is routinely noncompliant with his psychotropic medications. Frank is very religious and frequently reads the Bible for hours. He develops a belief that his mother has been taken over by Satan. Frank finds his father's firearm and shoots and kills his mother based on his delusional belief that he must kill Satan to save his mother. Frank's brother arrives home hours later and finds his mother dead with Frank praying over her. Will Frank be convicted of murdering his mother?

In this example, Frank committed a criminal act (actus reus), shooting and killing a person. At the time of his act, Frank's mental state was such that he intended to cause death (mens rea). The challenge for an evaluator, and ultimately for the court, will be to evaluate whether Frank should be legally excused by the affirmative defense of insanity because he perceived himself as killing Satan and not a human. Forensic mental health professionals are commonly called to evaluate such defenses because of their knowledge of and experience in evaluating mentally ill individuals and ability to evaluate a defendant's mental state at the time of the offense. This specialized expertise will be explored further in later portions of this chapter.

THE INSANITY DEFENSE

Legal insanity is an affirmative defense to the commission of a crime. The use of the insanity defense is generally overestimated [2] and misperceived by the public. The common misperception is that the insanity defense is frequently raised, frequently successful, and results in a mentally ill defendant released immediately back into society, free to re-offend. In reality, the NGRI defense is raised by approximately 1% of defendants charged with a felony [3, 4]. Of defendants who raise the insanity defense, 15%–25% are successful with the defense [3, 4]. Juries are much less likely to issue a verdict for insanity than judges [5]. The majority of insanity acquittals arise from plea agreements [6] or an agreement by the prosecution that insanity is an appropriate verdict. It is rare for a defendant to be adjudicated as legally insane when the prosecution disputes the insanity defense, or when mental health professionals disagree on the issue of insanity.

A defendant adjudicated NGRI is technically acquitted of the offense; the court may not punish defendants who are acquitted. Insanity acquittees are not sentenced to prison or probation because there is an element of punishment in these dispositions. Therefore, disposition of an insanity acquittee focuses on treating the defendant's mental illness and protection of the public from any risk that the defendant's mental illness may present. Although NGRI is an affirmative defense, a defendant acquitted by insanity may be committed to a hospital for additional evaluation or treatment until he or she is no longer dangerous due to mental illness [7]. Typically, defendants adjudicated as legally insane are civilly committed; experience lengthy psychiatric hospitalization; receive multiple and extensive risk assessments, and if released are subject to close monitoring and treatment provisions to minimize the risk of re-offense.

Persons with a clear history of mental illness account for the majority of insanity acquittals. Studies have identified that persons with a psychotic disorder have the highest rates of insanity acquittals [8, 9]. Mood disorders and mental retardation are lesser but significantly reported diagnoses supporting insanity [8]. Jeffrey et al. [10] similarly found that defendants with a diagnosis of Schizophrenia were more likely to be adjudicated NGRI in contrast to defendants with personality and substance use disorders. Callahan et al. [4] reported that 90% of successful insanity acquittees had a prior diagnosis of mental illness. Successful NGRI acquittees were also more likely to have been hospitalized in the past.

INSANITY DEFENSE HISTORY AND INSANITY STANDARDS

References to the insanity defense date to biblical times. The requirements for an insanity defense in many jurisdictions have changed over time in response to public opinion, changing attitudes, scientific advances, and high-profile criminal cases in which the insanity defense has been used. Although insanity defense standards may vary by jurisdiction, all state and federal insanity standards require the presence of a mental illness, disease, or defect as a condition of the insanity defense. However, persons adjudicated NGRI are not acquitted merely because of their mental disorder, but symptoms of their disorder must impair their ability to know or appreciate the wrongfulness of their action or some other capacity identified by law.

English law influenced insanity standards in the United States, the M'Naghten [11] case in particular. M'Naghten was a Scottish wood turner who had a delusional belief that the governing Tory Party, including one of its leaders, Sir Robert Peel, was persecuting him. He sought to kill Peel, but he instead mistakenly shot and killed Peel's secretary, Edward Drummond. M'Naghten pled insanity to a charge of Murder. At trial, psychiatric testimony was unanimous that M'Naghten was insane, and the jury rapidly returned a verdict of insanity. Due to public outrage at M'Naghten's insanity acquittal, however, 15 judges of the House of Lords reviewed the case and articulated a new insanity test which became known as the M'Naghten Rule:

> [T]o establish a defense on the ground of insanity, it must be proved that, at the time of the committing of the act, the party accused was laboring under such a defect of reason, from disease of the mind, as not to know the nature and quality of the act he was doing; or if he did know it, that he did not know he was doing what was wrong [11].

Many state jurisdictions retain a version of the M'Naghten Rule. Although the wording varies by jurisdiction, the basic rule requires the defendant to have a "defect in reason caused by a disease of the mind (mental illness), which impairs a person's ability to know the wrongfulness of one's conduct" [2 (p12)]. States have modified the original version by substituting terms for "know" (e.g., appreciate, understand); omitting the "nature and quality" language; or omitting the wrongfulness language [12].

The knowledge of wrongfulness issue used in the M'Naghten standard raises the question of knowledge of *moral wrongfulness* versus *legal* wrongfulness. Legal wrongfulness simply means knowledge that an act is illegal. Moral wrongfulness can be broken down further into subjective moral wrongfulness and objective moral wrongfulness. Subjective moral wrongfulness refers to a defendant committing an offense with knowledge that the act is illegal, but who proceeds because (as a result of mental disease or defect) he feels personally justified. Objective moral wrongfulness equates with a defendant who, as a result of mental disorder or defect, fails to know that society considers their acts wrong. Many jurisdictions using the M'Naghten standard do not specify which type of wrongfulness test is to be applied to the case, and leave this issue for the jury to decide. Modern English insanity standards specify that knowledge of legal wrongfulness is to be used. Some American jurisdictions specify that the term "wrongfulness" means moral wrongfulness or legal wrongfulness; however, many statutes are not specific and entrust the jury to interpret the issue of wrongfulness.

The definition of wrongfulness to be applied is an important distinction to clarify before conducting a forensic assessment. Consider, for example, a defendant who knew that his act was legally prohibited but believed that his act was morally right due to a delusional belief. The expert must realize that they are bound by the jurisdictional criteria and render their opinion accordingly.

The M'Naghten test focuses on the cognition of the defendant at the time of the offense. The M'Naghten test does not include any assessment of whether the defendant's mental state compromised his or her ability to conform their behavior to the rules of law. The Irresistible Impulse Test articulated in the 1840 English trial of Edward Oxford, in contrast, relied on the defendant's ability to control impulses or conform conduct: "If some controlling disease was, in truth, the acting power within him which he could not resist, then he will not be responsible" [13]. American support for this test is found in *Parsons v. State* (1886) [14] and later part of the American Model Penal Code insanity standard. Distinguishing between irresistible impulse and an impulse not resisted has proved challenging from a practical standpoint of applying this test.

The New Hampshire Supreme Court, expressing that the M'Naghten standard was too narrow, articulated the Product Test (*State v. Pike*, 1870) [15]: the defendant is insane if the "offense was a result of their mental disease or defect." The test gained notice when Judge David Bazelon in the District of Columbia adopted the standard in *Durham v. United States* (D.C. Cir. 1954) [16]. Today, only New Hampshire and the Virgin Islands retain this test.

In 1955, the American Law Institute (ALI) drafted the Model Penal Code (MPC), including a standard for insanity. The ALI/MPC test contains components of both the cognitive test from M'Naghten and the irresistible impulse test.

> "A person is not responsible for criminal conduct if at the time of such conduct as a result of mental disease or defect he lacks substantial capacity either to appreciate the criminality of his conduct or conform his conduct to the requirements of law (ALI, 1985)" [17].

The ALI/MPC test also adds qualifying language to exclude mental abnormality manifested only by repeated criminal or otherwise antisocial conduct.

The ALI/MPC insanity test was widely adopted by states and the federal government as an alternative to the M'Naghten standard prior to John Hinckley, Jr.'s assassination attempt on President Ronald Reagan. Although many states retain this standard, in the aftermath of the Hinckley trial, Congress enacted the Federal Insanity Defense Reform Act (FIDRA) of 1984 [18], which is used in federal jurisdictions today.

Under the FIDRA, a defendant is legally insane if "at the time of the commission of the acts constituting the offense, the defendant, as a result of a severe mental disease or defect, was unable to appreciate the nature and quality or the wrongfulness of his acts." This Act removed the irresistible impulse component, which had been adopted under federal law as part of the ALI/MPC standard. It is a cognitive test that adopted the more expansive term "appreciate" from the ALI/MPC test. The FIDRA states that the defendant's mental illness must be "severe" [19].

VIGNETTE 2

Consider, again, Frank from Vignette 1. Frank is charged with murdering his mother. He pleads NGRI. You are hired to evaluate Frank in a jurisdiction that uses the M'Naghten standard for insanity. It is established that Frank committed the voluntary act. What is your opinion?

The formal entry of an insanity plea triggers an order from the court for a psychiatric evaluation regarding sanity. Many courts have associated psychiatric clinics that provide these evaluations. The prosecution, as well as the defense, may request additional psychiatric assessments for the purposes of evaluating a possible insanity defense. All jurisdictions require the presence of a mental disease or defect to establish the insanity defense. Here, Frank has a diagnosis of Schizophrenia. At the time of act, he experienced symptoms of his illness and delusionally believed that his mother had been overtaken by Satan. The defense can likely demonstrate the first criteria of the insanity defense that Frank had a mental disease or defect at the time of the offense, based on his prior diagnosis of schizophrenia; that schizophrenia is a chronic relapsing mental disorder; Frank's psychotropic medication nonadherence; and his psychotic symptoms and behavior at the time of the offense. However, as outlined above, the presence of a mental disease or defect at the time of the offense is only the first step in evaluating Frank's insanity defense. The focus, then, turns on whether, as a result of his mental disease or defect, Frank lacked the ability to know the wrongfulness of his act.

The expert should determine any jurisdictional requirements for wrongfulness before rendering an opinion. Frank delusionally believed that he was killing Satan. Although Frank knew that he was killing something, one could argue that Frank did not know the legal wrongfulness of his actions because Frank believed that he was killing Satan and did not realize the he was killing a human being. Regarding moral wrongfulness, Frank perceived himself as helping his mother (and likely society) by killing Satan, indicating that Frank believed that he was doing the right thing by committing the acts underlying the offense.

DIMINISHED CAPACITY AND MENS REA DEFENSES

Jurisdictions may elect to eliminate the insanity defense because, currently, the defense is not required by the United States Constitution, as interpreted in 2006 by the United States Supreme Court in *Clark v. Arizona* [20]. Four states have abandoned the insanity defense: Idaho, Kansas, Montana, and Utah. An alternative to the defense of insanity is negating the mens rea component of the crime. These defense strategies are not synonymous. As described above, NGRI is an affirmative defense that excuses liability when the elements of the crime are established or accepted. A defendant acquitted by NGRI faces likely civil commitment. When one negates mens rea, in contrast, he or she refutes an element of the prosecution's case.

Diminished capacity is a mens rea defense available in some jurisdictions. As discussed above, the law recognizes different levels of mens rea (intent). In its basic form, the defense of diminished capacity allows the defendant to present mental state evidence to cast doubt on whether he or she had the ability to form the required mens rea for the crime. The focus is on the mens rea at the time of the act. In contrast to NGRI, there are no specific legal standards (like the *M'Naghten* standard of FIDRA) for diminished capacity, other than the principle that the defendant lacked the ability to form the requisite mens rea due to mental disease, mental defect, extreme emotional disturbance, or intoxication.

Consider, for example, a man who shoots and kills another while highly intoxicated. To succeed with a diminished capacity defense to the charge of Murder, the defendant must prove that he was so intoxicated when he fired the weapon that he could not form the intent to purposefully kill the victim. If successful, the defendant would be convicted of manslaughter, not murder.

The diminished capacity defense is controversial and often confusing because there are different jurisdictional versions. To add to the confusion is a related concept of using mental state evidence to mitigate punishment. This is commonly termed diminished responsibility. By way of illustration, consider a man who has been diagnosed with schizophrenia who shoots and kills a bus driver. Forensic evaluators agree that he does not meet the criteria for the jurisdiction's insanity defense. At sentencing, if this man's mental illness played a limited role in his crime, although not rising to the level required for an insanity defense, his penalty could be reduced.

Different jurisdictions allow mens rea defenses to move forward on a basis of a defendant's mental disorder, alcohol or substance intoxication, or extreme emotional distress. Approximately half of the states and the federal jurisdiction permit a defendant to introduce evidence of mental abnormality to negate mens rea. However, many states limit the admissibility of such evidence. For example, some states permit evidence of mental abnormality to negate only certain mental states, such as the premeditation as may be required in first-degree murder statutes. Some provisions are specific to a particular crime. Jurisdictions, by illustration, that have adopted the Model Penal Code's section on Manslaughter allow evidence of "extreme mental or emotional disturbance" (also called "heat of passion") to negate the mens rea of intentional homicides (murder) to the lesser offense of manslaughter [21 (p210)]. In contrast, other states prohibit all evidence of mental illness to rebut criminal intent. In *Clark v. Arizona* (2006) [20], the U.S. Supreme Court upheld Arizona's right to preclude mental health testimony on the issue of mens rea.

Likewise, states are divided in allowing evidence of voluntary alcohol or drug intoxication to be used to negate mens rea. The U.S. Supreme Court upheld a state's position to exclude mental status testimony related to the effects of voluntary intoxication. In *Montana v. Egelhoff* (1996) [22], the Court held that the defendant did not have a fundamental right to have a jury consider evidence of voluntary intoxication in determining whether he possess the specific intent required for the crime. Courts are more receptive to evidence of a defendant's involuntary intoxication (e.g., coerced or unknowingly became intoxicated). In some jurisdictions, such evidence supports a mens rea defense; in others, it is used as a basis for a version of the insanity defense.

As a result of criticism to the insanity defense, several states have now enacted legislation called Guilty but Mentally Ill (GBMI). Although GBMI is not a defense per se and is not related to negating mens rea, it is mentioned here to identify that it is considered by some to be an alternative to NGRI. In several states, both NGRI and GBMI provisions exist. Persons found GBMI are found fully culpable of the crime but have a mental disorder. In contrast to NGRI, GBMI does not require a causal finding between the defendant's mental state and criminal act. A defendant convicted as GBMI is identified for evaluation for mental health treatment, usually under the state's penal system.

IMPACT OF DSM-5 ON CRIMINAL RESPONSIBILITY AND MENS REA DEFENSES

Mental illness definitions and threshold

All state statues require a threshold mental illness for a successful insanity defense. In fact, the term "mental disease or defect" is commonly used in state insanity statutes as the requisite threshold mental illness. However, what is that threshold and who should define it—mental health professionals, legislators, or courts? These are challenging questions that illustrate the inherent tension between legal concepts and medical knowledge. Some have argued that medicine or science should guide any definitions of mental illness. Forensic psychiatrist Bernard Diamond [23] artfully articulated his position about this tension:

> I believe it is wrong to concede any threshold definition of mental illness other than that determined by scientific and clinical knowledge.... [I]t is not up to the law to establish the threshold for the existence of mental illness in a criminal defendant. But it is up to the law to determine the particular forms and degree of psychopathology it will recognize as exculpatory [23 (p26)].

However, courts have closely guarded their role in determining what satisfies legal concepts. Illustrative of this is the D.C. Court of Appeal's opinion in *McDonald v. U.S.* (1962) [24]:

> Our purpose now is to make it very clear that neither the court nor the jury is bound by the *ad hoc* definition or conclusions as to what experts state is a disease or defect. What psychiatrists may consider a 'mental disease or defect' for clinical purposes... may or may not be the same as mental disease or defect for the jury's purpose in defining criminal responsibility.

With this as background, terms such as "mental disease or defect" that are used in insanity statutes are legal terms of art, meaning that they reflect specific legal, not clinical, definitions. In contrast, DSM-5 contains diagnostic clinical criteria for "mental disorders." Accordingly, a "mental disease or defect" is not necessarily synonymous with a DSM-5 diagnosis. For example, the mental disorder pedophilic disorder is defined by DSM-5 criteria, but it is not recognized by statutory or case law as a "mental disease or defect" required for an insanity defense. Although some jurisdictions do define mental disease in terms of the DSM, this is not the norm [25]. Likewise, the definition of the mental disorder may differ from the same mental disorder's definition in the state's other laws relevant to mental health, such as civil commitment statutes.

Consistent with prior versions of the DSM, this principle is further reflected by the cautionary statement in DSM-5 [26] that the presence of a DSM-5 diagnosis does not in itself imply that the legal definition for a mental disorder nor criminal responsibility has been met. This statement also emphasizes that having a DSM-5 disorder does not suggest any particular underlying cause for the disorder nor does it suggest any relationship between a mental disorder and the individual's ability to control his or her own behavior[26 (p25)].

DSM-5's cautionary statement's specific reference to a diminished behavioral control is directly relevant to the insanity standards that have a volitional component or "irresistible impulse"-type of test. In those jurisdictions that have a volitional standard, the DSM-5 diagnostic category of Disruptive, Impulse-Control, and Conduct Disorders will likely be more relevant than in jurisdictions with strictly cognitive tests.

The definitions and severity of mental disease or defect vary by jurisdiction. Many jurisdictions attempt to narrow the threshold of mental illness. After the Hinckley case, a number of organizations supported a more limited definition for the purpose of insanity. The American Bar Association favored a cognitive definition of mental disease attributable to functional or organic impairment in contrast to deficits in character or passion, cautioning that the insanity defense should not apply to a normal defendant who becomes abnormally impassioned [27]. Likewise, the American Psychiatric Association advocated for a "serious" mental disease requirement for the insanity standard [27].

The FIDRA adopted language speaking to the severity of mental illness. To reiterate, the FIDRA requires the presence of a "severe" mental disease or defect to establish insanity. The legislative history of the FIDRA reflects that Congress added "severe" to exclude "non-psychotic behavioral disorders, such as an 'inadequate personality,' 'immature personality,' or a pattern of 'antisocial tendencies" (*US v Long* (5th Cir. 2009) [28]. A number of states have adopted this "severe" disease language [12]. Psychotic disorders, major depressive disorder, and bipolar disorder generally qualify as severe mental disease; other DSM diagnoses and other syndromes are not universally accepted.

Limiting illness eligible for NGRI consideration

Many jurisdictions identify specific exclusions to their statutory definitions of mental disease or defect. Consistent with the ALI/MPC insanity test, the most common of these relates to antisocial acts or Antisocial Personality Disorder. Few statutes name the disorder explicitly. The DSM-5 has retained the diagnosis of antisocial personality disorder. DSM-5 has also retained from DSM-IV language that emphasizes that even if an individual has a problem following societal rules, this aberrant behavior alone does not mean they have an actual mental disorder [26 (p20)].

Even where antisocial acts or Antisocial Personality Disorder is excluded from the jurisdiction's definition of mental disorder or insanity, an evaluator should assess for the presence of other mental disorders, which may have alternatively driven the behavior in question.

Some jurisdictions explicitly exclude other personality disorders as constituting a mental disease/defect for the purposes of an insanity defense (in addition to antisocial acts or Antisocial Personality Disorder). For example, Oregon excludes illness "constituting solely a personality disorder" [29]. The per se exclusion of personality disorders is not universally accepted.

Voluntary intoxication and certain substance use disorders are another category that some jurisdictions have legislatively excluded as a mental disorder from their insanity statutes. All states prohibit voluntary intoxication as a sole basis for insanity, and some states codify this in their statutory scheme. In contrast, involuntary intoxication (typically by coercion or mistake) is widely accepted in some version as a defense to criminal culpability. Finally, when chronic alcohol or substance use leads to a persistent mental condition, courts refer to this as "settled insanity" and may be the basis for NGRI.

Challenges presented by DSM-5

Given jurisdictional variation in defining mental disease or defect, and that these are legal terms not generally synonymous with DSM diagnoses, DSM-5 is not expected to radically modify the forensic evaluator's role in assessing criminal responsibility. One criticism of DSM-5 has been concern that certain diagnoses "medicalize" normal variations of human behavior. With this criticism flows the related concept that more persons are likely to meet criteria for such disorders and, because these disorders are recognized as legitimate psychopathology in DSM-5, more persons will attempt to use them to exculpate responsibility via a mental health defense, or in other medicolegal issues. Although this may be true for some forensic assessments, such as disability claims, it is less likely to be a major factor for criminal responsibility because the insanity tests require specific inabilities (e.g., inability to tell right from wrong) resulting from the mental disorder. A sampling of DSM-5 changes is discussed here in the context of criminal responsibility.

Intellectual disability

In DSM-5, intellectual disability replaces the term Mental Retardation. DSM-5 retains the specification for intelligence testing. However, intellectual disability disorder classifies severity as mild, moderate, severe, or profound and emphasizes adaptive functioning abilities (conceptual, social, and practical) in addition to IQ scores [26]. With the removal the multiaxial system in DSM-5, intellectual disability is no longer an Axis II disorder. These changes associated with the adaptive functioning criteria impact criminal responsibility and mens rea evaluations because they require mental health evaluators to more thoroughly assess these domains through their interview and use of collateral information. Take, for example, the case of a 17-year-old male, formerly diagnosed with Mental Retardation, who is charged with sexual assault against a 15-year-old girl at his group home. The boy's lawyer asserts that the boy did not have the ability to understand the age difference or lack of consent. Under DSM-5, the severity of intellectual disability is not be determined by IQ testing, but rather requires an assessment of adaptive abilities.

Schizophrenia spectrum and other psychotic disorders

With DSM-5, modest changes have been made to the diagnostic criteria for the various psychotic disorders. The main change is the emphasis on symptom severity that requires a "quantitative assessment" of psychotic symptoms [26 (p100)]. For each psychotic disorder, an evaluator may specify the diagnosis with a severity rating. Although DSM-5 does not require the use of any specific symptom severity scale to make a diagnosis, it includes the Clinician-Rated Dimensions of Psychosis Symptom Severity Scale, found in the Emerging Measures and Models section of the text. Mental health evaluators should familiarize themselves with the severity ratings because they may be tasked with specifically commenting on symptom severity retrospectively at the time of the criminal event. (See Chapter 3 for detailed information about this scale.)

Bipolar and related disorders

The main diagnostic change in DSM-5 to the Bipolar and Related Disorders is the addition of "persistently increased goal-directed activity or energy" for both mania and hypomania [26 (p124)]. This descriptor was added to make explicit that these are hallmark symptoms of the diagnosis. The change has forensic implications because the mental health evaluator will need to assess the duration of these particular symptoms to make the diagnosis.

Disruptive mood dysregulation disorder

DSM-5 added the diagnosis of disruptive mood dysregulation disorder to fill a gap for children with persistent mood dysregulation different than those with bipolar disorder. This diagnosis is likely to be applicable to juveniles using criminal responsibility defenses or mitigation. Mental health evaluators should be aware that the diagnosis requires repeated and extreme problems with anger management that are in marked excess to the underlying trigger for the behavior [26 (p156)]. Because nearly all juveniles have temper outbursts, the evaluator needs to distinguish between symptoms of the disorder and ordinary or volitional outbursts. The diagnosis cannot be made for the first time in persons age 19 or older. DSM-5 lacks guidance as to whether the diagnosis may be used by someone age 19 or older if he or she met criteria for the diagnosis before the age of 19.

Premenstrual dysphoric disorder

This diagnosis has moved from a category for further study in DSM-IV to the DSM-5 category of Depressive Disorders. The use of Premenstrual Dysphoric Disorder (PMDD) or premenstrual syndrome to excuse culpability has long been discussed in medical and legal articles [30]. The diagnosis requires symptom confirmation by daily symptom ratings for a minimum of two symptomatic menstrual periods [26 (p171)]. Accordingly, collateral information, such as gynecologic or other medical records, may be particularly useful in making the diagnosis. This diagnosis has been used successfully to excuse or mitigate responsibility in a limited number of cases in the United States [31]. Moving the disorder into the main text of DSM-5 legitimizes it as a disease of the mind rather than a hormonal or physiologic ailment. Accordingly, there may be increased interest by defendants and lawyers to assert the condition in an insanity defense. In jurisdictions following the M'Naghten standard, in particular, it will be difficult for the defendant to establish, because of PMDD, that she lacked knowledge of the wrongfulness of the act. The requirement remains that there is a nexus between the disorder, the criminal behavior, and not knowing the wrongfulness of the criminal behavior.

Hoarding disorder

Hoarding, often considered a subtype of Obsessive Compulsive Disorder (OCD), is a unique diagnosis in DSM-5. Classifying hoarding as a distinct disorder in DSM-5 has legal implications because some states have crimes related to hoarding, namely animal hoarding. Accordingly, defendants charged with crimes like animal hoarding are likely to plead NGRI or use other mens rea defenses on the basis of a hoarding diagnosis. The diagnosis requires sustained problems with giving up or separating from items that one has collected [26 (p247)]. Insight specifiers similar to OCD are available for the evaluator. One specifier is "with absent insight/delusional beliefs" [26 (p247)]. The mental health evaluator should use caution is assessing insight; lack of insight does not necessarily equate with lack of mens rea. Individuals with hoarding, for example, may have insight into their possessive behaviors but have difficulty in parting with possessions because of unreasonable ideas about the value of the possessions. The diagnosis requires that the symptoms are not better explained by another disorder. For persons with severe hoarding that appear to take on delusional proportions, another diagnosis (e.g., psychotic disorder) may need to be considered.

Posttraumatic stress disorder

Posttraumatic Stress Disorder (PTSD) has, although rarely, been used as the basis for the insanity defense. In DSM-5, PTSD has been reclassified from the Anxiety Disorders chapter in DSM-IV to the category of Trauma and Stressor-Related Disorders. The diagnostic criteria have changed. Most notably, the A criterion is more explicit in what qualifies as a traumatic event. With DSM-5, directly and witnessed traumatic experiences qualify as traumatic events, as does learning that a friend or family member experienced a nonaccidental trauma or being exposed during the course of one's job to emotionally distressing details about traumatic incidents to others [26 (p271)]. The subjective reaction criterion (A2) from DSM-IV has been eliminated. Concern has been raised that these more "liberal" A-criteria widens the door for more individuals to claim PTSD [32]. In DSM-5, dissociative reactions (flashbacks) are described on a continuum (criterion-B), hence defendants with only minimal dissociative reactions may satisfy this criterion for the diagnosis. Regardless, PTSD as a basis for NGRI has been viewed skeptically, and will continue to so, because of the subjective nature of the disorder, heavy reliance on evaluee self-report, and belief that it is relatively easy to imitate [33]. Military-related PTSD is highly comorbid with substance use disorders, adding to skepticism because of the difficulty in defining the degree of impairment from PTSD.

With DSM-5 diagnostic criteria for PTSD, defendants will continue to find difficulty in demonstrating lack of knowledge of wrongfulness as required under a M'Naghten-type standard. For example, the presence or absence of intense fear or horror (former A2 from DSM-IV) at the time of the traumatic event is unlikely to inform decisions of later wrongfulness. However, an argument for impaired cognition and awareness could be made if the defendant can establish that the crime occurred during a dissociative reaction (an element of criterion B). A nexus between PTSD and the crime may be easier to establish in an ALI/MPC jurisdiction where a dissociative reaction or, possibly, increased arousal (criterion E) would be relevant to the volitional arm of the insanity test.

Dissociative identity disorder

Defendants have raised this disorder in defense of a variety of criminal charges. However, relying on this disorder is often difficult because the defendant, essentially, asserts that more than one personality (or alter) exists in the single human body and that one personality committed a criminal act while the dominant personality was not aware. Courts vary in their approach to criminal responsibility of persons with this diagnosis and there is no consensus among states. A couple of changes to dissociative identity disorder (DID) in DSM-5 have medicolegal implications. First, this disorder now requires two or more fully distinct personalities, which may include an "experience of possession" (Criterion A) [26 (p292)]. The concept of "possession" is described as a state that most commonly presents as if a spirit or supernatural force has taken over the individual and as a result the individual talks or behaves in an obviously different manner than usual [26 (p293)]. It is not difficult to imagine defendants claiming that they were "possessed" in effort to avoid criminal responsibility. Mental health evaluators should assess whether a possession state may more aptly reflects a cultural or spiritual practice than a mental disorder.

Second, in DSM-5 memory lapses (Criterion B) may only affect recall of daily incidents in contrast to DSM-IV that required lapses involving a loss of memory for significant personal data. It is foreseeable that more people will qualify for DID with this change. Although more people may qualify for DID, the diagnosis has been—and will likely continue to be—controversial and viewed with suspicion due to concerns about malingering, difficulty obtaining information about the personality who allegedly committed the crime, and various theories about whether personalities should be considered distinct from persons in law.

Dissociative amnesia

Persons with dissociative amnesia lack the ability to recall personal information. In contrast to the DSM-IV, the new criterion explicitly identifies two types: localized or selective versus generalized. Given this, it is a disorder ripe for defendants to claim, for example, selective amnesia for the criminal event. Also new to DSM-5, the specifier "with dissociative fugue" is listed here rather than as a separate diagnosis [26 (p298)].

Nonrapid eye movement sleep arousal disorders

Sleep-related sexual behavior (sexsomnia or sleep sex) is a specialized form of sleepwalking, which is one of the nonrapid eye movement sleep arousal disorders. Sexsomnia is characterized by sexual behavior committed while in a sleeping state without conscious awareness of the behavior [26 (p401)]. Sexsomnia has been successfully raised as a defense to sexual assault charges, most notably in Canada [34]. In 2005, a defendant was acquitted of sexual assault charges based on expert testimony that the defendant was in the midst of a sexsomnia dissociative state when he engaged in unwanted sexual activity with a victim. The acquittal was upheld on appeal. Although only infrequently raised as a criminal defense, sexsomnia presents an interesting dilemma for forensic mental health and courts alike. Guidelines have been proposed to assist in the evaluation of this defense [35].

Disruptive, impulse-control, and conduct disorders

The disorders in this DSM-5 category are united by impairment in self-regulation. Retained in DSM-5 is the diagnosis of intermittent explosive disorder. Persons with this disorder have repeated problems with controlling their aggression (Criterion A) [26 (p466)]. In contrast to DSM-IV, which used referenced an inability to resist one's behavior, DSM-5 uses "failure to control" impulses, which can be manifested by verbal aggression or behavioral outbursts [26 (p466)].

The changes to Intermittent Explosive Disorder are expected to have little impact on insanity and mens rea evaluations. Because the diagnosis focuses on behavior, it will remain difficult for defendants to meet the standard for insanity in jurisdictions where a cognitive test (M'Naghten) is used. The diagnosis is more applicable in states using volitional insanity tests. For defendants with the diagnosis, it is important to recognize that any given act could be impulsive or defensive or premeditated. In a volitional NGRI assessment, the forensic evaluator is tasked with assessing whether the defendant had an irresistible impulse versus an impulse not resisted.

Substance-related and addictive disorders

An important change in DSM-5 is that the manual no longer distinguishes between "abuse" and "dependence," merging them into criteria sets for a "use disorder" for each class of drug. Other than simplifying diagnoses, the changes to the substance disorders are likely to have little impact on NGRI or mens rea assessments. Recall that all jurisdictions exclude acute voluntary intoxication as the sole basis for the insanity defense. In contrast, "settled" conditions (persistent mental symptoms based on chronic substance use) are generally allowed as the basis for an insanity defense. In cases where a defendant has both substance use and mental illness, the text of DSM-5 provides guidance on how to distinguish mental illness from comorbid substance intoxication. Another important change in DSM-5 is that gambling disorder (renamed from Pathological Gambling) has been moved to this chapter, rather than included with the impulse-control disorders. This change is expected to have little impact on criminal responsibility or mens rea assessments.

Mild neurocognitive disorder

Mild Neurocognitive Disorder is an example of a DSM-5 disorder that will now capture people who, under DSM-IV, would likely not have a formal psychiatric diagnosis. Although its intent is to identify persons for earlier focus of care, it labels as having illness individuals with "evidence of modest cognitive decline" [26 (p605)]. Included in the DSM-5 text is Table 1, which defines cognitive domains to aid an evaluator in diagnosis, severity level, and subtypes.

Because this diagnosis reflects deficits in cognitive function and most insanity tests have a cognitive component, it is foreseeable that this diagnosis may be the basis of an NGRI defense. However, it is unlikely that the inclusion of this diagnosis will lead to sweeping success for insanity acquittals because of the minimal level of impairment. The diagnostic criteria for mild neurocognitive disorder dictate that the symptoms of this disorder do not interfere with a person's independence or activities of daily living.

Paraphilic disorders

In DSM-5, Paraphilic Disorders have been separated into their own category. Previously, paraphilias had been embedded in the Sexual and Gender Identity Disorders Category in the DSM-IV. Despite debate regarding their inclusion as mental disorders, the DSM-5 commentary states that they are included in DSM-5 because of their frequency in the population and that some paraphilias entail actions with potential harm to others. Although DSM-5 workgroups proposed new categories for further study (e.g., hebephilia and paraphilic coercive disorder), these attracted prior criticism and were ultimately rejected [36]. New to DSM-5 is the addition of course specifiers "in a controlled environment" and "in remission" for all Paraphilic Disorders with the exception of pedophilic disorder. In the DSM-5 section titled "Highlights of Changes from DSM-IV to DSM-5," the text notes that the "in remission" specifier applies to all of the paraphilic disorders [26 (p816)]. This statement conflicts with the DSM-5 actual text defining pedophilic disorder, which does not include these specifiers. There is no expert agreement whether a chronic paraphilia can fully remit.

Retained from DSM-IV is the adoption of clinically significant distress criteria. The rationale is to distinguish paraphilias from paraphilic disorders. With DSM-5, a paraphilia corresponds to the A criterion (abnormal erotic focus). In contrast, a paraphilic disorder requires both the A criterion and B criterion (clinical distress). Although inclusion of the word "disorder" (as in Paraphilic Disorders) may legitimize for some these diagnoses as mental illness, it remains up to the jurisdiction to determine whether Paraphilic Disorders constitute mental disorders from a legal standpoint. The Oregon Supreme Court, in another context, ruled that Pedophilia qualifies as a mental disorder [37]. Of importance, as with DSM-IV criteria, forensic evaluators assessing for these conditions must be careful not to infer from criminal sexual behavior alone the existence of a paraphilic disorder.

Medication-induced movement disorders

DSM-5 has given Medication-Induced Movement Disorders their own chapter. These diagnoses may be used to describe adverse reactions or problems that patients may develop with medication administration. The DSM-5 text states that the conditions in the chapter "are not mental disorders" [26 (p22)]. Accordingly, it is important for the mental health evaluator to inquire whether these diagnoses qualify as mental disorders in the jurisdiction's insanity statues. Where they are not applicable, the defendant may nevertheless retain the ability to use these diagnoses to support an involuntary intoxication or mens rea defense in some jurisdictions.

When these diagnoses are used in criminal defense, the mental health evaluator should understand the types of symptoms commonly associated with the medication administration or withdrawal. The DSM-5 diagnosis of antidepressant discontinuation syndrome aptly describes the common symptoms, timeframe for onset, and symptom duration. For other medications, the evaluator may want to refer to other collateral sources, such as the Physician's Desk Reference or medication package insert for pharmacologic and other information. The mental health evaluator will also want to assess the defendant's mental state and symptoms before and after ingestion of the medication (or during withdrawal), how the medication was used, and any prior experience with the medication in evaluating for NGRI or mens rea defenses.

Most common mental disorders for insanity

The diagnoses expected to be most associated with insanity and mens rea evaluations include the Schizophrenia Spectrum and Other Psychotic Disorders, Bipolar and Related Disorders, and Depressive Disorders. There are relatively minor changes to these categories. Other than the specific changes discussed above, the changes in these categories are expected to have little impact on the assessment of criminal responsibility.

Impact on diminished capacity defenses

To date, there is little organized data relating to diagnoses and the success of a diminished capacity defense. Case law from several jurisdictions suggests that defendants have relied on numerous different DSM diagnoses and various mental syndromes in raising the defense. As with the insanity defense, a qualifying mental condition is subject to jurisdictional variation and the admissibility of mental condition evidence may not relate to whether the condition is a disorder recognized in the DSM. Cases from differing jurisdictions have held that evidence of Fetal Alcohol Syndrome, for example, is admissible for a defense based on diminished capacity [38]. In DSM-5, neurobehavioral disorder associated with prenatal alcohol exposure is included in the Appendix as a condition for further study.

Kischner and Galperin [39] assessed the characteristics of defendants in New York County who claimed "extreme emotional disturbance" in their defense to intentional murder or attempted intentional murder. In these cases, the defendant's psychiatric diagnosis did not substantially distinguish those defendants who would be successful with the defense. Instead, success was more likely when the trier of fact understood the defendant's behavior to be motivated by a reasonable fear that he or she (or a loved one) would be physically harmed if the defendant did not take action.

VIGNETTE 3

Recall Frank from Vignettes 1 and 2. Frank killed his mother due to a delusional belief that his mother was possessed by Satan. He used his father's firearm and killed her in the family home. Hours after the killing, Frank's father, George, learns of the details of his wife's death. In the weeks following his wife's death, George consumes himself with handling his wife's affairs and taking care of Frank's brother, who remains in the home. Seven months after her death, George begins having nightmares about his wife's death, avoids going into Frank's former bedroom, is forgetful, believes that no one can be trusted, and has restless sleep. Although George has returned to work, his performance review criticizes him for lack of concentration on tasks. George decides to speak with his supervisor about the status of his position. When his supervisor puts off their conversation, George flies into a rage. George pushes his supervisor, who falls and strikes his head. George is arrested and charged with Assault. His lawyer hires you to evaluate whether George had a qualifying mental disorder should he want to purse an insanity defense. The jurisdiction has recognized the DSM-5 as a basis for mental disorders in insanity cases. What do you think?

Here, George exhibited symptoms of PTSD due to his wife's traumatic death. The A criterion in DSM-5 is established because George learned that a traumatic event occurred to a close family member and the event was violent. He has the requisite symptoms from the four symptom clusters. Consistent with DSM-IV, DSM-5 has a specifier that indicates PTSD symptoms may not present immediately. DSM-5 has termed this specifier "with delayed expression," which is provided "if the full diagnostic criteria are not met until at least 6 months after the event..." [26 (p274)]. The "delayed expression" specifier is applicable here because George did not meet full criteria until seven months after the event. The diagnosis of PTSD has been used with the insanity defense. However, the validity of a PTSD diagnosis has been treated with skepticism in some cases due to the heavy reliance on a defendant's self-report and ease at identifying and reporting symptoms. In cases of "delayed expression" symptoms, the evaluator may find it more difficult to obtain collateral information demonstrating a nexus between the event and subsequent development of symptoms. In addition, intervening events that could cause the defendant's symptoms should be explored. As discussed above, the presence of a mental disorder at the time of the offense does not end the inquiry if George pursues an insanity defense, rather it is just one component to be evaluated. In this example the defense would bear the burden of proving how George's PTSD caused George not to know the wrongfulness of his actions as he assaulted his supervisor. This proposition is unlikely, unless George was in PTSD-induced dissociative state so extreme that he could not realize the wrongfulness of his actions. Instead, George would more likely be successful pursuing mitigation—that his PTSD was a factor (not exculpatory) in the criminal behavior.

EVALUATION GUIDELINES: ASSESSING MENTAL STATE AT THE TIME OF THE OFFENSE

Expert opinion is often critical in criminal responsibility cases because it aids the trier of fact in understanding the defendant's mental state at the time of the offense. The forensic evaluator is tasked with three major responsibilities: (1) ascertaining the exact legal standard for the specific jurisdiction, if a legal standard exists (e.g., for NGRI); (2) assessing the facts of the case through personal interview with the evaluee and collateral information; and (3) applying the legal standard to the facts of the case to render an expert opinion [40].

A criminal defendant's thinking and motivation behind his or her behavior is relevant to assessing any association between the person's mental condition and the crime. Recall, for example, Frank from Vignette 1. Had he killed his mother because they argued over finances, he would likely not qualify for any insanity defense despite his diagnosis of Schizophrenia. In this situation, there is no nexus between the mental state and the act for the purpose of the insanity defense. This is a very different situation than believing he had to kill his mother to absolve her from Satan.

Regardless of the jurisdictional law, the forensic evaluator should identify how the defendant does or does not meet the specific requirements of the insanity standard. As discussed above in the section on insanity tests, most jurisdictions have a cognitive component in their insanity test that calls into question the defendant's understanding of the wrongfulness of the criminal act at the time of the offense. It is appropriate to question the defendant about his or her knowledge of the criminality of the act and any reasons why the actions were justified. Extrinsic evidence also speaks to a defendant's knowledge of wrongfulness. Thoroughly assessing the descriptions of the defendant's statements and/or behavior at the time of the offense gives key insights into the defendant's mental state at the time of the offense, and the defendant's knowledge of the wrongfulness of their action. Evidence of wearing a disguise, discarding the murder weapon, or fleeing the scene implies that the defendant knew the wrongfulness of the behavior. Suggestive that the defendant did not know the wrongfulness are evidence that the defendant acknowledged the act or remained at the scene, or had no rationale alternative motive [40]. In Vignette 1, Frank did not flee the scene, he espoused a delusional moral justification for the act, and had no alternative rationale for the offense.

In jurisdictions that have an inability to refrain element to their insanity test ("inability to conform conduct to requirements of law" also known as the irresistible impulse test), the analysis is whether the defendant could not control his or her behavior as the result of a mental disease or defect. Could the defendant chose an alternative behavior other than the offense, or postpone the offense? Was any inability to refrain due to mental illness or rather an intoxicating agent or anger? Severe mania has been identified as fitting the volitional prong but the evaluator must be mindful that manic conditions can differ in severity.

SUMMARY

Although the transition to DSM-5 may bring anxiety to forensic experts due to relative inexperience with the new manual and anticipated critique by attorneys, overall these changes will have little impact on the evaluation of criminal responsibility because, in addition to the presence of a mental disorder at the time of the offense, there needs to be a connection (legally defined in insanity) between the mental condition and how the crime came to be committed. Key points from this chapter include the following:

- Insanity and mens rea defenses require retrospective assessment of the defendant's mental state at the time of the offense.
- Jurisdictions vary in their legal standards for the insanity defense and whether the psychiatric evidence may be used to negate mens rea.
- All insanity standards require a threshold mental illness.
- DSM-5 diagnoses are not necessarily synonymous with mental disease definitions in law.
- The presence of a DSM-5 diagnosis is insufficient alone to meet the criteria for an insanity or mens rea defense.
- The forensic evaluator should familiarize himself or herself with the jurisdiction's legal standards for mental disease as well as criminal responsibility.

REFERENCES

1. Stroud, DA. *Mens Rea or Imputability Under the Laws of England*. London, England: Sweet and Maxwell; 1914.

2. Steadman HJ, McGreevy MA, Morrissey JP, et al. *Before and After Hinckley: Evaluating Insanity Defense Reform*. New York, NY: Guilford Press; 1993.
3. Callahan L, Meyer C, Steadman HJ. Insanity defense reform in the United States—post Hinckley. *Ment Phys Dis L Repor* 1987; 11:54–59.
4. Callahan L, Steadman J, McGreevy MA. Rates of insanity acquittals and the factors associated with successful insanity pleas. *Bull Am Acad Psychiatry Law* 1991; 19:331–338.
5. Rogers JL, Bloom JD, Manson SM. Insanity defense: contested or conceded? *Am J Psychiatry* 1984; 141:885–888.
6. Melton GB, Petrila J, Poythress NG, Slobogin, C. *Psychological Evaluations for the Courts: A Handbook for Mental Health Professionals & Lawyers*. 3rd ed. New York, NY: Guildford Press; 2007.
7. *Foucha v Louisiana*, 504 US 71 (1992).
8. Warren JI, Fitch WL, Dietz PE, Rosenfeld BD. Criminal offense, psychiatric diagnosis, and psycholegal opinion: An analysis of 894 pretrial referrals. *Bull Am Acad Psychiatry Law* 1991; 19:63–69.
9. Cochrane RE, GrissoT, Frederick, R. The relationship between criminal charges, diagnosis, and psycholegal opinion among federal pretrial defendants. *Behav Sci Law* 2001; 9:565–582.
10. Jeffrey RW, Pasewark RA, Bieber S. Insanity plea: predicting not guilty by reason of insanity adjudications. *Bull Am Acad Psychiatry Law* 1988; 16:35–39.
11. M'Naghten's Case, 101 Cl. & F. 200, 8 Eng. Rep. 718 (H.L. 1843).
12. Giorgi-Guarnieri D, Janofsky J, Keram E, et al. *AAPL practice guidelines for forensic psychiatric evaluation of defendants raising the insanity defense. J Am Acad Psychiatry Law* 2002; 30(2 Suppl):S3–S40.
13. Smith R. Trial by Medicine. Edinburgh: University Press; 1981.
14. *Parsons v State*, 81 Ala. 577, 596 2 So. 854, 866 (1886).
15. *State v Pike*, 49 NH 399 (1970).
16. *Durham v United States*, 214 F.2d 862 (D.C. Cir. 1954).
17. American Law Institute, Model Penal Code, Sec. 4.01 (1985).
18. Federal Insanity Defense Reform Act, 18 USC sec. 17 (1984).
19. Uniform Code of Military Justice, 10 USCS. sec. 850a (2000).
20. *Clark v Arizona*, 548 US 735 (2006).
21. American Law Institute. Model Penal Code. Washington, DC: American Law Institute; 1962.
22. *Montana v Englehoff*, 518 US 37 (1996).
23. Diamond B. Reasonable medical certainty, diagnostic thresholds, and definitions of mental illness in the legal context. *Bull Am Acad Psychiatry Law* 1985; 13:121–8.
24. *McDonald v United States*, 312 F.2d 847 (D.C. Cir. 1962).
25. West. Va. Code Ann. Section 5-16-7 (2010).
26. American Psychiatric Association. *Diagnostic and Statistical Manual of Mental Disorders, Fifth Edition*. Arlington, VA: American Psychiatric Association; 2013.
27. American Bar Association. The insanity defense: ABA and APA proposals for change. *Ment Disab L Rep* 1983; 7:136–146, 210–211.
28. *United States v Long*, 562 F.3d 325 (5th Cir. 2009).
29. Oregon Revised Statute, section 16.295 (1983).
30. Solomon L. Premenstrual syndrome: the debate surrounding criminal defense. *Maryland L Rev* 1995; 54:571–600.

31. Brown DL. PMS defense successful in Va. drunken driving case. *Washington Post* June 7, 1991:A1.
32. Wortzel HS. The DSM-5 and forensic psychiatry. *J Psychiatr Pract* 2013; 19: 238–241.
33. Frierson RL. Combat-related posttraumatic stress disorder and criminal responsibility determinations in the post Iraq era: a review and case report. *J Am Acad Psychiatry Law* 2013; 41:79–84.
34. Zaharna M, Budur K, Noffsinger S. Sexual behavior during sleep: convenient alibi or parasomnia. *Current Psychiatry* 2008; 7:21–30.
35. Bornemann MA, Mahowald MS, Schenck CH. Parasomnias: clinical and forensic implications. Chest 2006; 130:605–610.
36. Zucker KJ. DSM-5: call for commentaries on gender dysphoria, sexual dysfunctions, and paraphilic disorders. *Arch Sex Behav* 2013; 42:669–674.
37. *Rios v Psychiatric Security Bd.*, 325 Ore. 151 (Ore. 1997).
38. *Dillbeck v State*, 643 So.2d 1027 (Fla. 1994).
39. Kischner SM, Litwach TR, Galperin GJ. The defense of extreme emotional disturbance: a qualitative analysis of cases in New York County. *Psychol Public Pol L* 2004; 10:102–133.
40. Resnick PJ, Noffsinger S. Competency to stand trial and the insanity defense. In: The Simon R, Gold LH, eds. *American Psychiatric Publishing Textbook of Forensic Psychiatry*. Washington DC: American Psychiatric Publishing; 2004:329–347.

CHAPTER 7

DSM-5 and Civil Competencies

INTRODUCTION

Psychiatrists and other mental health professionals are often asked to evaluate a person's mental capacity (competence) to perform important tasks, such as making medical decisions, executing a will, or managing their finances, among others. These assessments essentially ask the evaluator to consider (1) the requirements of the task in question and (2) whether the evaluee has the requisite mental and physical ability to carry out the task. These legally important tasks in the civil context are generally referred to as "civil competencies." The completion of the legal document is often known as "executing the instrument."

Forensic evaluators and others who conduct these assessments recognize that civil competence evaluations may require opinions of the evaluee's past, current, or future capacities. For example, individuals often create wills and durable powers of attorneys for healthcare to guide future decisions about these issues when they are no longer able to make them. However, the individual's capacity to execute the instrument may be called into question at a later date. In such cases, the evaluator is asked to opine on the evaluee's past ability to execute the instrument at the time it was signed. Examples of present-day competence assessments include the ability to make medical decisions and marry. Guardianship and conservatorship assessments are classic examples where an opinion on both contemporary and future capacity of the evaluee is required.

The Diagnostic and Statistical Manual of Mental Disorders, Fifth Edition (DSM-5) completed in 2013 [1] has resulted in significant changes to diagnostic criteria for many diagnoses that are likely to impact civil competence assessments. A threshold question in most civil competence assessments is whether the evaluee has a mental disorder. If so, the next step is to assess whether, given the disorder, the evaluee has the capacity

Table 7-1. ILLUSTRATIVE LIST OF CIVIL COMPETENCIES
Care for oneself/guardianship or conservatorship
Consent for research
Consent for voluntary hospitalization
Enter a contract
Provide informed consent for treatment/treatment refusals
Marry, divorce
Perform occupational duties
Give testamentary capacity, handle financial affairs, make a gift
Provide testimony in a civil case

to perform the civil competency raised. The presence of a mental disorder does not necessarily equate to incompetence for a specific function. In this chapter, we review the role of the mental disorder requirement in civil commitment and other civil assessments. We provide a sampling of types of common civil competence assessments and discuss how DSM-5 changes may impact assessments in these areas. Table 7-1 represents a list of common civil competences.

MENTAL DISORDER IN CIVIL COMPETENCIES

When psychiatrists and other mental health professionals perform evaluations involving civil competence, the use of psychiatric diagnoses plays an important role in this process. Some jurisdictions legally require the offering of a mental disorder if incompetence is the conclusion in designated evaluations [2]. Where the jurisdictional statutes require the presence of a mental disorder to determine a lack of civil competence, the statutes rarely specify which diagnostic classification system to use or the qualifying diagnoses. However, psychiatrists, along with other mental health professionals in the United States, have generally adopted the diagnostic nomenclature of the Diagnostic and Statistical Manual (DSM) since the appearance of its First Edition in 1952 [3]. As such, the transition from the previous DSM version, the DSM-IV-TR [4] from 2000 to the DSM-5 [1], brings along potential challenges, arguably as great as the transition from the Second Edition (DSM-II) [5] in 1968 to the Third Edition (DSM-III) in 1980 [6]. In this transition, DSM-III adopted the multiaxial diagnostic system along with more rigorous diagnostic criteria. In addition, DSM-III version represented the first attempt in the DSM series to achieve diagnostic interrater reliability [6]. The transition to DSM-5 has abandoned the multiaxial system and has introduced a dimensional focus in addition to the traditional categorical approach to diagnoses in its place.

The definition of mental disorder from DSM-IV-TR remained the same as had been presented in the Third Edition-Revised (DSM-III-R) [7] in 1987 and in the Fourth Edition (DSM-IV) [8] in 1994 . This definition emphasized the association of emotional or behavioral symptoms to the individual's experience of personal distress, impairment, or other form of suffering [4 (p xxxi)].

The DSM-5 definition of a mental disorder has been rewritten and focuses on the relationship of a person's difficulty in thinking, feeling, or behaving to an underlying impairment in the individual's growth and development, medical status, or psychological functioning. DSM-5 also notes that individuals suffering from a mental disorder usually experience some type of impairment or loss of functioning in important areas of their life. DSM-5 maintains DSM-IV's explanation that culturally appropriate responses to events and certain conflicts between individuals and society (e.g., political, religious, or sexual) are not considered mental disorders [1 (p20)].

The DSM-5 definition of a mental disorder retains the two key components from prior definitions, namely necessitating that there is a "clinically significant disturbance" and that such disturbances are associated with "significant distress" or "disability" [1 (p20)]. This definition infers a relationship to a mental disorder with "disability" or a parallel lack of ability or capacity, thereby supporting the importance of providing a diagnosis of a mental disorder when assessing civil capacities even if not explicitly legally required.

This chapter's exploration of the influence of the DSM-5 in the evaluation of civil competencies (or for those wishing to maintain the dichotomy between the legal and clinical systems, civil capacities) begins with a review of the most commonly evaluated civil competency involving involuntary civil commitment and then branches out to other civil competencies. A review of all civil competencies is beyond the scope of this chapter; instead, a sampling of civil competencies has been selected to illustrate principles and the role of DSM-5.

INVOLUNTARY CIVIL COMMITMENT

Each jurisdiction has its own definition of what constitutes grounds for involuntary hospitalization and for civil commitment and the specific procedures and judicial reviews required. In some jurisdictions, civil commitment does not technically commence until the initial period of involuntary hospitalization and observation expires and there is a judicial order, and these two terms are distinguished from each other in that context. However, for purposes of this chapter, involuntary hospitalization and civil commitment are not distinguished and often used interchangeably below for simplicity. Nonetheless, jurisdictions have a mental disorder criterion as a necessary antecedent before applying involuntary hospitalization/civil commitment criteria to the evaluation. States may or may not offer a statutory definition of what constitutes a mental disorder. For illustrative purposes, we will look at two states, Washington and California, to highlight the potential role of DSM-5 in a state with and a state without a statutory definition of mental disorder.

In Washington, initiation of the involuntary civil commitment process (via the initial 72-hour period of detention) requires: "...as a result of a mental disorder: (i) Presents a likelihood of serious harm; or (ii) is gravely disabled...." [9]. In Washington, "Mental disorder" means any organic, mental, or emotional impairment which has *substantial adverse effects* on a person's *cognitive or volitional functions* [emphasis added]" [10]. Washington law explicitly recognizes that persons who are "developmentally disabled, impaired by chronic alcohol or drug abuse, or suffering from dementia" have a mental disorder, but nonetheless they must meet the other civil commitment criteria to be involuntarily detained [11]. In other words, Washington defines what constitutes a mental disorder for civil commitment purposes.

Considering this definition in Washington, the diagnosis requires that there be "substantial adverse effects" on "cognitive or volitional functions." This suggests that such DSM-5 categories as the Schizophrenia Spectrum and Other Psychotic Disorders, Bipolar and Related Disorders, Depressive Disorders, and Neurocognitive Disorders would continue to qualify under the Washington statutory definition of a mental disorder as these categories or their equivalent forerunners in DSM-IV-TR of Schizophrenia and Other Psychotic Disorders, Mood Disorders, and Dementia, Delirium, and Amnestic and Other Cognitive Disorders. However, the Washington definition of mental disorder might continue to exclude Personality Disorders because the general definition and for this category of disorders has not changed from the DSM-IV-TR to the DSM-5.

However, DSM-5's deconstruction of the multiaxial assessment schema, present since 1980 when introduced with DSM-III, raises an interesting theoretical consideration in the case where an individual is considered to have only a Personality Disorder and no other co-occurring mental disorder. For example, an individual with Borderline Personality Disorder [1 (pp 664-666)] could qualify for involuntary commitment based on criteria 9, of a "transient, stress-related paranoid ideation or severe dissociative symptoms" that has led to or about to lead to an act of harm to self or others. Until now, civil commitment in Washington could avoid this by adding a co-occurring diagnosis of Psychotic Disorder Not Otherwise Specified or Mood Disorder Not Otherwise Specified in axis I, when attempting to involuntarily detain an individual who may technically qualify only for a diagnosis of Borderline Personality Disorder. It may now be necessary to add an equivalent DSM-5 diagnoses such as unspecified schizophrenia spectrum or other psychotic disorder or unspecified bipolar and related disorder or unspecified depressive disorder or alternatively to allow transient symptoms in patients with a personality disorder diagnosis to be sufficient. Most likely, the implications of DSM-5 changes in this context will not be significant.

In contradistinction to Washington, there is no definition of mental disorder for involuntary civil commitment purposes in Oregon [2]. This is also true of California. California is used to illustrate this dilemma because it has additional potential complexities in the definition of a mental disorder. The current involuntary hospitalization and civil commitment framework derives from the passage of the Lanterman-Petris-Short (LPS) Act from 1969. The legislative intent of the LPS Act included providing "prompt evaluation and treatment of persons with serious mental disorders or impaired by chronic alcoholism" [12]. Involuntary hospitalization requires that "...as a result of mental disorder, to be a danger to others, or to himself or herself, or to be gravely disabled..." [13, 14].

California neither defines what constitutes a "serious mental disorder (from the LPS Act's legislative intent)" [15] or a "mental disorder (from how the LPS Act is operationalized)" for the initial and subsequent involuntary hospitalization of adults [16]. Insofar as mental disorder is concerned, it would appear that any mental disorder as defined by DSM-5 would qualify, so long as the predicate is met, that is, the mental disorder is serious and it gives rise to dangerousness or grave disability. Some counties though decide to exclude dementia (major neurocognitive disorder in DSM-5) as a mental disorder for LPS purposes unless something like psychosis also is present. Ambiguities in the law in California and likely elsewhere in the absence of case law are interpreted differently from county to county. Of course, even though "chronic alcoholism" is a qualifying condition, its DSM equivalents, and in the case of DSM-5, alcohol use disorder, would not culminate in involuntary hospitalization because there have been no specialized alcohol or drug treatment facilities in California to treat these involuntary patients according to the LPS framework. Instead, clinicians have resorted to offering a diagnosis of an alcohol-induced psychotic or mood disorder in order to involuntary hospitalize those with "chronic alcoholism" in a mental health facility. DSM-5 would not be expected to remedy this dilemma or change the situation.

In the case of minors in California, involuntary commitment is governed by a different statute [17]. Although similar to involuntary commitment for adults [14], for the case of a gravely disabled minor, "intellectual disability, epilepsy, or other developmental disabilities, alcoholism, other drug abuse, or repeated antisocial behavior" are specifically excluded as qualifying conditions. This statutory language arguably eliminates the DSM-5 categories of Neurodevelopmental Disorders, Substance-Related and Addictive Disorders, and Conduct Disorders (from the Disruptive, Impulse-Control, and Conduct

Disorders category) as qualifying conditions for involuntary commitment unless they are determined in the courts to be equivalent.

It is important to note that outpatient civil commitment statutes also exist in most states [18]. As with traditional inpatient civil commitment schemes, the goal of outpatient civil commitment is to ensure psychiatric services to individuals who require supervision as well as treatment. The criteria for outpatient civil commitment are generally similar to traditional commitment in that they require the presence of a mental disorder and evidence of dangerousness or grave disability. Washington's statute [19] is illustrative:

> "If the court finds that a person, as the result of a mental disorder, presents a likelihood of serious harm, or is gravely disabled, but that treatment in a less restrictive setting than detention is in the best interest of such person or others, the court shall order an appropriate less restrictive course of treatment..."

In states that have defined mental disorder by statute, the same definition is generally used for both inpatient and outpatient civil commitment.

RIGHT TO REFUSE PSYCHIATRIC TREATMENT

Justice Cardozo famously wrote in the case of *Schloendorff v. Society of New York Hospital*: "[E]very human being of adult years and sound mind has a right to determine what shall be done with his own body" [20 (pp 129-130)]. A patient's right to accept or refuse treatment, as well as to provide informed consent, highlights the value of autonomy. However, in attempting to balance the competing interests between individual rights and societal interests, states have taken different approaches. In some jurisdictions, such as Washington and California, the right to make treatment decisions continues through civil commitment [21]. In other jurisdictions, such as Utah, involuntary commitment incorporates incompetence to make medical decisions [22].

By way of illustration, administering antipsychotic medication to someone who lacks capacity to consent to or refuse the medication varies by jurisdiction. The process for administering antipsychotic medication to civilly hospitalized persons in Washington is as follows: After an evaluation and determination that antipsychotic medication is medically necessary, the treating physician attempts to obtain informed consent from the patient. If the patient lacks the capacity to make such medical decisions or refuses the medication, the treating physician must opine that (1) failure to medicate may result in a likelihood of serious harm or substantial deterioration and (2) that there is no less intrusive means of treatment [23]. A second physician must then evaluate the patient and opine as to both (1) and (2). When both physicians agree, the patient may be medicated despite refusal for up to 30 days. Additional review is needed for medication administration beyond 30 days and may require a court hearing. In addition, patients may refuse any psychiatric medication, including involuntarily ordered antipsychotic medication beginning 24 hours before any initial or continued civil commitment hearing or involuntary medication hearing [24]. However, a specific reference to the presence of a mental disorder is not stated, but appears to be assumed from the mental disorder criterion required to initiate involuntary commitment in Washington.

According to California law, a patient who is involuntarily committed and refuses antipsychotic medication is entitled to review hearing(s) before the medication is administered in nonemergency situations [25]. In California, capacity to refuse medication hearings are commonly referred to as "Riese Petitions" after a prominent legal case that resulted in these hearings. In *Riese v. St. Mary's Hospital and Medical Center* [26], the court held that, absent judicial determination of incompetence, informed consent is required to administer antipsychotic medications to involuntary committed persons in no emergent situations. To assess capacity, the court in *Riese* stated that the decision maker should focus on whether the patient: (1) is aware of his or her situation (e.g., diagnosis); (2) is able to understand the benefits, risks, and alternatives to medications; and (3) is rationally able to understand and evaluate the medication information and participate in the treatment decision. After this 1991 decision, the California legislature enacted SB 665 and codified in the statutes [27–29], which requires informed refusal for psychotropic medications absent an emergency and capacity hearings for those thought to be lacking capacity for such informed refusal of these medications. In practice, there is no interest in California in conducting hearings on those who consent to medication but lack the capacity to give informed consent.

Under California law, a patient who is to be involuntary medicated must be proven to lack capacity by "clear and convincing evidence." In practice, a court-hearing officer listens to the testimony at the hospital facility and makes a determination about whether or not the patient will be forcibly medicated. There may be patients who are found detainable at probable cause hearings, but they are not permitted to be given involuntary administration of psychotropic medication as a result of the Riese hearing. The California State legislature has not specified which mental disorders are relevant to Riese Petitions, nor has it specified which diagnostic system should be used. However, as with involuntary civil commitment, the use of the current DSM edition (now DSM-5) has become the standard bearer. However, the central issue in determining whether to override a person's medication refusal is his or her lack of capacity to weigh the risks and benefits of psychotropic medication. Therefore, a serious mental disorder would usually be required to lead to a lack of this capacity. Some other states have similar procedures.

In light of which mental disorders are represented in those who are involuntarily civilly committed, the DSM-5 diagnostic categories of Schizophrenia Spectrum and Other Psychotic Disorders, Bipolar and Related Disorders, and Depressive Disorders, will likely dominate the "capacity" hearings for two key reasons: (1) these disorders often result in a lack of capacity when the person is symptomatic, and (2) these disorders have medications likely to treat active symptoms. Most hearing officers and judges will only order medications for those with serious mental disorders for which there are medications to remedy the problem.

"Capacity" hearings, regardless of the diagnosis, are likely to primarily involve antipsychotic medications, which is also a pragmatic issue because there are no intramuscular forms for the currently commonly used antidepressants or mood-stabilizers. However, an antipsychotic medication that also helps treat bipolar disorder symptoms could be administered as an intramuscular injection alternative when a patient refuses a mood stabilizer and meets criteria for involuntary treatment. The "Riese petition" asks the provider to describe active symptoms of the mental disorder. DSM-5 has included the "Clinician-Rated Dimensions of Psychosis Symptom Severity" [1 (pp 743-744)], which may begin to play a role in these hearings. This DSM-5 psychotic symptom rating scale has the appearance of a diluted Brief Psychiatric Rating Scale (BPRS) [30] or Positive and Negative Syndrome Scale (PANSS) [31] and carries with it potential validity and reliability challenges if introduced into the courtroom.

Psychiatric treatment refusals for inmates detained in a correctional facility or for individuals found incompetent to stand trial are guided by different laws than those articulated above for civilly committed patients. In these circumstances, absent emergency, administration of psychotropic medications generally requires incapacity or refusal and the addition of a compelling government interest, such as to prevent harm in the case of penal patients (see *Washington v. Harper* [32], *Sell v. US* [33]). In *Washington v. Harper* [32], the court held (among others) that the penal institution's procedure adhered to substantive due process because it was reasonably related to the state's legitimate interest in reducing danger posed by a violent, mentally ill inmate. The policy applied exclusively to mentally ill inmates [32 (219-227)]. In *Sell v. United* States, the question before the court was whether the "Constitution permits the Government to administer antipsychotic drugs to a *mentally ill* criminal defendant" to render the defendant competent to stand trial (emphasis added) [33 (p166)]. The Court answered in the affirmative when certain conditions are met: the treatment is medically appropriate, substantially unlikely to have side effects that may undermine the fairness of the trial, less intrusive alternatives to medications were considered, and forced medication is necessary to further important government interests. Neither court in *Harper* or *Sell* commented on whether specific mental disorders are necessary, nor whether any specific diagnostic system is required in these determinations. Because specific diagnoses are not identified as required in these treatment refusal settings, one can infer that DSM-5 changes are unlikely to have any impact in these particular situations.

CAPACITY TO MANAGE MEDICAL DECISIONS

Psychiatrists are often called to assess patients' medical decisional capacity in the setting of no emergent medical or surgical treatment. Central to these evaluations is the concept of informed consent. The court in *Canterbury v. Spence* defined informed consent as follows: "True consent to what happens to one's self is in the informed exercise of choice, and that entails an opportunity to evaluate knowledgeably the options available and the risks attendant upon each" [34 (p780)]. Except in rare circumstances, consent to medical treatment, when given voluntarily by a person with capacity to make medical decisions, must be honored even if not the best treatment unless the request is medically unsound. Likewise, a competent person is generally permitted to refuse medical care, even if the refusal could lead to the person's death.

Although courts usually yield to the decisions of a competent adult, the exceptions occur in cases where there is a "compelling state interest" after balancing the individual's rights against the state's interest (see e.g., *Roe v. Wade* [35]). Identified state interests include preservation of life, protection of interests of innocent third parties, prevention of suicide, and maintenance of the ethical integrity of the medical profession. This balancing test, by way of illustration, has been routinely applied in the context of right-to-die cases, where a person or family wishes to discontinue life-sustaining measures (e.g., *Cruzan v. Missouri Department of Health* [36], *Superintendent of Belchertown State School v. Saikewicz* [37], and *Matter of Welfare of Colyer* [38]).

However, there may be a time when a person is unable to appreciate the risks and benefits of a healthcare decision. When a person lacks such medical decision-making capacity, the issue becomes who should make the decision for him or her. In Washington (and California), two schemes are used to make such decisions in the absence of emergency. The first is advance directives. The second is the use of a surrogate decision-maker when the person does not have a relevant advance directive. State statute guides the order of priority for surrogate decision-makers, including any appointed guardian, power of attorney for healthcare decisions, and family [39].

Some jurisdictions, such as California, have identified by statute what abilities are necessary for decisional capacity in general [40] and in the context of healthcare decisions [41, 42]. In general, the California Probate Code requires that the person respond knowingly and intelligently about their medical treatment, have a rational thought process, understand the seriousness of the illness or defect, the recommended treatment, benefits of treatment, risks, and alternatives [41]. More succinctly, the California Probate Code section states: "Capacity" means a person's ability to understand the nature and consequences of a decision and to make and communicate a decision, and includes in the case of proposed healthcare, the ability to understand its significant benefits, risks, and alternatives [42].

However, the California statutes stop short of offering specific mental disorder criterion to opine a lack of competence, although negation of capacity would require the presence of a mental disorder with active symptoms in nearly all cases. Other states, like Washington, are devoid of such statutory guidance. Again although there is no statutory requirement that a person must have a mental disorder in order to be incompetent for medical decisions, it seems inconceivable to support an opinion of incompetence without the presence of a mental disorder. On the other hand, silence as to a requirement of a mental disorder criterion does not preclude a mental disorder diagnosis.

The most common mental disorders found in the civil commitment setting would also most likely be involved in the context of incapacity for medical decision-making. Namely, these include the DSM-5 categories of the Schizophrenia Spectrum and Other Psychotic Disorders, Bipolar and Related Disorders, Depressive Disorders, and Major Neurocognitive Disorders. However, the Anxiety Disorders, Obsessive-Compulsive and Related Disorders, and Trauma- and Stressor-Related Disorders may make an appearance if the anxious or phobic symptoms are especially severe.

Of the diagnostic categories above, the DSM-5 section on Neurocognitive Disorders has particularly noteworthy changes. The major change from prior DSMs has been the introduction of the category of mild neurocognitive disorder that usually but not always would not lead to a lack of decisional capacity except in the most complex decisions. The diagnosis may lead to better recognition of impairment in those with milder deficits since it does not have an analog from prior DSMs [43]. Those with pre-DSM-5 diagnoses of Delirium will still be diagnosed with delirium in DSM-5. Individuals previously diagnosed with Dementia would be subsumed by the DSM-5 major neurocognitive disorder. However, the major neurocognitive disorder category is broader than the previous Dementia diagnoses. For example, memory impairment is not specifically required (as it was with the DSM-IV diagnosis of Dementia) and thereby will be more relevant to younger people with disorders such as traumatic brain injury.

However, criticism has been raised that the threshold between mild and major neurocognitive disorders is artificial [43]. Although not included as diagnostic criteria, DSM-5's paradigm for distinguishing the mild and major neurocognitive disorders is based in the text discussion on whether the cognitive impairment is 1 or 2 standard deviations from the mean on an unspecified standardized test [1 (p607)]. The lack of a specified test could lead to potential misuse in the forensic settings by some being tempted to choose a test most likely to produce a desired result that may not even have norms for the relevant population. The DSM-5 does not endorse or recommend specific tests because of proprietary concerns and due to the likelihood that new tests will be developed in the future. Therefore, the standard deviation text commentary serves as a general guideline rather than a diagnostic requirement, an important distinction especially in forensic contexts. In the DSM-5, the distinction is made by unspecified neuropsychological testing, but a clinical assessment can substitute for that so long as it is quantified. For forensic purposes, this can still lead to abuse by some choosing the tests most likely to lead to a desired result without the test necessarily having norms for the relevant population.

The distinction between 1 and 2 standard deviations below appropriate norms may nonetheless be a meaningful boundary between mild and major neurocognitive disorder, but it also can lead to confusion and diagnostic controversy and misuse in forensic settings and only a specific capacity might be relevant for a specified forensic purpose and not a general lack of capacity assessed in making the diagnosis. Although a specific diagnosis does not automatically infer incompetence, arriving at a diagnosis of major neurocognitive disorder will likely carry great weight in arriving at an opinion supporting incompetence. From these perspectives, making a distinction between mild and major neurocognitive disorders based on the number of standard deviations from the mean may assume more significance than it probably should. An artificial dividing line between <2 and >2 standard deviations also conflicts with the DSM-5's attempt to support a dimensional measure in diagnoses in addition to the inherent categorical nature of a diagnostic system. Nonetheless, objective-type measurements that assist in distinguishing between major and mild neurocognitive function in the clinical domains could also serve to support a medical opinion regarding competence. Such use of tests is appropriate so long as the following principles are considered: (1) care is taken in the selection of specific tools, (2) tests are not selected to purposely skew the results in any desired direction, and (3) the dividing line between major and mild in not overly emphasized because the relevant issue is capacity or lack of it for a specific purpose and not a more general capacity and (4) there are norms for the test on the relevant population. Examples of tools that may assist in differentiating between a mild and major neurocognitive disorder and potentially serve to support an opinion involving competence or incompetence are found in Table 7-2.

The DSM-5 does give some examples that are helpful in making the distinction between major and mild neurocognitive disorder. Six cognitive domains to be considered are listed in a table. They are complex attention, executive function, learning and memory, language, perceptual motor, and social cognition. Examples are then given of deficits in each of these domains that would fall under major and mild neurocognitive disorder as well as examples of assessment methods that would help assess the degree of these deficits [1 (p594–595)]. This part of the DSM-5 criteria should prove very helpful in making this distinction for both clinical and forensic purposes. Another helpful distinguishing factor is in the area of independent functioning. The cognitive deficits under Criterion B for major neurocognitive disorder interfere with independence in everyday activities. In contrast, for mild neurocognitive disorder, they do not interfere.

To diagnose either major or mild neurocognitive disorder, there must be a decline from a previous level of functioning. However, in some instances in which there is not good data or a reliable source of evidence, it may become difficult if not occasionally impossible to demonstrate such a decline.

When it appears that a patient lacks capacity to make medical decisions, the treating physician generally raises the initial question of whether the patient is competent. In situations of treatment refusal by a hospitalized medical or surgical patient, the treating physician will often ask for a consultation, usually from a psychiatrist or mental health provider, for further assessment of the patient's abilities. Much has been written on assessing competence for medical decision-making. For example, Grisso [44] and Grisso and Appelbaum [45] have identified important factors to consider in assessing capacity to make treatment decisions: the patient can express a choice about treatment; understands information pertinent to the treatment decision; has the capacity to appreciate the treatment recommendation in context of one's own situation; and has the ability to weigh treatment options with a logical manner.

Table 7-2. COGNITIVE SCREENING TOOLS EXAMPLES

1. Mini Mental State Exam (MMSE)
2. Montreal Cognitive Assessment (MoCA)
3. Cognistat (formerly Neurobehavioral Cognitive Status Examination)
4. Addenbrookes' Cognitive Examination—Revised (ACE-R)
5. Blessed Orientation-Memory-Concentration (BOME) Test
6. General Practitioner Assessment of Cognition (GPCOG)
7. St. Louis University Mental Status (SLUMS) Exam
8. Short Test of Mental Status (STMS)

Several authors have conceptualized a "sliding-scale" approach to capacity to make medical decisions [46, 47]. This model presumes that the degree of risk inherent in the treatment decision is a key factor in the analysis. In this scheme, there is a low bar for competence when the risk of the patient's decision is low and the benefit is large. In contrast, under this approach, a patient must more clearly demonstrate competence when the risk of the treatment is high or the benefits limited (e.g., experimental surgery).

Healthcare decision making involving end-of-life decisions include Do Not Resuscitate Orders, Advanced Directives, or naming a healthcare proxy decision maker should the person become incompetent. These healthcare decisions require the person be competent at the time the decision is made, identical to any healthcare decision a person makes. However, in the case of Physician Assisted Suicide, diagnostic considerations can play a role. The 1997 Oregon Death with Dignity Act authorizes Physician Assisted Suicide under very limited circumstances for terminally ill individuals [48]. Besides various safeguards, including the person making a competent decision, there is the following safeguard regarding mental health [49]:

> Counseling referral. If in the opinion of the attending physician or the consulting physician a patient may be suffering from a psychiatric or psychological disorder or depression causing impaired judgment, either physician shall refer the patient for counseling. No medication to end a patient's life in a humane and dignified manner shall be prescribed until the person performing the counseling determines that the patient is not suffering from a psychiatric or psychological disorder or depression causing impaired judgment.

The broad language of the Oregon statute allows DSM-5 to potentially have increased importance in determining the permissibility of Physician Assisted Suicide. Insofar as DSM-5 in concerned, as mentioned earlier in this section, major neurocognitive disorder and sometimes even the new mild neurocognitive disorder may come into play here. Expansion of Physician Assisted Suicide to other states at some point in the future highlight the potential role of diagnoses, especially if the above Oregon model is adopted with its broad exclusionary language of "a psychiatric or psychological disorder or depression causing impaired judgment" [49].

The question here is whether Jack has the capacity for medical decision-making. He has a history of traumatic brain injury with likely diagnosis of major or mild neurocognitive disorder due to traumatic brain injury under the DSM-5. The presence of a DSM-5 diagnosis is just one factor in the capacity assessment. Even if Jack has "major" neurocognitive impairment, he may nevertheless have capacity to make this medical decision if other conditions are met. Based on the sliding-scale model, it is helpful to know that the risk of Jack's decision here is relatively low, with a resultant high threshold for finding lack of decisional capacity.

The inquiry will rest, given his DSM-5 disorder, on Jack's functional abilities. Although there may be jurisdictional requirements in law, the general inquiry calls for assessment of Jack's ability to express a choice about his

VIGNETTE 1

Jack is a 35 year-old man who fell from a ladder and sustained significant injuries to his head. He develops hemiparesis. As a result of his injuries, he needs assistance with many of his daily tasks. He lives in a residential group home and works in a sheltered workshop environment. When he is at work one day, he badly cuts his hand. He is taken to the local emergency room where his physicians recommend stitches and he refuses. His doctors, aware of his head injury, ask if he is competent to make this decision. You are asked to consult.

treatment, his understanding of the material information regarding the treatment, ability to appreciate treatment recommendations in the context of his situation, and weigh his options in a logical manner [44].

COMPETENCY TO MANAGE FINANCIAL AFFAIRS/CONTRACT/MARRY

Forensic evaluators are often asked to evaluate the capacity of individuals to contract and manage finances. These evaluations are typically assessments of present-day capacities, although there are situations when an evaluator is asked whether a person had the ability to contract at a prior date. Consistent with other civil competencies discussed here, the context of the capacity is important. Such evaluations require an assessment of any mental disorder and an evaluation of any resulting impairments on the skills necessary for managing finances or engaging in a contract. The complexity of the financial arrangements or contract is one factor in the assessment.

As an example, California statutes require that judicial determinations finding a person lacks the legal capacity to perform a specific act must be based on "a deficit in one or more of the person's mental functions" rather than a diagnosis of a mental or physical disorder [50]. The California statutes specifically mention various civil competencies of "contracting, conveying, marrying, making medical decisions, executing wills or trusts" [51]. The

California Probate Code [52] lists the following specific deficits in mental functions:

(1) Alertness and attention, including, but not limited to, the following:
  (A) Level of arousal or consciousness
  (B) Orientation to time, place, person, and situation
  (C) Ability to attend and concentrate
(2) Information processing, including, but not limited to, the following:
  (A) Short- and long-term memory, including immediate recall
  (B) Ability to understand or communicate with others, either verbally or otherwise
  (C) Recognition of familiar objects and familiar persons
  (D) Ability to understand and appreciate quantities
  (E) Ability to reason using abstract concepts
  (F) Ability to plan, organize, and carry out actions in one's own rational self-interest
  (G) Ability to reason logically
(3) Thought processes. Deficits in these functions may be demonstrated by the presence of the following:
  (A) Severely disorganized thinking
  (B) Hallucinations
  (C) Delusions
  (D) Uncontrollable, repetitive, or intrusive thoughts
(4) Ability to modulate mood and affect. Deficits in this ability may be demonstrated by the presence of a pervasive and persistent or recurrent state of euphoria, anger, anxiety, fear, panic, depression, hopelessness or despair, helplessness, apathy or indifference that is inappropriate in degree to the individual's circumstances.

As with all evaluations of competence, the above deficit in mental function has to "significantly" impair the person's "ability to understand and appreciate the consequences of his or her actions with regard to the type of act or decision in question" [53]. Because the specific listed capacities are independent of diagnosis, these criteria will diminish the impact from the DSM-5 diagnostic changes in California.

As with the capacity to make healthcare decisions discussed in the prior section, the role of DSM-5 is essentially identical to that described with medical decision-making earlier in this chapter for these other civil competencies. In general, financial capacity calls the forensic evaluator to assess whether the evaluee has the requisite knowledge and skills to manage his or her finances. Jurisdictions have various procedures—from payees, to guardians, to conservators—to aid persons who are adjudicated incompetent to manage their funds. These procedures vary from state to state. Likewise, when a person's contractual capacities are questioned, the forensic evaluator assesses whether the evaluee understands the nature of the contract, terms of the contract, scope, and reasonable consequences. Marriage is viewed as a form of contract. In some jurisdictions, if a person has a guardian, any contract entered by the ward may be voidable.

With an aging U.S. population, the DSM-5 diagnoses included in the new category of Neurocognitive Disorders are likely to be relevant to financial and contractual capacity assessments for many years to come. It can be expected that more individuals will meet criteria for a neurocognitive disorder under DSM-5 for the following reasons. First, the major neurocognitive disorder diagnosis does not require a memory deficit as required for a diagnosis of Dementia under DSM-IV. Second, other conditions will qualify for major neurocognitive disorder that may not have qualified for DSM-IV Dementia, such as cognitive impairments resulting from traumatic brain injury and other disorders not related to age or a degenerative process. Finally, DSM-5 has created a "mild" neurocognitive disorder that will likely expand the number of individuals diagnosed with some type of cognitive impairment. Although an evaluee may now have a DSM-5 diagnosis, where perhaps they would not have had a diagnosis under DSM-IV, the skills and abilities of the evaluee to perform the questioned task should be the primary focus of the forensic evaluator in performing capacity assessments.

Along these lines, neuropsychological or intelligence testing may be helpful for further assessment of cognitive abilities, particularly where comorbid conditions may be present or the clinical presentation is ambiguous. As with other screening tools, however, there is no clear correlation between the testing and a person's ability to manage their financial affairs or understand a particular contract. Of note, the psychological test may not focus on the specific relevant capacities for handling financial affairs. The use of intelligence testing, for example, may not be as useful for elderly evaluees because many tests were initially designed to predict academic performance [54]. Caution is needed when using tests to evaluate an individual's cognition. In particular, validity concerns may arise when administering objective assessment tools to individuals coming from population groups that have not been adequately normed, thereby increasing the likelihood that test scores will underestimate the person's actual cognitive ability such as with elderly people. Although these tests have a role and may be compelling as additional objective evidence of skills, the utility of the tests need to be considered within the context of the complete capacity assessment and for the specific function assessed.

Other DSM-5 diagnoses expected to be associated with questions of whether someone could manage their finances or enter a contract include the Schizophrenia Spectrum and Other Psychotic Disorders, Bipolar and Related

Disorders, and Depressive Disorders. Despite minor changes in these categories in comparison to DSM-IV, the changes are expected to have little impact on the assessment of these capacities.

Statutes can mention a specific diagnosis. In the California Probate Code section dealing with Powers and Duties of Guardian or Conservator of the Person, there is a specific reference to the diagnosis of "dementia," "as defined in the last published edition of the 'Diagnostic and Statistical Manual of Mental Disorders'" [55]. This statute allows the Conservator to make an appropriate placement for a person on a Probate Conservatorship who has dementia, lacks the capacity to give informed consent to placement, lacks general decision-making capacity, and benefits from placement in a "restricted and secure environment" [56]. Because DSM-5 specifically notes that major neurocognitive disorder is the essential equivalent to the DSM-IV diagnosis of Dementia, evaluators should have little difficulty clarifying for the court the similarities between these two diagnoses. In addition, as previously mentioned, the specific level of impairment in the various neurocognitive domains by clinical examination and use of the tools listed in Table 7-2 would have bearing for both the DSM-5 diagnosis and an opinion about competence. However, there is a difference insofar as major neurocognitive disorder, unlike dementia, does not require memory impairment. Until and unless statutes using the diagnosis of dementia are updated, explaining the diagnosis of major neurocognitive disorder may be needed when writing the forensic report or testifying to avoid misunderstandings.

TESTAMENTARY CAPACITY

A person's testamentary capacity, or the capacity to make a will, requires that a person is of sound mind when he or she executes the will. A person's testamentary capacity may be challenged before or after their death. All jurisdictions require testamentary capacity. Although the requirements are similar across states, each jurisdiction has its own specific requirements in law. For example, in Washington, any person 18 years of age and "of sound mind" can make a will [57]. Washington law does not identify any specific mental illness definition in this context. Presumably, then, any DSM-5 mental illness would be relevant to the assessment of whether someone is of sound mind.

California law defines persons who are not competent to make a will in the California Probate Code as follows [58]:

(a) An individual is not mentally competent to make a will

if at the time of making the will either of the following is true:

(1) The individual does not have sufficient mental capacity to be able to (A) understand the nature of the testamentary act, (B) understand and recollect the nature and situation of the individual's property, or (C) remember and understand the individual's relations to living descendants, spouse, and parents, and those whose interests are affected by the will.
(2) The individual suffers from a mental disorder with symptoms including delusions or hallucinations, which delusions or hallucinations result in the individual's devising property in a way which, except for the existence of the delusions or hallucinations, the individual would not have done

Similar to Washington, there is no specific language on mental illness included in the definition for this California statute. Nonetheless, part of the California statute [59] refers to the concept known as an "insane delusion." There are occasions when a will is invalidated, although the testator displays the cognitive abilities for will formation, because the testator cannot make a rationale disposition of assets due to a delusion. Take for example a situation where the testator mistakenly or delusionally believes that a spouse has purged certain assets of the testator. In such cases, the inquiry becomes whether formation of the will was a product of the delusions [60]. DSM-5 diagnoses most relevant to this situation include the Schizophrenia Spectrum and Other Psychotic Disorders, Bipolar and Related Disorders, Depressive Disorders, and Major Neurocognitive Disorders. DSM-5 Substance Use Disorders may also be relevant to this statutory provision and concept to the extent that psychosis may manifest in these conditions.

Scholarly articles and case law on the topic of testamentary capacity routinely identify four general requirements for testamentary capacity: (1) that the person understands that he or she is making a will; (2) the general nature and extent of their property; (3) the natural objects of their bounty; and (4) to whom and how their property is to be disposed [61]. Mental illness per se is not a predicate to incapacity to execute a will. Even the presence of a severe mental disorder alone does not negate capacity. For example, a person who commits suicide could have had testamentary capacity when their will was executed, and even someone with schizophrenia or major neurocognitive disorder might still retain these capacities.

When testamentary capacity is challenged after the testator's death, the forensic evaluator is unable to complete a customary in-person evaluation of the testator. In contrast, the forensic evaluator is called to rely on collateral information, including medical records, nursing home records, copies of prior wills, witnesses to the will, collateral information from people who knew the testator, and material about the nature of the estate. Of key importance in the assessment is whether the testator had symptoms of mental illness at the time of their will execution. If so, did the symptoms impact the testator's thought process or ability to rationally appraise the situation?

Many DSM-5 disorders are potentially relevant to testamentary capacity. Particular DSM-5 disorders, such as Schizophrenia Spectrum and Other Psychotic Disorders, Major Neurocognitive Disorders, Neurodevelopmental Disorders, Depressive Disorders, and Substance Use Disorders, should be explored but may not necessarily negate testamentary capacity. For the most part, the testamentary capacity assessment will change little from those under the DSM-IV.

As identified in earlier sections of this chapter, however, the Neurocognitive Disorders under DSM-5 have broadened the scope of the former DSM-IV Dementia diagnoses and, thus, might capture more individuals. Even with this expansion, however, most people with a mild neurocognitive disorder, and some even with a major neurocognitive disorder, may nevertheless be able to identify and discuss their estate, heirs, and wishes for dissolution of the estate.

A related concept not yet discussed in this chapter is the Global Assessment of Functioning Scale (GAF) that was present on Axis V of the multiaxial classification system in use for more than the past 30 years in the DSM-III through the DSM-IV-TR. Axis V has been removed from the DSM-5 and the GAF with it. Previously, the GAF could be used to measure overall functioning at a point in time and to provide reference points for comparison over time. With several disorders, review of a person's GAFs over time could be superimposed on the time of the event in question (i.e., execute a will) as an additional source of information for the evaluator. In the absence of the GAF, there may be need to be more reliant on descriptive terms for the person's condition, unless the psychiatrist chooses a cognitive screening tool (see Table 7-2 for examples) in the case of a neurocognitive disorder, or the BPRS, PANSS, or the DSM-5's "Clinician-Rated Dimensions of Psychosis Symptom Severity" in the case of a Schizophrenia Spectrum and Other Psychotic Disorder.

It is not uncommon for a person to create or change their will after one of their relative's dies. Under DSM-5, the DSM-IV bereavement exclusion for Major Depressive Disorder has been removed and the diagnosis may be made in the presence of grief. Although the diagnosis of major depressive disorder may be given in this context, it remains the evaluator's responsibility to explore all of the requirements of testamentary capacity and the possible need for delay until the bereavement subsides.

Finally, the related concept of undue influence arises in the setting of execution of a will. This situation arises when an individual is vulnerable to the influence of another person, usually a beneficiary of the estate. For undue influence, it must generally be established that that the person actually exerted influence over the testator; the influence rises to the level or coercion; and the influence caused the testator to execute a will that he or she would not have created absence the undue influence [62]. Forensic evaluators may be asked to assess the testator's vulnerability to undue influence. Factors for the forensic evaluator to consider include the testator's mental and physical disabilities as well as "when an individual keeps other family members away from the testator; tells tales about other heirs to alienate them from the testator; and controls personal access, mail, and phone calls from relatives to the testator" [63]. Although not likely to be relevant in other aspects of testamentary capacity as the mental disorders listed above in the testamentary capacity section, mild neurocognitive disorder may not infrequently play a role in susceptibility to undue influence.

Under DSM-5, the diagnosis of Schizophrenia has changed modestly. The subtypes have been removed, and the two A criteria are required. Fred's mental disorder is relevant because testamentary capacity requires one to be of "sound mind" at the time of will execution. His diagnosis is one factor in the inquiry of testamentary capacity. Here, Fred displays the cognitive abilities generally required for testamentary capacity. However, his symptoms suggest that he is suffering from an "insane delusion." The inquiry becomes whether formation of the will was a product of the delusions [60]. This is likely true here because the delusions triggered Fred to execute a will that would not have been created absent the delusion.

VIGNETTE 2

Fred is a 45 year-old man with history of schizophrenia. His symptoms had been well controlled for several years. A few years ago, he married. At the time of marriage, he created a will leaving his assets to his wife. Now, several years later, he abruptly changes his will.

Fred understands the concept of a will and tells you that he inherited previously under his grandfather's will. Although he has few assets, he identifies the property that his grandfather left him and his personal belongings. He knows that his wife would naturally inherit should he die. You learn that he abruptly changed his will because he overheard a friend say that his wife "is an alien from outer space disguised as a human." He left his assets to the CIA because "they can track her and keep her from harming anyone." He has been hearing voices from the CIA instructing him to monitor her. Did he have capacity to execute a new will?

Fred has a history of schizophrenia.

EVALUATION GUIDELINES

As illustrated by the range of topics that fall under the broad category of civil competencies, the assessment of any one particular competence is guided by the knowledge and skills required to carry out the particular task. In this sense, competence assessments are context specific. A consulting psychiatrist or forensic examiner is called to assess an evaluee's cognitive, psychiatric, and emotional state and opine whether any limitations in these areas reasonably prevent the evaluee from participating in the task.

A prerequisite, then, for assessing a person's capacity for a task is an understanding of the underlying task and the necessary elements of that task. As alluded to above, sometimes jurisdictions, by statute or other provision, outline requirements necessary for the competence. The California statutory requirements for medical decision-making is illustrative. Where jurisdictional guidance is not available, the evaluator is tasked with identifying the requisite requirements. The question posed to the evaluator can be vague (e.g., understand the consequences of marriage), requiring the evaluator to operationalize a definition or set of skills for the task.

Foubister and Connell [31] have outlined a "general assessment approach" for medical decisions that is useful in variety of civil competence contexts. Their approach focuses on background information typical of a standard psychiatric assessment and "on the individual's capacity or incapacity... rather than on an ultimate declaration of competence... The ultimate competence judgment may rest on balanced consideration of the severity of consequences and the individual's capacities, a decision that involved moral or 'values' considerations and may best be made by the court" [64 (p508)]. Likewise, Grisso [44] put forth a model for evaluation of competencies with the following key elements: functional, causal, interactive, judgmental, and dispositional. These models are useful in helping to characterize the nature of more general capacity impairment. They may be relevant in situations of extreme capacity deficiencies demonstrating lack of capacity for all or almost all purposes. However, it is important to recognize that legal capacities are specific to the purpose in question, and evaluators need to have the specific capacities for that purpose in mind when performing an evaluation. A person may lack a specific capacity although retain general capacity for most purposes. Or a person can lack general capacity but retain a specific capacity so except in extreme cases they may be less useful. If general capacity tests are used, it is essential not to lose sight of the need to assess and focus on how any impairment(s) affects the particular legal capacity in question.

For many common civil competencies, a body of literature exists that helps inform the evaluation. Assessments tools are also available to aid in several civil competence evaluations, particularly for medical decision-making and guardianship. Although not exhaustive, identified in Table 7-3 are several assessment tools for civil competencies adapted in part from Grisso [44] and Drogin and Barrret [65].

SUMMARY

Psychiatrists and forensic evaluators are often called to assess for civil competencies. These assessments can be both challenging and interesting due to their varied nature of required tasks. Evaluators doing this type of work will want to familiarize themselves with any jurisdictional requirements for the competency being evaluated. Likewise, evaluators will want to identity any jurisdictional definitions of mental disorder. This is particularly true in the area of civil commitment. Working with DSM-5, one should be mindful whether a DSM-5 diagnosis comports with any mental disorder definition

Table 7-3. ILLUSTRATIVE LIST OF COMPETENCE ASSESSMENT TOOLS

Aid to Capacity Evaluation (ACE)	Medical decision-making
Assessment of Consent Capacity for Treatment (AACT)	Medical decision-making
Capacity Assessment Tool (CAT)	Reasoning in medical decisions
Community Competency Scale (CCS)	Daily living skills
Decision-Making Instrument for Guardianship (DIG)	Guardianship
Direct Assessment of Functional Status (DAFS)	Daily living skills
Everyday Problems Test for Cognitive Challenged Elderly (EPPCE)	Performance of daily activities
Functional Independence Measure (FIM)	Predictive of need for caregiver
Hopemont Capacity Assessment Interview (HCAI)	Medical decision-making
Independent Living Scaled (ILS)	Cognitive skills for independent living
MacArthur Competence Assessment Tool for Treatment Decisions (MacCAT-T)	Medical decision-making
MacArthur Competence Assessment Tool for Clinical Research (MacCAT-CR)	Clinical research participation
Multidimensional Functional Assessment Questionnaire (MFAQ)	Daily functioning and resource allocation
Perceptions of Disorder Instrument (POD)	Medical decision-making
Philadelphia Geriatric Center Multilevel Assessment Inventory (MAI)	Behavior and activities of daily living
Thinking Rationally About Treatment (TRAT)	Medical decision-making
Understanding Treatment Disclosures	Medical decision-making

necessary for the specific capacity or competence. Although the presence of a DSM-5 diagnosis alone is not sufficient to establish incompetence, a DSM-5 diagnosis can have utility in reporting and conveying helpful information about the evaluee and the longitudinal course and prognosis of an illness. However, an accurate assessment of a person's specific symptoms and skills will provide more forensic utility than the diagnosis. Key summary points from this chapter include the following:

- Be familiar with any local laws regarding the competency definitions and procedures.
- Know your jurisdiction's mental disorder criterion.
- Remember that civil competencies are task-specific and are assessed based on the requirements of the specific task.
- Assess how symptoms of DSM-5 disorders affect legal criteria.
- Understand that DSM-5 has made changes to facilitate communicating information. However, in doing so, not only has there been an improvement in calling attention to areas of impairment, there are also drawbacks because the new criteria may differ from DSM-IV-TR nomenclature and criteria and sometimes thereby can lead to confusion or give the mistaken impression of more or less impairment than actually is the case.
- Avoid over interpretation in regard to the scientific validity of certain tests merely because the results can be quantified.
- Appreciate that although DSM-5 was designed for clinical purposes, the changes in many diagnostic criteria DSM-5 are likely to impact civil competence assessments nonetheless. The presence of a DSM-5 disorder does not equate with civil incompetence but is relevant to the evaluation.

REFERENCES

1. American Psychiatric Association. *Diagnostic and Statistical Manual of Mental Disorders, Fifth Edition*. Arlington, Virginia: American Psychiatric Association; 2013.
2. Bloom JD, Rogers JL. The legal basis of forensic psychiatry: Statutorily mandated psychiatric diagnoses. *Am J Psychiatry* 1987; 144:847–853.
3. American Psychiatric Association. *Diagnostic and Statistical Manual of Mental Disorders, First Edition (DSM-I)*. Washington, DC: American Psychiatric Association; 1952.
4. American Psychiatric Association. *Diagnostic and Statistical Manual of Mental Disorders, Fourth Edition, Text Revision (DSM-IV-TR)*. Washington, DC: American Psychiatric Association; 2000.
5. American Psychiatric Association. *Diagnostic and Statistical Manual of Mental Disorders, Second Edition (DSM-II)*. Washington, DC: American Psychiatric Association; 1968.

6. American Psychiatric Association. *Diagnostic and Statistical Manual of Mental Disorders, Third Edition (DSM-III)*. Washington, DC: American Psychiatric Association; 1980.
7. American Psychiatric Association. *Diagnostic and Statistical Manual of Mental Disorders, Third Edition-Revised (DSM-III-R)*. Washington, DC: American Psychiatric Association; 1987.
8. American Psychiatric Association. *Diagnostic and Statistical Manual of Mental Disorders, Fourth Edition (DSM-IV)*. Washington, DC: American Psychiatric Association; 1994.
9. Revised Code of Washington 71.05.150(1).
10. Revised Code of Washington 71.05.020(26).
11. Revised Code of Washington 71.05.040.
12. California Welfare and Institutions Code 5001(b).
13. California Welfare and Institutions Code 5008(f).
14. California Welfare and Institutions Code 5150(a).
15. California Welfare and Institutions Code 5001 et seq.
16. California Welfare and Institutions Code 5150 et seq.
17. California Welfare and Institutions Code 5585 et seq.
18. Anfang SA, Appelbaum PS. Civil commitment: the American experience. *Isr J Psychiatry Relat Sci* 2006; 43:209–218.
19. Revised Code of Washington 71.05.240.
20. *Schloendorff v. Society of New York Hospital*, 211 N.Y. 125 (1914).
21. Revised Code of Washington 71.05.360.
22. Utah Code 62A-15-631 (10).
23. Revised Code of Washington 71.05.215.
24. Revised Code of Washington 71.05.210.
25. California Welfare and Institutions Code 5332.
26. *Riese v. St. Mary's Hospital and Medical Center*, 209 Cal.App.3d 1303, 271 Cal. Rptr. 199 (1987), petition for review granted 751 P.2d 893, 245 Cal.Rptr. 627 (1988), petition dismissed 774 P.2d 698, 259 Cal.Rptr. 669 (1989).
27. California Welfare and Institutions Code 5008.
28. California Welfare and Institutions Code 5325.5.
29. California Welfare and Institutions Code 5333-5337.
30. Overall JE, Gorham DR. The brief psychiatric rating scale. *Psychol Rep* 1962; 10:799–812.
31. Kay SR, Fiszbein A, Opler LA. The positive and negative syndrome scale (PANSS) for schizophrenia. *Schizophr Bull* 1987; 13:261–276.
32. *Washington v. Harper*, 494 U.S. 210 (1990).
33. *Sell v. U.S.*, 539 U.S. 166 (2003).
34. *Canterbury v. Spence*, 464 F.2d 772 (D.C. Cir. 1972).
35. *Roe v. Wade*, 410 U.S. 113 (1973).
36. *Cruzan v. Missouri Department of Health*, 497 U.S 261 (1990).
37. *Superintendent of Belchertown State School v. Saikewicz*, 370 N.E.2d 417 (Mass. 1977).
38. *Matter of Welfare of Colyer*, 660 P.2d 738 (Wash. 1983).
39. Revised Code of Washington 7.70.065.
40. California Probate Code 810-812.
41. California Probate Code 813.
42. California Probate Code 4609.

43. Blazer D. Neurocognitive disorders in DSM-5. *Am J Psychiatry* 2013; 170:585–587.
44. Grisso T. *Evaluating Competencies: Forensic Assessments and Instruments.* 2nd ed. New York, NY: Kluwer Academic; 2003.
45. Grisso T, Appelbaum PS. *Assessing Competence to Consent to Treatment: A Guide for Physicians and Other Health Professionals.* New York, NY: Oxford University Press; 1998.
46. Roth LK, Meisel A, Lidz CW. Tests of competency to consent to treatment. *Am J Psychiatry* 1977; 134:279–284.
47. Cahana A, Hurst SA. Voluntary informed consent in research and clinical care: an update. *Pain Practice* 2008; 8:446–451.
48. Oregon Revised Statutes 127.800-995.
49. Oregon Revised Statutes 127.825 §3.03.
50. California Probate Code 810(c).
51. California Probate Code 810(b).
52. California Probate Code 811(a).
53. California Probate Code 811(b).
54. Krauss IK, Popkin SJ. Competence issues in older adults. In: Hunt T, Lindley CJ, eds. *Testing older adults: A Reference Guide for Geropsychological Assessments.* Austin, TX: Pro-Ed, 1989.
55. California Probate Code 2356.5.
56. California Probate Code 2356(b)(1-4).
57. Revised Code of Washington 11.12.010.
58. California Probate Code 6100.5(a).
59. California Probate Code 6100.5(a)(2).
60. In re Estate of Scott, 128 Cal. 57 (1900).
61. Melton GB, Petrila J, Poythress NG, et al. *Psychological Evaluation for the Courts: A Handbook for Mental Health Professionals and Lawyers.* 3rd ed. New York, NY: Guilford Press; 2007.
62. Beyer GE. *Wills, Trusts, and Estates.* New York, NY: Aspen Law & Business; 1999.
63. Gutheil TG. Common pitfalls in the evaluation of testamentary capacity. *J Am Acad Psych Law* 2007; 35:514–517.
64. Foubister N, Connell M. Competency to consent to treatment. In: Drogin EY, Dattilio FM, Sadoff RL, Gutheil TG, eds. *Handbook of forensic assessment: Psychological and Psychiatric Perspectives.* Hoboken, NJ: John Wiley & Sons; 2011.
65. Drogin EY, Barret CL. *Evaluation for Guardianship.* New York, NY: Oxford University Press; 2010.

CHAPTER 8

DSM-5 and Personal Injury Litigation

INTRODUCTION

Civil litigation is a major aspect of the legal system in the United States, marked by a vast number and variety of cases. According to census data from 2008, more than 19 million civil cases were filed in state trial courts in that year alone. In the U.S. District Courts, 285,215 civil cases were filed in 2010, with 87,256 of those involving tort actions [1, 2]. Even if cases involving psychiatry represent only a small percentage of these civil actions, they nevertheless encompass a significant number of evaluations in which a forensic evaluator's expertise is vital. It stands to reason that changes in how mental disorders are diagnosed portend significant implications for assessing how alleged harms are assessed under tort law.

Tort law governs the legal resolution of complaints regarding medical treatment and alleged personal injury. A tort is a civil wrong. Tort law seeks to financially compensate individuals who have been injured or who have suffered losses due to the conduct of others. Intentional torts are those where the individual or agency intends harms or knows harm will result from his or her actions [3]. In contrast, unintentional torts involve those situations in which the individual's behavior unintentionally causes an unreasonable risk of harm to another [3]. Depending on the type of civil litigation, claims of emotional distress can include a claim of intentional infliction of emotional distress and/or a claim of negligent (i.e., unintentional) infliction of emotional distress.

When evaluating alleged emotional damages arising during the course of civil litigation, the evaluator generally considers the elements summarized in Table 8-1.

This chapter summarizes how DSM-5 diagnostic changes may impact the assessment of claims of emotional distress and psychiatric injury in medical

Table 8-1. RELEVANT QUESTIONS TO CONSIDER WHEN EVALUATING EMOTIONAL DISTRESS CLAIMS

1. Does the person meet criteria for a recognized mental disorder?
2. If the person does not meet criteria for a recognized mental disorder, is there evidence that the individual genuinely experienced some type of emotional distress?
3. Is there evidence that the person is malingering?
4. Does the evidence support that the alleged stressor is solely responsible for the reported symptoms?
5. Is there evidence that the person has a preexisting mental disorder?
6. If the person has a preexisting mental disorder, does the evidence indicate that the alleged stressor is nevertheless solely responsible for the reported symptoms?
7. If the person has a preexisting mental disorder, does the evidence support that the alleged stressor aggravated the preexisting mental disorder?
8. Are there other factors that are causally related to the reported symptoms independent of the alleged stressor?

malpractice and personal injury litigation. In addition, the impact of DSM-5 substance use disorder criteria on civil litigation involving "addiction" is highlighted.

MEDICAL MALPRACTICE CLAIMS

Overview

Medical malpractice claims can involve intentional or unintentional torts. Examples of intentional torts that involve mental healthcare include assault (an attempt to inflict bodily injury), battery (touching without consent), false imprisonment, and violation of a person's civil rights. In some circumstances, failure to give informed consent regarding a medication's potential side effects can be considered a battery because the person's body was "touched" without their consent.

Negligent torts are often referred to as claims of malpractice (i.e., medical negligence). Negligent torts are the most common type of malpractice claim that involves patient care. The four elements required to establish medical negligence are generally known as the "four Ds." These are a *Dereliction* of *Duty* that *Directly* results in *Damages*. A duty is most commonly established for a clinician when the patient seeks treatment and treatment is provided. Dereliction of duty is usually the most difficult component of negligence for the plaintiff to establish. Two aspects of causation generally cited as establishing negligence in medical malpractice cases include the foreseeability of the harm and the clinician's role in directly causing the harm. *Damages* are the amount of money the plaintiff is awarded in a lawsuit.

DSM-5 and civil litigation related to risk assessment

Many malpractice claims involve an allegation that the patient was not appropriately diagnosed, which could be a dereliction of duty if proved true. Practitioners who fail to utilize the DSM-5 may face allegations (justly or unjustly) that they fell below the standard of care in making a diagnosis. In particular, a failure to appropriately diagnose may be linked to failures to identify and potentially treat mental health risk factors associated with an increased risk of suicide or violence. In DSM-IV, many disorders, such major depressive disorder and schizophrenia, included descriptions of suicide risk under the subheading "Associated Features and Disorders." This focus is expanded in DSM-5, with a separate subheading labeled "Suicide Risk" for 25 different mental disorders. Suicide risk was *not* emphasized in many of these disorders in DSM-IV. The subheading of Suicide Risk is different for each disorder, but it typically includes information about the level of risk associated with the disorder, common risk factors for suicide, and comorbid disorders that may further increase suicide risk. This information may impact civil litigation, particularly malpractice cases, because it demonstrates a greater focus in the DSM-5 on considering suicide risk in clinical practice and provides some guidance that attorneys may use as evidence of the "standard of care."

Although suicide risk was separated into a new subheading, discussions of violence risk remain relatively unchanged in DSM-5 compared to DSM-IV. Certain disorders, such as schizophrenia, provide information about violence risk in the subheading "Associated Features Supporting Diagnosis." These descriptions of violence risk are less consistently documented in the DSM-5 text and provide less guidance for the clinician or forensic evaluator than the text describing suicide risk.

DSM-5 and civil litigation related to prescribed medications

DSM-5 diagnostic categories specific to potential harms that may be caused by medications include medication-induced mental disorders and medication-induced movement disorders. These diagnostic categories are reviewed below, because they represent potential sources of malpractice claims against medication prescribers.

Medication-induced mental disorders

In DSM-5, there are two different types of medication-induced disorders described: those considered mental disorders (called substance/medication-induced) and those not considered as mental disorders (called medication-induced movement disorders and other adverse effects of medication). The medication-induced mental disorders include substance/medication–induced psychotic disorder, bipolar and related disorder, depressive disorder, anxiety disorder, obsessive-compulsive and related disorder, sleep disorder, and sexual dysfunction. Many of the medication-induced mental disorders were included under the "Substance-Induced" diagnostic category in DSM-IV.

In both DSM-IV and DSM-5, Criterion A describes mental health symptoms that must be present to make the diagnosis. Compared with other non-substance/medication-induced disorders in the same diagnostic categories, the substance/medication-induced mental disorders and their DSM-IV counterparts generally require fewer symptoms to establish the diagnosis. For example, the DSM-5 diagnosis of substance/medication-induced depressive disorder requires only that the person have a depressed mood or decreased enjoyment in most aspects of their life [4 (p175)]. As a result, fewer symptoms are needed to establish a substance/medication induced depressive disorder diagnosis compared with the Criterion A of major depressive disorder, which requires five depressive symptoms.

DSM-5 also retains the suggestion that medications may *cause* a mental disorder, an important element in civil litigation. The previous diagnosis of "Substance-Induced" mental disorder in DSM-IV included medications as a potential substance that may cause symptoms, but DSM-5 brings the word "medication" into the title of the diagnosis. Although many similarities exist between the previous diagnoses and the ones present in DSM-5, there are also multiple criteria changes that may impact their use in forensic psychiatry.

The first change in substance/medication-induced mental disorders is in the diagnostic categories themselves. DSM-5 separates obsessive-compulsive and related disorders out from anxiety disorders and similarly separates bipolar and related disorders and depressive disorders into their own categories, instead of using the general mood disorders designation. Because these are now separate entities, the substance/medication-induced mental disorders in these categories reflect a different diagnosis for each.

Second, in the transition from DSM-IV to DSM-5, some of the language of Criterion A in the substance/medication-induced mental disorders has changed, mainly to add or subtract mention of clinical significance of symptoms. Many of these changes are not particularly significant because both the DSM-IV and DSM-5 versions of these diagnoses retain Criterion E, which requires clinically significant distress or impairment. The exception to this is the diagnosis of substance/medication-induced psychotic disorder. In DSM-IV, if the person was aware that their substance use caused their hallucinations, then such hallucinations were not considered as one of the diagnostic criterion of substance-induced psychosis [5 (p342)]. However, this statement is not retained in DSM-5, indicating an expansion of the criteria to include hallucinations that the individual knows are caused by the substance or medication. DSM-IV also did not include Criterion E (i.e., impairment that negatively impacts an individual's clinical presentation or course) for the diagnosis of substance-induced psychotic disorder, but this criterion is present in the DSM-5 version.

The third major change is perhaps the most relevant to forensic psychiatry. In DSM-IV, Criterion B for the substance-induced mental disorders required only one of the following criteria:

1. The development of symptoms within 30 days of intoxication or withdrawal from substance use; *or*
2. The symptoms are considered causally connected to the substance use [5 (p409)].

DSM-5 now requires that the substance used must be able to cause the symptoms *and* to result in the development of symptoms within a brief period of time after substance use [4 (p175)].

These changes may affect the diagnosis of substance/medication-induced mental disorders in a significant way. A forensic evaluator now needs to provide both evidence of a medication's capability of producing a symptom and evidence that the symptom occurred around the time of exposure to the medication. Case reports alone are generally insufficient evidence by themselves to conclude that a medication causes a particular symptom.

The last major change in substance/medication-induced mental disorders is noted in Criterion C. Both the DSM-IV and DSM-5 use Criterion C to provide instructions as to how one may distinguish a substance or medication induced mental disorder from a primary mental disorder. However, DSM-5 removes the DSM-IV instruction that emphasized the need to consider the dose and duration of the substance to the symptom presentation [5 (p483)]. Unfortunately, this deletion ignores the reality that the dose and duration of the medication is often very relevant in considering the ability of the medication to induce symptoms.

Medication-induced movement disorders

The other set of medication-induced disorders described in DSM-5 are medication-induced movement disorders and other adverse effects of medication. This category was present in DSM-IV (called medication-induced movement disorders), although it was placed in the section labeled "Other Conditions That May Be a Focus of Clinical Attention." In DSM-5, the category of medication-induced movement disorders and other adverse effects of medication has been moved into its own section. Diagnoses in this section include neuroleptic-induced parkinsonism, other medication-induced parkinsonism, neuroleptic malignant syndrome, medication-induced acute dystonia, medication-induced acute akathisia, tardive dyskinesia, tardive dystonia, tardive akathisia, medication-induced postural tremor, other medication-induced movement disorder, and antidepressant discontinuation syndrome.

DSM-5 clearly documents that these medication-induced movement disorders are not mental disorders, which differentiates them from substance/medication-induced mental disorders. In addition, both DSM-IV and DSM-5 emphasize that attributing the symptoms of a movement disorder to medication use is challenging, particularly because some of these same movement disorders are observed in patients who have never taken a medication [4 (p709)].

The language used can be a critical distinction for a forensic evaluator, because the diagnosis alone does not necessarily mean the medication *caused* the symptoms described. This approach differs from substance/medication-induced mental disorders, which presume that the medication causes the described symptoms when making the diagnosis.

DSM-5 adds a new diagnosis to this section called antidepressant discontinuation syndrome. This diagnosis involves a cluster of specific symptoms that can present after a person has taken their antidepressant medication for at least 30 days without interruption and then suddenly stops taking the medication or significantly lowers the medication dose. DSM-5 also describes that these discontinuation symptoms usually occur within two to four days after stopping the medicine [4 (p712)].

DSM-5 notes that frequently reported symptoms of antidepressant discontinuation syndrome include experiencing flashes of light, "electric shock" sensations, nausea, a heightened sensitivity to noises or lights, nonspecific anxiety, and feelings of dread [4 (p713)]. DSM-5 emphasizes that to establish the diagnosis of antidepressant continuation syndrome, the evaluator should assess whether the reported symptoms were present before the antidepressant dosage was reduced and whether or not reported withdrawal symptoms are alleviated by restarting the same medication or starting a different medication that has a similar mechanism of action. In the diagnostic features section, DSM-5 indicates that unlike withdrawal syndromes from other substances, antidepressant discontinuation syndrome has no distinct symptoms, which distinguishes it from other substance withdrawal disorder diagnoses.

PERSONAL INJURY CLAIMS

Personal injury claims are wide-ranging and can involve claims that a person experienced emotional distress or a psychiatric injury (such as a mental disorder or diagnosis) as a result of an accident, sexual harassment, discrimination, or exposure to a toxic agent. The following vignette presents a typical case involving a person reportedly injured in a motor vehicle accident with the subsequent application of new DSM-5 criteria to consider when assessing his claims.

VIGNETTE

Mark is a 45-year-old married computer software sales representative who is leaving work when he is rear-ended by another car that is going less than 35 miles per hour. Mark is wearing his seat belt but his air bag does not deploy. He is able to get out of the car without assistance. He calls his wife to tell her that he has been in an accident and she becomes immediately emotionally distraught, wrongly believing that Mark was nearly killed and suffered great injuries. Mark is fully alert without evidence of any injury and with a Glasgow Coma Score of 15. Mark is taken to the emergency room where a computed tomography scan of the head is normal and his physical examination is completely unremarkable. He tells the emergency room physician that he did not lose consciousness or hit his head. Mark complains of back and neck pain and he is diagnosed with "neck and back strain." He is discharged home with instructions to follow up with his primary care provider, and a 10-day supply of diazepam and hydrocodone is provided. Over the next several days, Mark reports increasing back and neck pain with numbness and tingling in his legs. Over the subsequent two-year period, he undergoes repeated tests and various scans that do not find a cause for his leg numbness and weakness. One magnetic resonance imaging scan shows some potential narrowing of the vertebral columns, and Mark is told that he may have sustained "damage to his spinal cord." He believes this finding explains all of his symptoms, and he becomes extremely worried about its implications. He reports persistent severe pain, despite physical therapy and various medication trials. He spends a great deal of time visiting doctors and surgeons, and he is anxious he will never "return to normal." Mark is reluctant to go out with his family to dinner due to fear that he will "strain his back" and his pain will worsen.

Mark does not have any known prior history of mental health disorders. A review of Mark's history indicates that at the time of the accident, he also had multiple other life stressors, including serious marital problems. On the afternoon of the accident, just moments before he got into the car to leave work, he learned that his job was in jeopardy due to corporate downsizing.

Mark sues the insurance company of the driver who hit him for severe emotional distress. In his complaint, he alleges that he suffers severe pain, fatigue, dizziness, depression, nightmares of the accident, fear of driving, persistent headaches, numbness and tingling in his legs, and marked problems with his concentration and memory. He also reports that there has been a significant change in his personality, to include marked irritability and sudden mood changes. Mark recently resumed working in a job similar to his prior job, but he emphasizes that he has to exert greater effort to successfully perform his job duties.

Mark's reported symptoms are commonly seen in personal injury accident litigation and encompass a wide range of potential diagnoses. Those DSM-5 diagnoses that are particularly relevant when considering Mark's legal complaint are summarized below with a focus on DSM-5 diagnostic changes and/or additions to the DSM-IV.

Depressive disorders

Major depressive disorder criteria are essentially unchanged from DSM-IV, and the DSM-5 diagnosis of persistent depressive disorder includes the DSM-IV diagnoses of chronic major depressive disorder and dysthymic disorder. Although the evaluator will need to carefully determine whether Mark meets criteria for a DSM-5 depressive disorder, DSM-5 does not make substantial changes to this diagnostic category that warrants further discussion here.

Somatic symptom and related disorders

DSM-IV emphasized that somatoform disorders were characterized by the presence of physical symptoms when an underlying medical condition could *not* be determined. DSM-5 abandons this approach. Instead, the DSM-5 somatic symptom and related disorders focus on the distress or life disruption caused by the person's physical illness or their worries of becoming physically ill, *with or without* an identified medical cause. The DSM-IV diagnoses of somatization disorder, hypochondriasis, pain disorder, and undifferentiated somatoform disorder are replaced in DSM-5 by newly named or newly included disorders, which are summarized below and applied to Mark's case.

Somatic symptom disorder

In somatic symptom disorder, Criterion A describes that the person experiences one or more physical symptoms that cause distress or significant life disruption. Although persons with somatic symptom disorder often have multiple somatic symptoms, the DSM-5 highlights that the diagnosis can also be made if "only one severe symptom, most commonly pain, is present" [4 (p311)]. DSM-5 specifically notes that even if a medical cause cannot be found to explain the person's reported symptom, their presentation should nevertheless be considered as genuine. This particular statement does not take into consideration situations when there is no underlying medical condition and the person is malingering or feigning their physical symptoms. In this situation, their suffering would *not* be authentic, and the forensic evaluator needs to make this clear in their assessment. Furthermore, for unclear reasons, DSM-5 does not list either malingering or factitious disorder in the differential diagnosis of somatic symptom disorder, although both were noted in the differential diagnosis for the DSM-IV diagnoses of somatization disorder, undifferentiated somatoform disorder, and pain disorder.

Criterion B focuses on whether or not the person has experienced "excessive thoughts, feelings, or behaviors related to their somatic symptoms or associated health concerns" [4 (p311]. The qualifier "excessive" is not defined and is likely to have different subjective interpretations by examiners. In Mark's case, if he has been told that his narrowing of his vertebral columns is the cause of his pain, at what point does his spending time and energy to achieve pain relief become "excessive"? DSM-5 provides three presentations that indicate the individual is demonstrating "excessive" thoughts, feelings, or behaviors. These presentations include having a sustained and significant worry about one's medical condition, demonstrating a concern about the significance of one's health that is out of proportion to the clinical situation, and spending a large amount of time and effort related to one's perceived medical situation [4 (p311)].

When reviewing the above three presentations, both forensic evaluators and clinicians should attempt to quantify how much a person thinks about their symptoms, how much time and energy they spend related to their symptoms, and how much they worry about their symptoms. Structured assessments that rate the degree of anxiety a person experiences (e.g., Beck Anxiety Inventory [6]) may be useful adjuncts to the clinical examination.

DSM-5 includes the specifier "with predominant pain" for somatic symptom disorder [4 (p311]. As a result, the diagnosis of "somatic symptom disorder with predominant pain" is the effective equivalent of the DSM-IV pain disorder diagnosis. Based on Mark's presentation, he will likely qualify for somatic symptom disorder, with predominant pain if the evaluation indicates that he is not malingering or feigning.

Illness anxiety disorder

In contrast to somatic symptom disorder, the newly added DSM-5 illness anxiety disorder. Characteristics of this disorder include a person who becomes overly concerned with having a significant medical illness, even though he or she has minimal, if any, actual physical symptoms. In addition, the person's preoccupation with their risk for becoming ill is "clearly excessive or disproportionate" [14 (p315)]. As with somatic symptom disorder, the determination of when a person's preoccupation is "excessive" or "disproportionate" will likely involve some subjective interpretation. For example, consider the case of Jane, a 26-year-old woman who works in a fertilizer plant and is potentially exposed to toxic fumes after a plant explosion. Although her physical examination is normal, she repeatedly checks her body for any "rashes and lesions" and becomes highly anxious about her health, despite no evidence or symptoms to suggest she is ill. Would all examiners assess her behaviors as excessive and disproportionate? How does one determine the dividing line between normal concern and excessive worry?

In Mark's case, he will not likely meet criteria for illness anxiety disorder because he has multiple significant health complaints that are above and beyond the minimal somatic symptom limitation noted in illness anxiety disorder.

Conversion disorder

In DSM-5, conversion disorder is also named "functional neurological symptom disorder." In both the DSM-IV and DSM-5, individuals with conversion disorder typically present with symptoms that suggest altered motor or sensory function. However, DSM-5 has three important changes that impact how conversion disorder is now diagnosed. First, DSM-5 eliminates DSM-IV's requirement that the presenting symptoms must be related to an underlying psychological factor [5 (p498)]. No longer does the evaluator need to opine that a psychological factor, such as an overwhelming emotional stress, resulted in the person's sensory/motor loss. DSM-5 recognizes that conversion disorder symptoms may be associated with stress or trauma but specifically states that the diagnosis can be made even if no associated psychological issues is uncovered [4 (p320)]. Second, DSM-5 abandons the DSM-IV requirement that presented symptoms are not intentionally produced or feigned because of concerns that feigning cannot be reliably detected [4 (p320)]. However, unlike the diagnoses of somatic symptom disorder and illness anxiety disorder discussed above, DSM-5 includes factitious disorder and malingering in the differential diagnosis for conversion disorder. Third, DSM-5 emphasizes that to make a diagnosis of conversion disorder, the evaluator must establish that the symptom presentation is not consistent with any known medical or neurological disorder [4 (p318)]. To establish this criterion, the evaluator should carefully evaluate any presentation inconsistencies, particularly in civil litigation cases. Such inconsistencies include varying statements from the individual about the onset and nature of reported symptom, contradictory symptom presentations in the medical records, and inconsistent presentation of symptoms during the examination.

DSM-5 provides two specifiers for conversion disorder: "with psychological stressor" and "without psychological stressor." Although the use of the "with psychological stressor" specifier suggests that the stressor may have *caused* the conversion disorder, the DSM-5 text reads, "the *potential* etiological relevance of this stress or trauma may be *suggested* by a close temporal relationship" [4 (p320)] [emphasis added] The fact that there *may* be a potential relationship between a stressor and emotional outcome is not the same as establishing an *actual* causal relationship. Therefore, the examiner should not automatically assume that the litigated stressor caused the conversion disorder if one is diagnosed. In Mark's case, his marital stress and recent potential job loss could also account for his somatic and conversion disorder symptoms.

Psychological factors affecting other medical conditions

This disorder is newly placed in the DSM-5 chapter on Somatic Symptom and Related Disorders. In DSM-IV, this disorder was included under "Other Conditions that May be the Focus of Clinical Attention." Its move to Section II of DSM-5 elevates this condition to the status of a fully recognized mental disorder. In DSM-IV, this diagnosis emphasized how the presence of one or more psychological or behavioral factors could adversely impact a "general medical condition" [5 (p731)]. The DSM-5 text also comments that a connection between a person's medical presentation and underlying emotional issues should be logically linked, even if an actual association cannot be established [4 (p323)].

In the forensic context, this text indicates that the evaluator should have some credible data to link how psychological factors impact the person's medical condition. In Mark's case, it is unclear if and how psychological factors adversely affect his somatic symptom presentation. To help make this distinction, the evaluator assesses whether Mark's pain worsens *after* he experiences some psychological or behavioral symptom (such as being depressed, irritable, or angry). DSM-5 notes that in situations in which the person's psychological or behavior reaction occurs *in response to* the medical condition, the more appropriate diagnosis would be adjustment disorder. However, in

Mark's case, his intense focus and worry about his somatic symptoms and pain are more consistent with a diagnosis of somatic symptom disorder as opposed to an adjustment disorder alone.

The DSM-IV text focused on recognized medical conditions from a broad range of disease categories that may be adversely impacted by psychological factors. In contrast, DSM-5 Criterion A adds that a reported medical symptom alone is sufficient for purposes of making this diagnosis. As a result, this diagnosis is greatly expanded and includes not only specific medical disorders, such as asthma or stomach ulcers, but also general medical complaints, such as becoming easily tired, experiencing pain, or feeling light headed [4 (p322)]

Under this broadened definition, *unexplained* fatigue or pain is now considered a medical condition. To distinguish this presentation from somatic symptom disorder, DSM-5 notes that the individual suffering from the diagnosis of "psychological factors affecting other medical condition" does not present with excessive worries or anxious behaviors in regard to their physical complaint.

Factitious disorder

In DSM-IV, Factitious Disorder had its own separate chapter. DSM-5 has moved this disorder into the Somatic Symptom and Related Disorders chapter because of the predominance of somatic symptom complaints and presentation of the individual in medical settings. In addition, DSM-5 adds a D criterion, which emphasizes that factitious disorder cannot be diagnosed if the person meets criteria for another diagnosis, such as schizophrenia [4 (p324)]. Although Mark has sought out treatment with multiple medical personnel, there is no evidence from the record that he is taking surreptitious actions to cause his symptoms making a diagnosis of factitious disorder highly unlikely.

Trauma- and stressor-related disorders

Posttraumatic stress disorder

Traumatic events are a widespread phenomenon, with the vast majority of Americans exposed to at least one throughout their life [7]. In civil litigation, a plaintiff's exposure to a stressor is often alleged to have caused posttraumatic stress disorder (PTSD) or some other type of emotional distress or disorder. In reality, PTSD is an uncommon outcome for persons exposed to a traumatic stressor. In one study, only 23.6% of persons exposed to a traumatic event went on to develop PTSD [8].

PTSD was formally introduced as a diagnosis in the DSM-III [9]. PTSD Criterion A defines what constitutes a traumatic event, and this definition has evolved in its scope and language with the release of each DSM edition. Altering the definition of a traumatic stressor can change what type of trauma is sufficient to warrant a PTSD diagnosis. In the DSM-III, Criterion A describes that the stressor should not be one typically experienced in life and when experienced should be significantly upsetting to virtually all exposed [9 (p238)]. This definition was considered an "objective" standard because the traumatic event required to produce PTSD had to be distressing to most people (as opposed to a single individual). In contrast, the DSM-IV Criterion A highlights that the person is exposed to a situation that *they* believe could cause harm to themselves or others [5 (p467)]. This definition is considered a "subjective standard" because the focus is on how an individual person, not a group at large, perceives an event. Ameringen et al. [10] reviewed the impact of the DSM-IV altering the DSM-III A criterion and found that this wording change led to a 2% increase in the rate of PTSD diagnosis.

If past revisions to the DSM criteria can change the prevalence of PTSD, how might such changes impact the resulting legal aspects of being diagnosed with PTSD? Dr. Alan Stone famously stated that, "No diagnosis in the history of American psychiatry has had a more dramatic impact on law and social justice than post-traumatic stress disorder" [11]. Stone [11] proposed that the diagnosis of PTSD has far reaching aspects in both the criminal and civil arenas. For instance, Stone [11] writes that in civil litigation, the adding of PTSD to the DSM-III opened the door for damages of "purely psychic injury," whereas courts were previously reluctant to award damages without an accompanying tangible physical injury [11]. If the introduction of PTSD as a new mental disorder had such far reaching consequences, then what might be the impact of DSM-5's new PTSD diagnostic criteria on the frequency of PTSD claims in civil litigation? The following sections outline key criterion changes that the DSM-5 makes to the diagnosis of PTSD, which is now included in a separate section titled "Trauma- and Stressor-Related Disorders."

DSM-5 PTSD Criterion A: The traumatic stressor defined

Although there are multiple changes from DSM-IV to DSM-5, the presence of a trauma preceding symptoms continues to be a required criterion of PTSD. However, the definition of what constitutes a trauma has evolved with DSM-5 in meaningful ways. First, DSM-5 removes the requirement that the person experiences some intense emotional reaction or shock at the time of the event Friedman writes that presence or absence of a person's reaction is not predictive of PTSD outcome and therefore irrelevant in making a PTSD diagnosis [12].

Second, Criterion A adds "sexual violence" as a stressor in addition to the DSM-IV stressors that involved facing potential death or significant physical harm [4 (p271)]. Gone, however, is DSM-IV's wording that allowed a person to qualify as being exposed to a traumatic event if he or she experienced a "threat to the physical integrity of self or others" [5 (p467)]. This deletion may impact how frequently PTSD can be diagnosed in civil litigation cases that involve a sexual harassment claim. For example, under DSM-IV, a plaintiff alleging sexual harassment could claim that the alleged harasser represented a threat to their "physical integrity," even if there was no actual or threatened death or serious injury. Because the DSM-5 wording indicates that there must be actual or threatened death, serious injury, or sexual violence, cases in which this level of trauma exposure is not present (as is often seen in sexual harassment cases) will *not* likely qualify for PTSD. Furthermore, DSM-5 has added a diagnosis titled "Other problem related to employment" in the section titled "Other Conditions that May be a Focus of Clinical Attention" (a section that includes diagnoses that are *not* mental disorders). DSM-5 provides a range of work conditions considered as employment-related problems, and "sexual harassment on the job" is included among them [4 (p723)]. As a result of these DSM-5 diagnostic changes, an employee who reports emotional distress related to sexual harassment will more easily meet criteria for the diagnosis of "Other problem related to employment," as opposed to PTSD.

A third, and quite robust, change is the addition of two exposures that may qualify as a traumatic event (in addition to directly experiencing or witnessing the trauma). First, becoming aware that a close friend or family member experienced an incident that involves trauma or violence now qualifies as a potential exposure that can lead to PTSD. Second, individuals whose work may expose them to horrific outcomes of traumatic incidents may also qualify as having been exposed to a PTSD causing trauma, even if they were not personally in harm's way [4 (p271)]

These new trauma categories expand situations that qualify as a traumatic event and may lead to an increased number of individuals diagnosed with PTSD. With these new criteria, an individual can be diagnosed with PTSD without ever being present at the traumatic event. In Mark's case, the evaluator will try to determine if during his accident Mark was genuinely exposed to actual or threatened death or serious injury. With the new DSM-5 criteria, Mark's wife may now claim that when she learned of Mark's accident, she believed that his life had been threatened and he might die. Although DSM-5 expands the types of trauma exposures that qualify for a diagnosis of PTSD, these expansions are not without limits. In the case of learning about a traumatic event that occurred to a close family member or friend, the event must have been violent or traumatic. This restriction excludes the majority of deaths from natural causes; had this exclusion not been included, the number of individuals qualifying for traumatic event in Criterion A of DSM-5 would likely be much greater.

DSM-5 Criterion B: Presence of one or more intrusion symptoms

DSM-5 provides some changes in the criteria related to intrusive thoughts, which are enumerated in Criterion B, both in DSM-IV and DSM-5. In DSM-5, the DSM-IV term "distressing memories" is changed to "distressing recollections." DSM-5 specifies that these recollections are "involuntary" (a descriptor not included under DSM-IV), indicating that voluntary reflection of a traumatic event does not qualify as a PTSD symptom. DSM-5 rewords how distressing dreams are manifest, effectively expanding the range of dreams that satisfy this criterion. In particular, DSM-5 alters the description of recurrent, distressing dreams; previously, DSM-IV specified that the dreams were of the traumatic event. In DSM-5, the content and/or affect of the dreams are *related* to the traumatic event(s). This change expands the criteria to include dreams that have some relationship to the traumatic event, but dreaming only about the event itself is no longer required.

Flashbacks, a symptom that many associate with PTSD, are retained in DSM-5 as Criterion B3. In DSM-IV, flashbacks were described as acting or feeling as if the traumatic event was recurring, along with a sense of reliving the experience, illusions, and hallucinations. Interestingly, DSM-IV also included that flashbacks and the other symptoms in Criterion B3 could occur when the person awoke or when they were under the influence of a substance [5 (p468)]. By removing the description that symptoms could occur when intoxicated, DSM-5 further attempts to separate PTSD from comorbid substance use disorders. DSM-5 also emphasizes that flashbacks can range from mild to severe, and in their most extreme presentation, the person may no longer be aware of their actual environment [4 (p271)].

DSM-5 also broadens the definition of psychological distress when a person is confronted with reminders of the trauma In DSM-IV, psychological distress was required to be "intense" [5 (p468)]; DSM-5 describes that the distress can be "intense or prolonged" [4 (p271)]. This change extends the criteria to consider not only the intensity of the psychological distress, but also the time course.

Although DSM-5 widens some criteria that may result in PTSD being more easily diagnosed, there is also new wording that seems to narrow some criteria. For example, under DSM-IV, Criterion B5 required that the individual have some degree of physical reaction when exposed to traumatic reminders [5 (p468)]. DSM-5 adds the descriptor "marked" to the level of physiological activity, clearly indicating that a physical response upon trauma exposure must be significant rather than minimal or mild [4 (p272)].

DSM-5 Criterion C: Persistent avoidance of stimuli associated with the traumatic event(s)

DSM-5 includes only two avoidance symptoms under Criterion C, in contrast to DSM-IV, which included seven. The two remaining DSM-5 symptoms focus on a person's avoidance of upsetting "memories, thoughts, or feelings" that are associated with the trauma and avoidance of outside reminders that are associated with the trauma [4 (p271)]. Both of these symptoms are very similar to the first two avoidance symptoms listed under Criterion C in DSM-IV. However, DSM-5 eliminates the DSM-IV requirement that the individual feels numb and instead the focus is solely on evaluating the person's persistent avoidance of stimuli.

DSM-5 Criterion D: Negative alterations in cognition and mood

Although this criterion is new to DSM-5 and was not delineated under DSM-IV, five of the seven listed symptoms were included under DSM-IV's Criterion C. The five DSM-IV symptoms now moved to DSM-5 Criterion D include having trouble remembering key aspects of the trauma, continued or lasting pessimistic views about oneself or the surrounding world, decreased involvement in important life interests, and a sustained restricted ability to communicate pleasant feelings (such as caring for someone). The two newly added criteria include experiencing sustained adverse feelings (e.g., personal embarrassment related to the trauma) (and sustained altered thoughts and beliefs about factors resulting in the trauma or its outcome [(4 (p272)].

When reviewing the new DSM-5 criteria, several important comparisons between DSM-IV and DSM-5 become apparent. First, DSM-5 criteria D1, D5, and D6 are nearly identical to their DSM-IV Criterion C counterparts. Second, the DSM-IV equivalent to the DSM-5 D2 criterion described that the individual sensed they had a foreshortened future. The revised DSM-5 version expands such negative beliefs *beyond* the individual and now includes negative thoughts about others and the "the world" at large. However, the modifier "persistent" has been added when evaluating these beliefs, and this addition indicates that such thoughts are not brief or fleeting. Third, Criteria D3 and D4 are completely new to the DSM-5. Evaluators should now ask the individual about their personal feelings of guilt or responsibility related to the trauma and any persistent negative emotions they have experienced after the trauma. Finally, the DSM-5 D7 criterion modifies its DSM-IV equivalent by adding the modifier "persistent" when evaluating the extent of the individual's inability to experience positive emotions [(4 (p272–273)].

DSM-5 Criterion E: Marked alterations in arousal and reactivity

DSM-5 alters the arousal section to also include reactivity as part of the overall criterion, as well as noting that the arousal must be "marked." DSM-5 also clarifies that Criterion E symptoms must be related to the traumatic event; in DSM-IV, this relationship was not specified, but rather the symptoms simply had to begin after the trauma occurred. This change focuses the evaluation so that only deficits in arousal and reactivity that are specifically related to the trauma can be counted toward a PTSD diagnosis. As a result, the evaluator should carefully determine which reported symptoms are preexisting or unrelated to the traumatic event. Finally, DSM-5 adds self-harmful behaviors to this section, which was not previously present in DSM-IV [(4 (p272)].

Other DSM-5 PTSD components

DSM-5, like DSM-IV, requires that symptoms last at least one month to qualify for a PTSD diagnosis. In addition, DSM-5 maintains the DSM-IV requirement that PTSD difficulties impair a person's functioning in some aspect of their life [4 (p272)]. DSM-5 includes a new criterion that emphasizes that PTSD can not be diagnosed if the symptoms are due to an underlying medical illness or side effects of a substance. DSM-5 removes the specifiers of "acute" and "chronic" from the criteria for PTSD. Instead, DSM-5 adds a "with dissociative symptoms" specifier, which is used when an individual experiences ongoing or repeated symptoms of depersonalization or derealization. DSM-5 renames the specifier "with delayed onset" to "with delayed expression" [4 (p272)]. In the new criteria, delayed expression is given when the person does not meet full diagnostic criteria for PTSD until at least six months after the event. This change reflects that some PTSD symptoms may occur immediately but full expression of symptoms can be delayed. DSM-5 includes separate descriptors for PTSD for children six years or younger. Finally, for unclear reasons, DSM-5 has removed DSM-IV's consideration of malingering in the differential diagnosis of PTSD. Considering that PTSD is one of the most common diagnoses alleged in civil litigation, this elimination is ill advised, and the forensic evaluator should continue to carefully evaluate for the possible exaggeration or feigning of symptoms, particularly in a forensic context.

Acute stress disorder

Acute stress disorder is also listed in the Trauma-and Stressor-Related Disorders section and has the same A criterion as the DSM-5 diagnosis of

PTSD. DSM-5 made the following changes to the DSM-IV diagnosis of Acute Stress Disorder, in addition to the PTSD Criterion A change, outlined above. First, DSM-5 is much more specific in identifying specific symptoms that characterize acute stress disorder. Second, DSM-5 requires at least nine of 14 symptoms from any of the five identified categories (intrusion, negative mood, dissociation, avoidance, and arousal) that begin or worsen after the trauma exposure in order to make an acute stress disorder diagnosis. DSM-5 does not require a specific number of symptoms from *each* of the five categories-only a *total* of nine symptoms is required. As a result, a person can experience *no* arousal symptoms yet still meet criteria for acute stress disorder if they have sufficient symptoms in the other categories. Likewise, under this new diagnostic scheme, a person can experience *no* intrusion symptoms (e.g., distressing dreams, flashbacks, or prolonged distress upon exposure), yet still meet criteria for acute stress disorder. The forensic and clinical implication of this change is clear: there will likely be many different presentations of acute stress disorder when using DSM-5 diagnostic criteria.

In contrast, DSM-IV required at least three dissociative symptoms, at least one intrusion symptom, evidence of marked avoidance of stimuli that arouse recollections of the trauma, and marked symptoms of anxiety or increased arousal. DSM-IV was not as precise as DSM-5 in the specific number of symptoms necessary to make the diagnosis; however, DSM-IV required at least some symptom evidence in each category of dissociation, intrusion, avoidance, and anxiety or arousal. Third, the DSM-5 version removes the DSM-IV symptom that emphasized a decrease in emotional responsivity [5 (p471)] and replaces it with a "negative mood" symptom characterized by a sustained inability to have positive feelings, such as caring for others [4 (p281)]. Finally, under DSM-5, the duration of the symptoms must last at least three days (and no longer than one month) after trauma exposure, whereas DSM-IV only required that the symptoms last for two days (and no longer than one month).

Adjustment disorders

Adjustment disorders are now included in the "Trauma and Stressor-Related Disorders" section, whereas in DSM-IV they had their own chapter. The diagnostic criteria are essentially the same despite the geographic move to another chapter. However, two important changes in the text are noteworthy considerations. First, DSM-5 adds that a sustained and painful medical condition can be viewed as an ongoing stressor even if the trigger event (such as an automobile accident) has resolved [4 (p287)]. Second, DSM-5 more clearly states that an adjustment disorder can include symptoms typically considered associated with PTSD or acute stress disorder.

This newly added language specifically includes symptoms of either PTSD or acute stress disorder that do not meet criteria for either disorder [4 (p288)]. In Mark's case, he would likely meet criteria for an adjustment disorder (with mixed anxiety and depressed mood) in addition to somatic symptom disorder. In particular, he has some PTSD symptoms (i.e., nightmares) but not enough PTSD symptoms to meet the diagnosis. He also has depressive symptoms related to his unresolved pain that he believes is connected to the accident.

Neurocognitive disorders

As with many accidents that involve alleged head trauma, the possibility of a neurocognitive disorder must be carefully considered. DSM-5 lists two types of Neurocognitive Disorders: major neurocognitive disorder and minor neurocognitive disorder. Major neurocognitive disorder is the DSM-IV equivalent of Dementia. In DSM-IV, Dementia specified that the person had to have both memory impairment and at least one of four identified impairments (e.g., aphasia, apraxia, agnosia, or disturbances in executive functioning) to qualify for a diagnosis. In contrast, DSM-5 is less precise in how cognitive impairment is defined. For example, in regard to the diagnosis of major neurocognitive disorder, Criterion A notes that there must be a substantial decrease in at least one area of the person's functioning, such as their ability to learn or sustain attention [4 (p602)]. According to DSM-5, this cognitive decline must involve concern by the patient, someone who knows the patient, or the clinician that there has been a "significant decline in cognitive function" and a "substantial impairment in cognitive performance" [4 (p602)]. DSM-5 suggests that this impairment be documented by standard neuropsychological testing or another quantified clinical assessment, but it does not require any specific test. Under the DSM-5 structure, if cognitive deficits are identified, they must interfere with independence in everyday activities to qualify as a major neurocognitive disorder. Mark has not undergone any neuropsychological testing that indicates substantial impairment in cognitive performance, and he has been able to resume work, despite his complaints of pain. He is not likely to meet the criteria for major neurocognitive disorder.

Mark may meet criteria for the new DSM-5 diagnosis of mild neurocognitive disorder. In particular, he complains of memory loss and problems concentrating. In contrast to major neurocognitive disorder, mild neurocognitive disorder requires only a "modest" (as opposed to a substantial) cognitive decline and the cognitive deficits do not interfere with the person's capacity for independence in everyday activities. The evaluator will need to assess whether Mark's reported symptoms are genuine, result from another DSM5 disorder (such as depression), or are malingered. The evaluation to make this determination will likely involve a combination of neuropsychological testing, instruments designed to assess malingered cognitive impairment, and a structured clinical interview.

Personality change due to another medical condition

The DSM-5 diagnosis of personality change due to a medical condition is virtually identical to the DSM-IV diagnosis called "Personality Change Due to a General Medical Condition," and there are no new forensic implications for this diagnosis. The only minor change noted is the shift of this diagnosis from the DSM-IV section titled "Mental Disorders Due to a General Medical Condition" to the DSM-5 section titled "Personality Disorders."

SUBSTANCE USE DISORDERS AND CIVIL LITIGATION

Important DSM-5 changes related to substance use disorders are highlighted in Chapter 2. To quickly review, DSM-IV established a hierarchical relationship between the diagnosis of Substance Dependence and Substance Abuse, that is, a diagnosis of Substance Dependence excludes the diagnosis of Substance Abuse. It has been pointed out that this hierarchy has resulted in assumptions that Abuse is a milder form of Dependence, that all cases of Dependence also meet criteria for Abuse, and/or that Abuse is the prodrome of Dependence [13].

In DSM-5, the DSM-IV diagnoses of Substance Abuse and Substance Dependence are collapsed into one diagnosis called substance use disorder. DSM-5 codes substance use disorders according to their severity. Severity is based on the number of symptom criteria endorsed with a *mild* substance use disorder suggested by the presence of two to three symptoms, *moderate* by four to five symptoms, and *severe* by six or more symptoms [4 (p484)].

"Addiction," rather than "substance use disorder," is the term commonly used in a variety of medicolegal contexts. In civil litigation, examples include personal injury and wrongful death actions alleging that negligent prescribing practices or use of a manufactured product caused addiction, addiction-related comorbidity and death, accidental overdose, and suicide. Damage assessments in a wrongful death due to any cause may include consideration of the presence of addiction in the deceased and consideration of the person's potential future had the individual not died. Malpractice cases may allege impairment due to the physician's addiction, with resulting negligence causing damages. In addition, Medical Board actions against physicians can be based upon impairment resulting from addiction. Fraudulent nondisclosure of addiction may be alleged in a life-insurance case involving denial of benefits. Termination of parental rights, child custody, and parental access cases may be influenced by the diagnosis of addiction in a parent. Eligibility to adopt children may be harmed by an addiction diagnosis in a prospective parent. In employment settings, there may be allegations of wrongful termination or failure to accommodate on the basis of an addiction diagnosis, for example, to alcohol. Medical records including a diagnosis of addiction may create problems for job applicants to various governmental agencies and may undermine suitability to obtain security clearance in government or civilian occupations.

With so much attention to addiction in a variety of civil lawsuits, where in DSM-5 is the clinical disorder commonly referred to as "addiction"? The title of the overall section, "Substance-Related and Addictive Disorders," suggests that addiction is a diagnosis therein. For many years, the DSM-IV diagnosis of Substance Dependence has been conceptually and practically used as the equivalent of addiction. There is a long history of the disease or disorder of addiction described as a "dependence syndrome" [14–16]. Collapse of the DSM-IV Abuse and Dependence diagnoses into one diagnosis implies that the resulting DSM-5 Substance Use Disorder diagnosis is not the equivalent of "Substance Dependence" or "addiction." Perhaps to provide conceptual and practical continuity, DSM-5 offers some guidance in its text under the Substance Use Disorders section because it emphasizes that the word *addiction* is used in many countries to reflect the type of "severe problems" caused by the continued use of a substance [4 (p485)].

Based upon this text, the DSM-5 diagnosis equivalent to "addiction" would appear to be "severe substance use disorder."

Does a DSM-5 substance use disorder meet the manual's own definition of a distinct "mental disorder?" In its "Use of the Manual" section, DSM-5 notes that to establish a DSM-5 mental disorder, the person must actually meet the established criteria for a mental disorder. DSM-5 defines a mental disorder as "a syndrome characterized by clinically significant disturbance in an individual's cognition, emotion regulation or behavior." In addition, the DSM-5 highlights the importance of a "generic diagnostic criterion," which emphasizes that the mental disorder usually results in some type of impairment in the person's life [4 (p21)]. This "generic diagnostic criterion" is included as a requirement for many diagnoses (e.g., major depressive disorder, generalized anxiety disorder, PTSD, etc).

In exploring this issue for a DSM-5 substance use disorder, the descriptive text makes no mention of clinically significant distress or impairment. In the listings of criteria for the substance-specific use disorders, "Criterion A" refers to a "problematic pattern of alcohol use leading to clinically significant impairment or distress, *as manifested by* at least two of the following, occurring within a 12-month period" [4 (p490)] (emphasis added). Does this wording suggest that the presence of at least two of the criteria occurring within a 12-month period is, in and of itself, manifest evidence of clinically significant impairment of distress? This interpretation would seem to elevate the risk of false-positive diagnosis, if the criteria present are simply added up and the total compared with a threshold number. Alternatively, in addition to identifying the presence of the threshold number of criteria, must the diagnostician assess whether the disturbance causes clinically significant impairment or distress? This approach would appear to be in keeping with the DSM requirement that the diagnosis should meet the DSM-5 actual definition of a mental disorder. Guidance has been provided in an editorial by one of the Work Group members [17], who writes: "It is important to note that even the mild substance use disorder...can only be diagnosed in the context of significant impairment in life functioning or distress to the individual or those around them" [17 (p662)]. Thus, the presence of two or more criteria, assessed to be unaccompanied by clinically significant impairment or distress, would *not* be sufficient to make the diagnosis of a substance use disorder in DSM-5.

In judicial and legislative contexts, the diagnostic and conceptual discontinuity between DSM-IV and DSM-5 approach to substance use disorders may present problems, given that the previous DSM editions, including the DSM-IV, have been cited in court opinions more than 5500 times and in legislation more than 320 times [18]. Unlike the DSM-IV diagnosis of Substance Dependence, which has been more thoroughly researched and has been demonstrated to have excellent reliability and validity, the same is not yet true for the DSM-5 diagnosis of a substance use disorder. It has been noted that the DSM-5 field trials did not compare the DSM-IV and the DSM-5 prevalence rates for the same disorder through head-to-head diagnosis by the same clinician. Instead, the field trials relied primarily on academic medical centers with the most severe cases, rather than typical outpatient settings. Furthermore, there was an extraordinarily high rate of attrition among clinicians approved to participate in the field trials, no tests of predictive validity of the DSM-5 diagnoses were undertaken, planned tests of convergent validity were abandoned, and the threshold requirement for interrater reliability was lowered substantially [19, 20]. It has been predicted [21] that experts adopting the latest edition "will encounter criticisms related to the newness of and inexperience with DSM-5," whereas experts who choose to stick with the DSM-IV "will likely experience aspersions suggesting that their practice is antiquated and outdated" [21 (p240)]. Therefore, regardless of choice, the forensic expert may need a working knowledge of the issues relevant to DSM-IV and DSM-5, including the changes, rationale, research, criticisms, and the relationship of the new substance use disorder diagnosis to "dependence" and "addiction."

SUMMARY

DSM-5 has reorganized, added, and altered multiple diagnoses in the transition from the DSM-IV. Many of these changes may impact how claims of psychiatric injuries (to include emotional distress) are evaluated in malpractice, personal injury, and "addiction" civil litigation cases. Key summary points for this chapter include the following:

- Medication-induced mental disorders imply causation by virtue of the diagnosis, whereas medication-induced movement disorders may not.
- Somatic symptom disorder is an expansion of previous Somatoform Disorders and does not require the presence or absence of a medical condition to make the diagnosis.
- DSM-5 both expands and restricts different criteria for PTSD, which will likely affect different types of personal injury claims in various ways.
- Revisions to substance use disorders may not easily fit into previous concepts of addictions in the legal system, and the presence of clinically significant impairment is a factor evaluators may need to consider in using these diagnoses.

REFERENCES

1. US Census Bureau, Law Enforcement, Courts, and Prisons. *Total Incoming Caseloads in State Trial Courts by Case Category: 2008*. Washington, DC: US Census Bureau, Statistical Abstract of the United States; 2012.
2. US Census Bureau, Law Enforcement, Courts, and Prisons. *US District Courts—Civil Cases Filed, Terminated, and Pending by Basis of Jurisdiction and Nature of Suit: 2009 and 2010*. Washington, DC: US Census Bureau, Statistical Abstract of the United States; 2012.
3. Schubert FA. *Grilliot's Introduction to Law and the Legal System*. Boston, MA: Houghton Mifflin; 1996: pp 537–541.
4. American Psychiatric Association. *Diagnostic and Statistical Manual of Mental Disorders, Fifth Edition*. Arlington, VA: American Psychiatric Association; 2013.
5. American Psychiatric Association. *Diagnostic and Statistical Manual of Mental Disorders, Fourth Edition*, Text Revision. Washington, DC: American Psychiatric Association; 2000.
6. Beck AT, Epstein N, Brown G, Steer RA. An inventory for measuring clinical anxiety: Psychometric properties. *J Consult Clin Psyc* 1988; 56:893–897.
7. Breslau N. The epidemiology of trauma, PTSD, and other posttrauma-disorders. Trauma, *Violence, Abuse* 2009; 10:198–210.

8. Breslau N, Davis GC, Andreski P, Peterson E. Traumatic events and posttraumatic stress disorder in an urban population of young adults. *Arch Gen Psychiatry* 1991; 48:216–222.
9. American Psychiatric Association. *Diagnostic and Statistical Manual of Mental Disorders, Third Edition*. Washington, DC: American Psychiatric Association; 1980.
10. Ameringen MV, Mancini C, Patterson B. The impact of changing diagnostic criteria in posttraumatic stress disorder in a Canadian epidemiologic sample. *J Clin Psychiatry* 2011; 72:1034–1041.
11. Stone A. Post-traumatic stress disorder and the law: critical review of the new frontier. *Bull Am Acad Psychiatry Law* 1993; 21:23–36.
12. Friedman MJ. Finalizing PTSD in DSM-5: getting here from there and where to go next. *J Trauma Stress* 2013; 26:548–556.
13. Hasin DS, O'Brien CP, Auriacombe M, et al. DSM-5 criteria for substance use disorders: recommendations and rationale. *Am J Psychiatry* 2013; 170:834–851.
14. WHO Technical Report Series, No. 273, 1964 (Thirteenth report of WHO Expert Committee on Addiction-Producing Drugs).
15. Edwards G, Gross MM. Alcohol dependence: provisional description of a clinical syndrome. *Brit Med J* 1976; 1:1058–1061.
16. American Psychiatric Association. *Diagnostic and Statistical Manual of Mental Disorders, Third Edition*, Revised. Washington, DC: American Psychiatric Association; 1987.
17. Schuckit MA. Editor's corner: DSM-5—ready or not, here it comes. *J Stud Alcohol Drugs* 2013; 74:661–663.
18. Slovenko R. The DSM in litigation and legislation. *J Am Acad Psychiatry Law* 2011; 39:6–11.
19. Welch S, Klassen C, Borisova O, Clothier H. The DSM-5 controversies: how should psychologists respond. *Canadian Psychol* 2013; 54:166–175.
20. Jones KD. A critique of the DSM-5 field trials. *J Nerv Ment Dis* 2012; 200:517–519.
21. Wortzel HS. The DSM-5 and forensic psychiatry. *J Psychiatr Pract* 2013; 19:238–241.

CHAPTER 9

DSM-5 and Disability Evaluations

INTRODUCTION

Mental health providers are often asked to evaluate a person's disability, either in their role as a treatment provider or as a forensic evaluator. The definition of "disability" varies depending on the circumstances and context of the evaluation; in other words, there is no one unifying definition of what mental health symptoms make a person "disabled." When conducting psychiatric disability assessments, the evaluator should understand what type of disability evaluation is being requested, how disability is defined in that particular context, and what diagnostic tools or structured assessments, if any, are required for the examination.

Despite the range of disability definitions, they generally have one factor in common: a reliance and emphasis on using the Diagnostic and Statistical Manual (DSM). This chapter focuses on the relationship of the Diagnostic and Statistical Manual, Fifth Edition (DSM-5) to three common types of disability evaluations: workers' compensation claims, Americans with Disability Act (ADA) claims, and Social Security Disability Insurance (SSDI) evaluations. Many of these principles will also be relevant to private disability insurance evaluations, but these evaluations are not a focus of this chapter.

DSM-5 AND WORKERS' COMPENSATION CLAIMS

Similar to personal injury evaluations described in Chapter 8, workers' compensation evaluations require the evaluator to provide an opinion about a person's mental disorder in a legal setting. In contrast to personal injury evaluations, however, workers' compensation evaluations instruct the evaluator to provide opinions regarding several specific aspects of the injured worker's case, from determining whether the alleged psychiatric injury meets the state's criteria for causation, to assisting in the determination of the award to be given to the injured worker if a compensable permanent disability is present. Each component of assessment in workers' compensation requires the evaluator to understand the definitions as dictated by the state's Labor Code. This section describes the origin of the workers' compensation system in the United States, the necessary components required by the evaluator to assess the "claimant" who has filed a legal claim through the system, and the impact of DSM-5 on workers' compensation evaluations.

VIGNETTE

Mary Jones is a 45-year-old Caucasian woman, who has no previous history of mental illness. For 20 years, she has been working as an administrative executive for Global Exchange, a company that assists smaller companies with local and regional distribution of their products. Her duties include supervision of other administrative assistants in their activities, as well as some other administrative duties for managers in the company. Approximately six months ago, Ms. Jones suffered a physical injury at work, after falling on the ground while she was trying to sit in a chair that subsequently collapsed. She could not get up from the floor, and she was eventually transferred to a local hospital, where it was determined she had suffered from damage to her spine at L4-L5. She was taken off of work, and she received physical therapy, pain medication, and steroid injections to her back. Despite medical intervention, she continues to suffer from significant and continual pain, and a subsequent inability to return to work. She endorses that her "reason for living is work," and begins to suffer from symptoms consistent with major depressive disorder after she is no longer able to return to her job. She reports symptoms including daily feelings of depressed mood and loss of interest in activities, sleep impairment due to sadness, energy and concentration impairment, feelings of worthlessness, and thoughts of wanting to die. She has not received any treatment for her symptoms of depression.

Workers' compensation overview

Workers' compensation has been described as the nation's oldest social insurance program [1]. According to Mackenzie et al. [2], workers' compensation systems were developed to compensate employees for work-related injuries or illnesses. Compensation includes not only the cost of medical treatment but also temporary payment for lost wages and permanent disability payment for injuries that result in a decreased ability to compete in the job market.

Prior to the implementation of workers' compensation laws, individuals who suffered a work injury rendering them unable to work and requiring medical care had to sue their employer in civil court for compensation of lost wages and medical care [2]. Under this paradigm, the individual had to prove in court that the employer acted negligently against the employee and that this negligence was the predominant reason that the employee was injured. The employee faced significant hurdles under this course of action to include paying costly legal fees, finding compelling evidence to argue that the employer's negligence was responsible for the injury, and defending against claims that the employee contributed to their own injury. In the case vignette, Ms. Jones would have difficulty proving that her employer negligently caused her to fall from her chair and injure herself.

As an alternative to the civil litigation approach, each state developed workers' compensation programs that did not require the employee to overcome the hurdles described above. Instead, workers' compensation represents a "no fault" system that does not require the employee to establish that the employer was liable for their injury. This compromise approach guarantees employees compensation for injuries arising from and during their work and minimizes the employer's risk of costly litigation and unexpected financial awards [3]. Liability through the state workers' compensation system, then, is not a necessary standard to prove, and workers' compensation laws allow for the employee to file a claim without the need of an attorney.

However, the employee must still prove that they have suffered an injury as defined by the workers' compensation laws implemented in the employee's state. In California, Labor Code 3208.3 indicates that a qualifying injury is "any injury or disease arising out of the employment" [4]. In defining compensable mental health injuries, this Labor Code reads, "A psychiatric injury shall be compensable if it is a mental disorder which causes disability or need for medical treatment... in order to establish that a psychiatric injury is compensable, an employee shall demonstrate by a preponderance of the evidence that actual events of employment were predominant as to all causes combined of the psychiatric injury" [4].

In looking at Ms. Jones' situation, rather than attempting to prove her injury was the result of her employer's negligence, it would be easier for her to provide evidence that she suffered from a physical injury directly related to falling from her chair, and that her major depressive disorder predominantly arose from her physical injury.

PSYCHIATRIC CLAIMS UNDER WORKERS' COMPENSATION

There are three major types of psychiatric claims that an employee can bring under workers' compensation; these are summarized in Table 9-1.

Table 9-1. TYPES OF PSYCHIATRIC WORKERS' COMPENSATION CLAIMS

Claim	Definition
Physical-Mental	Physical injury (slip and fall) and resulting impairment causes mental illness (e.g., major depressive disorder).
Mental-Physical	PTSD from traumatic event (clerk being robbed at gunpoint) causes physical illness (heart attack).
Mental-Mental	Repeated stress from work (sexual harassment by a coworker) causes mental illness (generalized anxiety disorder).

The case vignette of Ms. Jones exemplifies one type of psychiatric claim commonly filed by workers' compensation claimants, that of "physical-mental" injury. In a physical-mental injury claim, the employee reports that a physical injury (i.e., Ms. Jones falling from her chair causing a back injury) leads to a mental injury (i.e., Ms. Jones' major depressive disorder). Physical-mental injuries are generally recognized as compensable workplace injuries [5]. In contrast to physical-mental injuries, mental-physical injuries occur when an employee experiences a stressful or emotional situation that results in a mental disorder with physical consequences [3]. An example of a mental-physical injury is illustrated in the case of an employee who experiences substantial anxiety after a major explosion at work that results in a heart attack and subsequent physical disability.

Mental-mental claims represent the third major type of psychiatric claim. Unlike the two prior examples of psychiatric claims, the mental-mental claim does not involve an actual physical injury [5]. Many states limit the scope of mental-mental claims under workers' compensation. For example, California restricts mental-mental claims by not allowing compensation "for a psychiatric injury if the injury was substantially caused by a lawful, nondiscriminatory, good faith personnel action" [4]. Noncompensatory good faith personnel actions include investigating possible employee misconduct, counseling the employee through meetings or memoranda, increasing workloads, reducing personnel, or changing management [6]. In California, if an employee alleges they suffer from generalized anxiety disorder as a result of having an increased workload and the increased workload is deemed a "good faith personnel action," the injured worker would not receive compensation.

Limitations of mental-mental claims are similar in other states. For example, Washington State Medical Examiner's Handbook notes that, "stress-related conditions (such as stress from financial difficulties, employment, claim management) are not compensable" [7]. According to the Colorado Mental Impairment Rating, mental-mental claims are compensable when they are caused by "a psychologically traumatic event that is generally outside of a worker's usual experience and would evoke significant symptoms of distress in any worker in similar circumstances" [8]. According to the State of Florida Labor Statute, "nothing... shall be construed to allow for payment of benefits... for mental or nervous injuries without an accompanying physical injury requiring medical treatment" [9].

Whether a mental-mental claim is accepted under specific requirements, or whether it is accepted at all, depends on the state in which the claim is filed. Therefore, the evaluator should review the labor code section of their state to find the definitions of compensability for this type of claim.

In addition to providing an opinion on whether the employee meets the statutory definition for a mental claim, the evaluator must address several additional issues, which are summarized in Table 9-2.

An opinion regarding temporary disability must be present, because individuals determined to be suffering from temporary impairment are entitled to temporary disability benefits [2]. If the claimant has received treatment for their symptoms, an opinion regarding whether the individual has received maximum medical improvement from treatment is necessary. Maximum medical improvement, also known as a determination that the individual is "permanent and stationary," is a finding in which the injured worker's condition has medically stabilized and the employee is not expected to improve further [2]. Those claimants assessed as having reached

Table 9-2. ISSUES TO ADDRESS IN WORKERS' COMPENSATION EVALUATIONS

Issue	Definition
Causation	Whether the injury was the predominant cause of the alleged injury.
Permanent and stationary	Also known as Maximum Medical Improvement (MMI). Whether the claimant has received maximal benefit from treatment.
Temporary disability	If the claimant has not reached MMI, whether they are currently temporarily or completely unable to work while they receive treatment.
Permanent disability	If the claimant has reached MMI, whether they suffer from a permanent partial or total disability that will not improve and will keep them partially or fully unable to work.
Apportionment	If the claimant has a permanent disability, whether factors either preexisting (prior mental illness) or subsequent issues (death in family after work injury) exacerbate the permanent injury and therefore should reduce permanent disability award value.
Future medical care	Whether additional psychiatric care will be needed to stabilize the permanent disability.

maximum medical improvement are no longer temporarily disabled, and they either have the ability to return to work or suffer from some amount of permanent disability. The Sixth Edition of the American Medical Association Guides to The Evaluation of Permanent Impairment notes that a condition is rated "permanent" when it is "not expected to change significantly over the next 12 months" [10 (p353)].

State workers' compensation programs have established instructions for the evaluator to assign a "disability rating" to quantify the employer's permanent disability presentation, which helps establish how much compensation the injured worker should receive. Each state varies as to how they approach assessing disability. Many states adopt the disability rating system as defined in the American Medical Association's Guides to the Evaluation of Permanent Impairment, Sixth Edition (AMA Guides), which uses three scales; the Brief Psychiatric Rating Scale (BPRS), the Global Assessment of Functioning Scale (GAF), and the Psychiatric Impairment Rating Scale (PIRS) [10]. After evaluating impairment based on all three scales and assigning a numerical impairment score for each, the evaluator is instructed to use the median (middle) value of the BPRS, GAF, and PIRS impairment scores, to determine a final impairment percentage. The final percentage, in turn, is used by the workers' compensation system to calculate a Whole Person Impairment number, which directly translates to a monetary amount.

California has adopted a different model for rating permanent disability. Adopted in January 2005, the California Schedule for Rating Permanent Disabilities [11] is a scale that translates the employee's GAF score to a Whole Person Impairment number (WPI). The WPI number is then used to determine a disability award.

Assuming Ms. Jones has received maximum medical improvement in regard to treatment, but she continues to suffer from psychiatric symptoms including continued depressed mood and loss of interest, and she is not able to perform chores around the house or interact appropriately with her husband, children, and friends, her current GAF could be considered to be 60. According to the California Schedule of Rating, then, her Whole Person Impairment would be 15, and the workers' compensation system would use this number to calculate Ms. Jones' permanent disability award.

Impact of DSM-5 on workers' compensation claims

DSM-5 has added approximately 15 mental disorders and has broadened the diagnostic criteria of some of the DSM-IV disorders. DSM-5 critics argue that these changes may over classify individuals in the general population and workplace as mentally ill when they are not [12]. When considering the impact of DSM-5 on workers' compensation claims, it is important to remember that the claimed mental disorder must have arisen out of and in the course of employment. Mental disorders that are typically not considered as causally related to the work environment include chronic psychotic disorders (e.g., schizophrenia), bipolar disorder, and neurodevelopmental disorders. The potential impact of DSM-5's diagnostic changes as related to those mental disorders typically used in workers' compensation claims is summarized below.

Adjustment disorders

Some states allow consideration of an adjustment disorder diagnosis in a workers' compensation claim. Under DSM-5, adjustment disorders no longer have a separate chapter and instead they are included in the section titled "Trauma- and Stressor-Related Disorders." Although DSM-5 diagnostic criteria for adjustment disorders are very similar to DSM-IV criteria, there are some interesting changes to the criteria that outline what symptoms and behaviors must be present in reaction to the stressor (e.g., B1 and B 2 criterion). In DSM-IV, the B1 criterion reads that symptoms and behavior are clinically significant when individual's emotional reaction is greater than anticipated based on the triggering incident [13 (p683)]. In DSM-5, the B1 criteria maintains most of this DSM-IV definition but also emphasizes that the evaluator should consider the impact of culture and environment on the individual's symptom course [14 (p286)]. The modified language in DSM-5 allows more subjective interpretation in evaluating an employee's distress by emphasizing contextual and cultural issues that may play a role in the employee's presentation. It is unclear how examiners will interpret this new diagnostic language and whether this new wording will result in an increase or decrease in those diagnosed with an adjustment disorder. Another text change is noted in criterion B2. In DSM-IV, B2 reads that the symptoms or behavior are clinically significant if they result in "significant impairment in social or occupational (academic) functioning" [13 (p683)], whereas DSM-5 B2 criterion adds "other important areas of functioning" to social or occupational impairment [14 (p286)]. This addition allows a more liberal consideration of other potential impairments, such as impairment in recreational activities or general activities of daily living. As a result, employees will more easily meet criteria for an adjustment disorder.

Somatic symptom and related disorders

DSM-5 made significant changes to DSM-IV mental disorders characterized by the presentation or concern about physical symptoms. Because many workers' compensation claims involve a workplace injury with a resulting or accompanying mental health component, the three following changes are particularly relevant when considering workers' compensation claims that involve physical symptoms. First, DSM-5 no longer includes the DSM-IV diagnosis of Pain Disorder. Instead, employees who experience injury pain that becomes a predominant focus of their attention will likely be diagnosed with a somatic symptom disorder. Somatic symptom disorder is a completely new DSM-5 diagnoses that may increase the number of compensable psychiatric injuries in the workplace [15]. According to the newly created diagnostic criteria, if an individual has one physical symptom for more than six months and is highly anxious about this symptom, he or she can be diagnosed with somatic symptom disorder [14 (p311)]. Somatic symptom disorder is most similar to the DSM-IV diagnosis of Hypochondriasis, which was not included in the DSM-5. Hypochondriasis required the *absence* of a known medical condition to make the diagnosis. In contrast, somatic symptom disorder can be diagnosed whether or not the person has an underlying condition. To illustrate, consider the case of Joe, an employee who experiences back pain for six months after he lifts a heavy box at work. If Joe becomes distressed and very anxious about his pain, he could be diagnosed with somatic symptom disorder and pursue workers' compensation for his associated mental injuries. The specifier "with predominant pain" would be given if pain is Joe's only symptom.

Second, DSM-5 has created a new diagnosis named "illness anxiety disorder." Characteristics of this disorder include a person who becomes overly concerned with having a significant medical illness, even though he or she has minimal, if any, actual physical symptoms [14 (p315)]. An employee who becomes fearful they may have been exposed to toxins in their work environment, and for six months is extremely anxious about developing cancer, would likely qualify for this diagnosis. Even if these fears are unreasonable, this employee may qualify for compensation.

Third, the diagnosis "psychological factors affecting other medical conditions" has been added as a mental disorder to DSM-5. The cardinal feature of this disorder is the presence of "one or more clinically significant psychological or behavioral factors that adversely affect a medical condition" [14 (p322)]. In DSM-IV, this diagnosis was listed under the section titled "Other Conditions that May Be a Focus of Clinical Attention" and was therefore not considered an actual mental disorder. Although a superficial review may suggest little difference between how this disorder is defined by the two manuals, there are some important wording changes. For example, DSM-5 notes that one way psychological or behavioral factors may adversely impact the individual is the development of "well-established" health risks [14 (p322)]. In contrast, DSM-IV required only that the person have "additional" health risks caused by psychological factors. As a result, the workers' compensation evaluator must determine whether the employee's associated health risks resulting from psychological or behavioral factors are ones that are "well established." Unlike DSM-IV, DSM-5 notes that this disorder *cannot* be made if the person's presentation is better accounted for by another DSM - 5 mental disorder [14 (p322)]. Therefore, the qualified medical examiner should also determine whether other diagnoses, such as panic disorder, major depressive disorder, or posttraumatic stress disorder, account for the employee's symptoms.

Posttraumatic stress disorder

DSM-5 changed several of the DSM-IV Posttraumatic Stress Disorder (PTSD) criteria, and additional details about these changes are provided in Chapters 2, 8, and 11. Under DSM-IV, an individual was diagnosed with PTSD only if they had experienced, witnessed, or were confronted with a traumatic event, and only if they experienced some adverse emotional response at the time the trauma occurred. The individual was also required to suffer from a specific number of symptoms from each of three additional criterion categories: one "re-experiencing" symptom, three or more "avoidance and numbing" symptoms, and two "arousal" symptoms [13]. In contrast, DSM-5 has expanded the definition of exposure to trauma, to include the situation in which an individual has received "aversive details of a traumatic event" [14 (p272)]. The need for a response of fear, helplessness, or horror in reaction to a stressor has been eliminated, and symptoms of "negative beliefs" and "angry outbursts" have been added [14].

These diagnostic changes allow presentations that would not have previously qualified for PTSD and may result in an increased number of employees diagnosed with PTSD as a result of their work environment. For example, a social worker who repeatedly hears details of child abuse from other social workers, experiences distressing dreams of child abuse, has difficulty sleeping, attempts to avoid exposure of child abuse reports by avoiding work, expresses negative beliefs about the world, and becomes physically aggressive towards others at work, may now be diagnosed with PTSD according to the DSM-5 criteria. Furthermore, as result of the diagnostic changes, problematic work behavior, characterized by missing work and physical aggression, could be characterized as a symptom of PTSD.

Mild neurocognitive disorder

The new DSM-5 disorder titled "mild neurocognitive disorder" carries the potential of labeling normal memory loss that occurs with aging as a mental illness [16]. An individual meets criteria for this disorder when there is clinical evidence of modest cognitive impairment and concern by the individual (or others) that a mild decline in cognitive function is present. According to the mild neurocognitive disorder diagnostic criteria, cognitive deficits must not be severe and must *not* interfere with the ability to do everyday tasks, such as paying bills or taking one's medication [14 (p505)]. Under this new diagnosis, the requirement for objective evidence of cognitive impairment is minimal. It is a reasonable conclusion that many employees will be able to claim they suffer from mild neurocognitive disorder with minimal difficulty. However, to receive workers' compensation, the employee will need to demonstrate how this disorder arose from their work environment. Cognitive deficits due to normal aging would not be expected to qualify.

Evaluating workers' compensation disability under DSM-5

The second major impact of DSM-5 on evaluating workers' compensation claims involves how permanent disability will be rated under this new diagnostic manual. DSM-5 has eliminated the GAF score as a disability rating measure. In those states that use the GAF scale for rating permanent disability, DSM-5 dramatically changes the way disability resulting from mental disorders can be measured. Evaluators who use DSM-5 in workers' compensation evaluations and are statutorily required to use the GAF rating system are faced with the dilemma of what to use in its absence. Evaluators who use the AMA Guides Sixth Edition for assessing and rating disability are also restricted because these AMA Guides specifically dictate that the GAF must be used in conjunction with the BPRS and PIRS to generate a percentage value.

DSM-5's elimination of the GAF scale may result in states that currently require a GAF score for workers' compensation evaluations ultimately changing this statutory requirement. Although this process is evolving, examiners are faced with three imperfect options. First, the examiner could use DSM-5 diagnostic criteria in rendering a diagnosis and report a GAF score, noting that the GAF is no longer included in DSM-5. Second, the evaluator could continue to use DSM-IV diagnostic criteria, which allows the use of a GAF score. Although the continued use of DSM-IV seemingly contradicts the need to use the most updated DSM, this option may be allowable in some jurisdictions depending on the statutory language. For example, California Labor Code §3208.3 reads,

> A psychiatric injury... is diagnosed using the terminology and criteria of the American Psychiatric Association's Diagnostic and Statistical Manual of Mental Disorders, Third Edition-Revised, or the terminology and diagnostic criteria of other psychiatric diagnostic manuals generally approved and accepted nationally by practitioners in the field of psychiatric medicine [4].

The direction for the evaluator to use "other diagnostic manuals" is presumably included to reflect allowance of future DSM volumes; however, as the law is specifically written, "other diagnostic manuals" could be interpreted to include the continued use of the older, "accepted" DSM-IV. Documented guidance from other state systems could also suggest that DSM-IV *should* be used. According to the Washington State Department Medical Examiners' Handbook, evaluators are instructed to "follow the format of all five Axes of the current Diagnostic and Statistical Manual of Mental Disorders (DSM) to report your diagnosis" [7]. Because an explicit instruction to use the DSM-5 is not currently present in workers' compensation laws, the evaluator could reasonably interpret existing and nonspecific laws as permitting the use of DSM-IV.

Second, the examiner could consider using DSM-5's proposed disability measure known as the World Health Organization Disability Assessment Schedule (WHODAS) 2.0. DSM-5 does not provide an officially adopted assessment of impairment to replace the GAF. Instead, DSM-5 has included the WHODAS 2.0 as a disability measurement proposed for future use. The WHODAS 2.0 is a self-report instrument that asks the individual to rate their level of disability in six life domains. According to the DSM 5, the WHODAS was included in Section III because "further study" was necessary [14 (p16)]. The statement that the WHODAS 2.0 needs to undergo "further study" indicates that it is not an official measurement of disability for individuals who suffer from psychiatric impairment.

However, investigation of the WHODAS 2.0 indicates that its use may be limited, even if it is eventually adopted by a future DSM. A significant concern involves the fact that the answers to the disability questions on the WHODAS are self-reported with answers indicating disability readily apparent [17]. If the examiner uses the WHODAS 2.0 self-report rating on disability, they must acknowledge the limitations of this instrument for the purposes of determining disability under workers' compensation.

Third, the examiner could utilize an alternate disability-rating instrument and explain why they chose to do so. Some states already allow for alternative methods of evaluating disability independent of a GAF score, and a detailed description is provided to assist evaluators looking for other approved disability evaluation schemes. For example, according to the Colorado Department of Labor and Employment's Permanent Impairment Rating Guidelines [18], once the evaluator has determined that a psychiatric permanent disability is present, four elements are to be rated. These areas include the employee's ability for Activities of Daily Living; Social Functioning; Thinking, Concentration and Judgment; and Adaptation to Stress. A numerical rating from 0 to 6, reflective of the level of severity of impairment, is assigned to each element, based on the evaluator's assessment of impairment severity of each element. After generating four numbers, the evaluator then takes the average of the two highest subcategory ratings to calculate a final number that represents overall impairment. Finally, the evaluator uses the number on the provided Category Conversion Table, to come up with the corresponding percentage that represents overall permanent impairment [18].

Regardless of how states modify their instructions for the evaluator to determine a disability rating, it is highly likely that a viable alternative strategy will eventually be implemented. Perhaps DSM-5's move away from using the GAF in impairment ratings will provide evaluators, and workers' compensation systems, an opportunity to improve upon disability rating in general.

THE AMERICANS WITH DISABILITIES ACT

The Americans with Disabilities Act (ADA) is federal legislation enacted in 1990 to protect the civil rights of individuals with disabilities in employment, State and local government services, public accommodations, commercial facilities, and transportation. The ADA provides a unique definition of disability. According to the ADA, a person is disabled when they have a "physical or mental impairment that substantially limits one or more major life activities of such individual; a record of such an impairment; or being regarded as having such an impairment" [19]. Under this definition, if a person has a qualifying current mental impairment, past mental impairment, or is wrongly believed to have a mental impairment, the ADA protects him or her from employment discrimination.

Mental impairment under the ADA

The ADA defines mental impairment as "any mental or psychological disorder, such as mental retardation, organic brain syndrome, emotional or mental illness, and specific learning disabilities" [20]. More recently, the ADA replaced the term "mental retardation" with the term "intellectual disability." The Equal Employment Opportunity Commission (EEOC) has an important relationship in both the enforcement of the ADA and in providing guidance for how the ADA definition of disability should be interpreted. The EEOC specifically notes the importance of using the DSM when evaluating mental impairment under the ADA. For example, in a document titled "EEOC Enforcement Guidance on the Americans with Disabilities Act and Psychiatric Disabilities," the EEOC writes, "The *current* [emphasis added] edition of the American Psychiatric Association's Diagnostic and Statistical Manual of Mental Disorders...is relevant for identifying these disorders" [21]. In addition, the EEOC has provided the following examples of "mental impairments" that qualify for disability consideration under the ADA: major depression, bipolar disorder; anxiety disorders (which includes panic disorder, obsessive compulsive disorders, and posttraumatic stress disorder); schizophrenia; and personality disorders [21]. The EEOC specifies that not all DSM conditions will qualify as a mental impairment for ADA purposes. For example, personality traits, such as poor judgment or a quick temper, will *not* qualify unless they are a manifestation of an underlying mental impairment.

Congress prohibits certain DSM diagnoses from ADA eligibility consideration. These excluded diagnoses include psychoactive substance use disorder resulting from current illegal use of drugs, compulsive gambling, kleptomania, pyromania, transvestism, transexualism, pedophilia, exhibitionism, voyeurism, gender identity disorder not resulting from physical impairments, and other sexual disorders [22]. In addition, the EEOC has commented that brief impairments due to an Adjustment Disorder may not be considered an impairment [21] nor do psychosocial problems (V and Z codes) qualify [23].

Employers may be concerned that new DSM-5 diagnoses or changes in prior DSM-IV diagnoses will greatly expand employee discrimination claims under the ADA. Some of the DSM-5 diagnostic changes most likely to impact future ADA evaluations are briefly summarized below.

Intellectual disability

The ADA utilizes the definition of intellectual disability provided by the American Association on Intellectual Association and Developmental Disabilities (AAIDD) [24]. According to the AAIDD, intellectual disability consists of three components: (1) an IQ below 70–75; (2) significant limitations in adaptive skill areas (e.g., conceptual, social, and practical adaptive skills); and (3) onset prior to age 18 [25]. DSM-5 defines intellectual disability as a disorder characterized by deficits in intellectual and adaptive functions that begin during the developmental period [14 (p33)]. Although these two definitions may seem nearly identical upon casual glance, there is in important distinction. In particular, DSM-5's definition does not require any cutoff IQ score to determine intellectual disability, in contrast to the definition of intellectual disability currently recommended for use by EEOC under the ADA. The DSM-5 text recognizes that intellectual functioning is usually measured with intelligence tests. However, under the new DSM-5 definition, a person could score *above* a recognized cutoff score to determine intellectual disability on testing but still be diagnosed with intellectual disability. In explaining this new approach, the DSM-5 emphasizes that IQ test scores are only estimates of a person's ability to function in real-life situations, and even those individuals with test scores above 70 may nevertheless experience significant problems with functioning in everyday life activities [14 (p37)].

DSM-5's definition of intellectual disability is significantly broader than DSM-IV's definition and the current definition provided by the ADA. Now employees who do *not* score below a recognized cutoff score for intellectual disability on testing may nevertheless be diagnosed with intellectual disability if they present evidence of impairment in at least one domain of adaptive functioning. DSM-5 provides conflicting guidance as to how extensive impairments in adaptive functioning must be to establish an intellectual disability diagnosis. In the outline of diagnostic criteria, DSM-5 notes that the adaptive deficits must limit functioning "across" "*multiple* environments", [14 (p33)] [emphasis added]. In contrast, the DSM-5 text notes that deficits in adaptive functioning are present when "at least *one* domain of adaptive functioning" is impaired to the degree that the person requires additional support to function" [14 (p37)].

For the person evaluating an ADA claim involving an intellectual disability, two important questions arise. (1) Which definition of intellectual disability is correct when evaluating an ADA claim-the ADA definition or the DSM-5 definition? As noted above, prior EEOC guidance states that the *current* DSM is relevant when making a diagnosis. However, DSM-5's diagnostic criteria conflicts with the EEOC's definition of intellectual disability used under the ADA. (2) If the evaluator uses DSM-5, must deficits in adaptive deficits limit functioning in one *or more than one* setting? These important questions are currently unanswered and likely to result in diagnostic confusion and contradictory results.

Social pragmatic communication disorder

Social pragmatic communication disorder (SPCD) is a new disorder in DSM-5 and included in the Neurodevelopmental Disorders section. This disorder is characterized by ongoing problems in the "social use of verbal and nonverbal communication" [14 (47)]. Would an employee who has difficulty with their verbal and nonverbal communication with others in the workplace potentially qualify for SPCD? Answer: likely not. In fact, the employee will have a relatively high hurdle to overcome to demonstrate that their interactions are due to SPCD. First, employees have to show they have deficits in *all* four of the following areas: social communication; problems with changing how one communicates based on the unique aspects of the listener; problems adhering to basic conversational principles (such as waiting one's turn to speak); or difficulties in making inferences or understanding vague nuances of language [14 (p47–48)]. To successfully make this claim, the employee will need to demonstrate that the symptoms began in the early developmental period and resulted in functional limitations in at least one major life activity. Individuals thought to be verbally clumsy or shy are unlikely to qualify for SPCD because the required communication impairment is more significant than being socially awkward or withdrawn.

Attention-deficit/hyperactivity disorder

Under DSM-5, employees are more likely to qualify for a diagnosis of Attention-Deficit/Hyperactivity Disorder (ADHD). For example, DSM-IV noted that to have a diagnosis of ADHD, there must be evidence of numerous inattentive or hyperactive symptoms prior to age seven [13 (p92)]. In contrast, DSM-5 only requires that inattentive or hyperactive symptoms are present prior to age 12 [14]. This easing of the diagnostic criteria allows more individuals to be diagnosed with ADHD and as a result may increase the number of employees who can now more easily pursue an ADA claim.

Depressive disorders

There are two diagnoses in DSM-5's section on Depressive Disorders that are particularly relevant to potential ADA claims: major depressive disorder and premenstrual dysphoric disorder. DSM-5 criteria for major depressive disorder are essentially the same as the DSM-IV criteria. However, DSM-5 has eliminated the DSM-IV "bereavement exclusion," which prevented one from being diagnosed with Major Depressive Disorder if his or her depressive symptoms were better accounted for by Bereavement. DSM-IV noted that bereavement involved a reaction to the death of a loved one and as a result, some individuals could have a psychiatric presentation similar to a Major Depressive Episode" [13 (p740–741)]. DSM-IV also stated that the diagnosis of Major Depressive Episode was not made unless the person continued to experience symptoms longer than two months following the loss. DSM-5 essentially eliminates this bereavement exclusion. As a result, employees who experience the death of a loved one with associated symptoms of depression within the first two months can be diagnosed with major depressive disorder. Because the ADA excludes V and Z codes from consideration as a qualifying mental impairment, employees previously diagnosed with bereavement would *not* have qualified as disabled under the ADA. Now, an employee can claim that their diagnosis of major depressive disorder, even when it results from the loss of a loved one, is a protected disability under the ADA. Whereas an employee with bereavement may have been granted only a relatively short time off of work based on the DSM-IV bereavement exclusion, the *same* employee with the *same* symptoms may now request an ongoing ADA accommodation for major depressive disorder.

Premenstrual dysphoric disorder (PMDD) is a completely new mental disorder in DSM-5. Women who suffer from at least five delineated symptoms for the majority of their menstrual cycles and experience "clinically significant distress" in one or more life activities can qualify for PMDD. Furthermore, DSM-5 specifically notes that PMDD may result in "decreased productivity and efficiency at *work*, school or home" [14 (p172)] [emphasis added]. It is unknown whether this new DSM-5 diagnosis will qualify as a protected disability under the ADA, and, if it does, what reasonable accommodations will be provided.

Hoarding disorder

Hoarding disorder is also new to DSM-5 and is included in the section titled "Obsessive-Compulsive and Related Disorders." Diagnostic criteria for hoarding disorder highlight that the individual has ongoing problems getting rid of their possessions and becomes upset when attempts are made to do so. DSM-5 provides specifiers that describe the person's level of insight into their hoarding behavior, ranging from "good or fair insight" to "with absent insight/delusional beliefs" [14 (p247)]. Imagine an employee whose desk becomes increasingly cluttered with numerous old documents that need to be discarded. The employee's workspace becomes an office eye sore and his supervisor repeatedly tells him to "clean up his mess." The employee ignores all instructions and his "mess" accumulates. The supervisor calls the employee into the office to initiate disciplinary action. Moments before doing so, the employee reports that he has been diagnosed with hoarding disorder, wishes to enter into the interactive process, and requests accommodations under the ADA. Because the EEOC includes Obsessive Compulsive Disorder as a possible disability under the ADA, this vignette outcome is not impossible to envision.

Posttraumatic stress disorder

DSM-5 diagnostic changes to PTSD have been outlined in detail in Chapters 2, 8, and 11 of this book and in the above section addressing workers' compensation claims. One additional point to review involves another aspect to the changed definition of traumatic stressor. In DSM-IV, PTSD required that the traumatic event involved exposure to "actual or threatened death or serious injury, or a threat to the physical integrity of self or others" [13 (p467)]. Under this definition, an employee could complain that he or she believed that they were exposed to workplace discrimination or sexual harassment that *threatened* their physical integrity. In contrast, DMS-5 notes that the exposure must be to "actual or threatened death, serious injury, or sexual violence" [14 (p271)]. This new language makes unpleasant, harassing, or difficult work situations alone unlikely to qualify as a PTSD traumatic stressor under the new DSM-5 criteria.

Binge-eating disorder

One new eating disorder, binge-eating disorder, may have interesting implications for possible future ADA claims as highlighted in the following vignette.

> VIGNETTE
>
> Michael is an overweight man with a body mass index (BMI) of 28 (normal BMI is 25 or less). He is not diagnosed as obese, which is generally defined as having a BMI of 30 or higher. However, Michael's doctor has told him he needs to lose weight for health reasons. He informs his employer that he would like additional time off of work to go to the gym and attend Weight Watchers meetings for his disability of being "overweight." His employer refuses noting that being overweight is not a recognized ADA disability. Although morbid and severe obesity (defined as greater than 100% of normal body weight) has been recognized as an ADA disability, being overweight has not [26].
>
> Michael is reading the DSM-5 over lunch one day when he realizes he may likely have a new mental disorder not excluded by the ADA, binge eating disorder. He tells his primary care physician that every Friday for the last three months, he has eaten more food compared to his coworkers when they go out for a weekly Friday lunch/work meeting at a local "all you can eat" Italian restaurant. He relates that he "woofs down his pasta" faster than he typically does at home, feels "stuffed," and when he returns to the office he is embarrassed and disgusted about his overeating. His doctor diagnoses him with binge eating disorder, and he submits documentation to his employer requesting accommodations for his disability.

Does Michael have a disability that now qualifies under the ADA? Under DSM-5, he may. Binge eating disorder is diagnosed when a person has repeated episodes of binge eating that occur at a minimum of once a week for at least three months. An episode of binge eating is characterized by eating more food in a distinct timeframe compared to what most people would eat in a similar timeframe and feeling an inability to control how much one eats when binging. In addition, the binge-eating episode must have at least three of the following four symptoms or behaviors: eating faster than usual; eating so much that the person feels uncomfortable; eating a lot of food even when the person has no appetite; and feeling ashamed or repulsed after the binge-eating episode. In contrast to bulimia nervosa, a person with binge-eating disorder does not take actions to prevent weight gain, such as using laxatives or inducing vomiting [14 (p350)]. The DSM-5 specifically notes that binge-eating disorder is usually associated with being overweight and obesity in persons who seek treatment [14 (p351)].

Based on Michael's presentation and his new diagnosis of binge-eating disorder, Michael could conceivable request that his employer provide him a reasonable accommodation for his new disability.

Substance use disorders and the ADA

As noted above, psychoactive substance use disorders resulting from current illegal use of drugs are excluded from coverage under the ADA. However, an employee who is no longer using illegal drugs and has completed a rehabilitation program or has been rehabilitated successfully from some other method would be protected by the ADA [27]. The EEOC also states that former drug addicts who have been successfully rehabilitated may be protected by the Act [28].

In contrast to illegal drug use, an employee who currently uses alcohol is not automatically excluded from ADA coverage. The EEOC Technical Assistance Manual includes a section titled "alcoholism" that explains this position. The EEOC Manual reads,

> While a current illegal user of drugs has no protection under the ADA if the employer acts on the basis of such use, a person who currently uses alcohol is not automatically denied protection simply because of the alcohol use. An alcoholic is a person with a disability under the ADA and may be entitled to consideration of accommodation, if s/he is qualified to perform the essential functions of a job. However, an employer may discipline, discharge or deny employment to an alcoholic whose use of alcohol adversely affects job performance or conduct to the extent that s/he is not "qualified" [28].

The language used by the ADA and EEOC that relates to substance use includes terms such as "drug addicts," "illegal user or drugs," and "alcoholic." Under the DSM-IV diagnostic scheme, Alcohol Dependence was an approximate equivalent for an "alcoholic" as was Drug Dependence for a drug addict. DSM-5 no longer separates substance abuse from substance dependence and instead combines the two into a single diagnosis of substance use disorder. In addition, DSM-5 specifically rejects the term "addiction" to be used as part of a DSM-5 substance use disorder diagnosis due to its unreliable definition and potential for establishing a negative bias against individuals [14 (p485)].

Although there are three severity ratings (i.e., mild, moderate, and severe) based on the number of diagnostic criteria met, what level of severity translates to a protected disability under the ADA? For example, does a mild or moderate alcohol use disorder equate with "alcoholism" protected by the ADA or must the individual have a severe alcohol use disorder? To date, the EEOC has not provided clarification on how the new DSM-5 criteria will translate into qualifying substance use disorders under the ADA.

Of additional interest is how the new diagnoses of cannabis withdrawal and caffeine withdrawal may result in an ADA claim. For example, because caffeine is not an illegal drug, would an employee who experiences caffeine withdrawal because they can not drink as much coffee at work as they do at home qualify for disability protection under the ADA? Would a reasonable accommodation from the employer include providing more coffee breaks? Likewise, in those states where cannabis is now legal to use, will some employees qualify as having a federally protected disability, whereas others do not based primarily on where they live?

Mild neurocognitive disorder

The new DSM-5 diagnosis "mild neurocognitive disorder" has been reviewed in multiple chapters in this book (e.g., Chapters 2, 7, and 11). In brief, this disorder requires a "modest cognitive decline" in previous functioning in one or more areas of cognition (such as learning or memory). Although these deficits may not interfere with the ability to complete complex activities, the DSM-5 notes, "greater effort, compensatory strategies, or accommodation may be required" [14 (p605)]. The Age Discrimination in Employment Act (ADEA) bans discrimination in the hiring practices of individuals 40 or older but does *not* require accommodations to accommodate older worker's cognitive deficits due to aging [29]. Perhaps employers will be required to provide assistance to employees with this "new diagnosis" whose difficulties with performing the essential functions of their job are related to normal effects of aging.

Evaluating ADA claims

Even if an employee meets criteria for an identified ADA *impairment*, a qualifying impairment alone does not establish that the worker has an ADA *disability*. As noted in the above statutory definition, the recognized impairment must

Table 9-3. QUESTIONS TO ASSESS ADA DISABILITY

1. Does the employee have an ADA qualifying impairment?
2. If yes, does this impairment substantially limit a major life activity?
3. If yes, what major life activity is limited and how is it impacted by the disability?
4. What are the essential functions of the employee's job?
5. Is the employee qualified for the job he or she has?
6. Is there a reasonable accommodation that can help the employee perform the essential functions of his or her job?
7. Can the employee do his or her job without an accommodation?
8. Can the employee do his or her job only with an accommodation?
9. What are specific accommodations that may assist the employee?

also substantially limit a major life activity. According to the EEOC, "substantially limits" is a lower standard than "severely or significantly restricts" or "prevents" [30]. In addition, the Americans with Disability Act Amendments Act of 2008 (ADAAAA) clarified that a substantial limitation in only *one* major life activity is required to meet the disability threshold [22]. The EEOC has provided a list of major life activities that include (but are not limited to) activities such as caring for oneself, performing manual tasks, seeing, hearing, eating, sleeping, speaking, learning, reading, concentrating, thinking, communicating, working, and interacting with others [30]. Table 9-3 provides questions that can assist the evaluator in assessing important components that constitute the definition of disability under the ADA. Finally, concerns about the use of the WHODAS 2.0 outlined in Chapter 3 and in a previous section of this chapter are also relevant when evaluating ADA claims.

DSM-5 AND SOCIAL SECURITY DISABILITY INSURANCE CLAIMS

The Social Security Administration (SSA) provides disability insurance through two programs: Supplemental Security Income (SSI) and Social Security Disability Insurance (SSDI). SSI is a means tested social welfare program designed to provide financial assistance to the needy, aged, blind, and disabled regardless of their work history. SSDI provides benefits to individuals who cannot work because they have a medical condition that is expected to last at least one year or result in death [31, 32]. This section focuses solely on DSM5's impact on SSDI disability claims.

In contrast to other types of disability compensation programs (e.g., workers' compensation and ADA claims), SSDI benefit eligibility requires that the person is *totally* disabled [32]. The SSA lists nine categories of mental disorders for adults and 11 categories for children that can be considered for SSDI eligibility. The SSA relies on the DSM in their listing of mental disorders for both adults and children. In their 2003 notice to address the revision of medical criteria for evaluating mental disorders, the SSA recommended the adoption of the most *current* DSM, which at that time was the DSM-IV-TR. This notice emphasizes the importance of the DSM in SSDI evaluations as illustrated in the following text:

> Many of our rules for adults are based on the American Psychiatric Association's Diagnostic and Statistical Manual of Mental Disorders, Third Edition . . . also called the DSM-III. That manual has been updated three times over the years since we first published comprehensive revisions of the adult mental disorder listings. Our childhood listings are based on the revision of the Third Edition (the DSM-III-R) . . . We want to update the terms in our listings so they are consistent with current medical terminology [33 (p12640)].

Further evidence of DSM's importance in regard to how the SSA defines mental disorders is demonstrated when SSA changed the diagnostic category named "mental retardation" to "intellectual disability." Among several reasons to explain this change, the SSA writes,

> The American Psychiatric Association (APA) is responsible for naming, defining, and describing mental disorders. In the fifth edition of the Diagnostic and Statistical Manual of Mental Disorders (DSM-5), the APA replaced "mental retardation" with "intellectual disability" . . . [34 (p46500)].

The SSA's specific citation of the DSM-5 indicates the likely importance that the DSM-5 will have moving forward with future claims. Although the SSA has previously commented that they want their diagnostic listings to be consistent with current terminology, their diagnostic listings for both adult and children do not yet match general diagnostic categories in the DSM-5 and still retain terms found in the DSM-III and the DSM-IIR. Table 9-4 outlines the nine SSA adult diagnostic categories with corresponding DSM-5 diagnoses.

When determining whether the SSDI applicant is eligibility for disability, the evaluator first determines whether the person has a mental health diagnosis that is included in the SSA's list of qualifying disorders. If so, the evaluator provides a description of the disorder (known as "Paragraph A") and lists functional limitations (known as "Paragraph B"). Four categories of functional limitations that require assessment under Paragraph B include: restriction of activities of daily living; difficulty in maintaining social functioning; deficiencies of concentration, persistence, or pace; and episodes of decompensation (each of extended duration). A final consideration involves a review of additional criteria ("Paragraph C") provided for certain disorders if the individual does not meet the severity requirements for "Paragraph B."

Table 9-4. SSA ADULT DIAGNOSTIC CATEGORIES AND PARALLEL DSM-5 DISORDERS

SSA Mental Disorder Listing	Parallel DSM-5 Mental Disorder
Organic Mental Disorder	Neurocognitive Disorder
Schizophrenia, paranoid, and other psychotic disorders	Schizophrenia Spectrum and Other Psychotic Disorders
Affective Disorders	Bipolar and Related Disorders
	Depressive Disorders
Intellectual Disability	Intellectual Disability
Anxiety-related disorders	Anxiety Disorders
	Obsessive-Compulsive and Related Disorders
	Trauma- and Stressor-Related Disorders
Somatoform disorders	Somatic Symptom and Related Disorders
Personality disorders	Personality Disorders
Substance addiction disorders	Substance-Related and Addictive Disorders
Autistic disorder and other pervasive developmental disorders	Neurodevelopmental Disorders

Will DSM-5's removal of the GAF significantly impact how an applicant's functioning is assessed for disability purposes? Unlikely. In fact, in their Administrative Message issued July 22, 2013, the SSA notes the following:

> We consider a GAF rating as opinion evidence. As with other opinion evidence, the extent to which an adjudicator can rely on the GAF rating as a measure of impairment severity and mental functioning depends on whether the GAF rating is consistent with other evidence, how familiar the rater is with the claimant, and the rater's expertise [35].

With the SSA's emphasis on maintaining currency with the most recent DSM-5 edition and the DSM-5's abandonment of the GAF to rate disability, the future use of the GAF in this setting seems somewhat limited. However, evaluators should continue to use specific evidence to support identified functional limitations rather than an over emphasis on any one rating tool. As outlined in the workers' compensation and ADA discussion, the WHODAS 2.0 has not been formally adopted by the DSM-5. An evaluator who uses this instrument should be aware of its strengths and limitations in rating a person's disability.

SUMMARY

Disability evaluations involve multiple considerations that are often unique to the specific type of disability assessment. However, for the majority of disability evaluations, they have one feature in common: they rely on the DSM for purposes of making a diagnosis. This chapter reviews potential implications of DSM-5 on workers' compensation evaluations, ADA evaluations, and SSDI evaluations. Key summary findings include the following:

- Workers' compensation is based on specific definitions of the individual states' Labor Code.
- Many states continue to require the use of the GAF score for determining a disability rating in workers' compensation evaluations, despite its abandonment by the DSM-5.
- Disability under the ADA requires not only the presence of a qualifying mental impairment, but also the demonstration that the impairment substantially limits the person in a major life activity.
- The WHODAS 2.0 is not a reasonable alternative to use in rating disability.
- The addition of new DMS-5 diagnoses and expansion of other diagnoses will potentially increase disability claims.

REFERENCES

1. Barth PS. *Compensating Workers for Permanent Partial Disabilities.* US Social Security Administration Office of Policy Social Security Bulletin 65(4). Washington, DC; 2003/2004.
2. MacKenzie D, Pitts R, Nagelberg S, et al. *State of California Department of Industrial Relations Industrial Medical Council Physician's Guide, 3rd ed.* San Francisco, CA: State of California Industrial Medical Council; 2001.
3. Drukteinis A. Workers' compensation evaluations. In: Gold LH, Vanderpool DL, eds. *Clinical Guide to Mental Disability Evaluations.* 1st ed. New York, NY: Springer Science+Business Media; 2013: pp 215–239.
4. Cal Labor Code §3208-3208.3, section (h) through (j).
5. Copeley L. Applicability of workers' compensation acts to mental disabilities: the plaintiff's perspective. Available at: http://cjglawfirm.com/wp-content/uploads/pdf/mental_disabilities_leto_copeley.pdf. Accessed 30 May 2014.
6. Schroth SN. Defending against the psychiatric injury claim-board panel defines "good faith personnel action" by employer. *The Workers' Compensation Newsletter.* October 1998. Available at: http://www.lflm.com/assets/files/pdf-articles/wcn1098b.PDF. Accessed 30 May 2014.

7. Washington State Department of Labor & Industries. Medical examiner's handbook. Available at: http://lni.wa.gov/IPUB/252-001-000.pdf. Published July 2013. Accessed 30 May 2014.
8. Colorado State Mental Impairment Rating, 2009. Available at: http://-coworkforce.com/dwc/physaccred/level%20ii%20accreditation/level%20ii/mental_impairment.pdf. Accessed 30 May 2014.
9. Fla Rev Stat ch 440, Title XXXI.
10. Rondinelli R, Genovese D, Katz R, et al., eds. *Guides to the Evaluation of Permanent Impairment. 6th ed.* Chicago, IL: American Medical Association; 2008: p 353.
11. California Labor Work Force and Development Agency, Department of Industrial Relations, Division of Workers' Compensation. Schedule for rating permanent disabilities under the provision of the labor code of the State of California. Available at: http://www.dir.ca.gov/dwc/pdr.pdf. January 2005. Accessed 30 May 2014.
12. Employers beware: psychiatry's latest diagnostic manual (DSM-5) creates new mental disorders, expands others. Available at: http://www.huntonlaborblog.com/2013/05/articles/ada-title-iii-and-state-disabl/employers-beware-psychiatrys-latest-diagnostic-manual-dsm5-creates-new-mental-disorders-expands-others. Updated May 20, 2013, Accessed 30 May 2014.
13. American Psychiatric Association. *Diagnostic and Statistical Manual of Mental Disorders.* 4th ed Text Revision. Washington, DC: American Psychiatric Association, 2000.
14. American Psychiatric Association. *Diagnostic and Statistical Manual of Mental Disorders.* Fifth Edition. Arlington, VA: American Psychiatric Association; 2013.
15. Chapman S. Somatic Symptom Disorder could capture millions more under health diagnosis. Available at: http://dxrevisionwatch.com/2012/05/26/somatic-symptom-disorder-could-capture-millions-more-under-mental-health-diagnosis/. Updated May 26, 2012. Accessed 30 May 2014.
16. Frances A. Opening Pandora's box: the 19 worst suggestions for DSM5. Psychiatric Times. February 11, 2010. Available at: http://www.psychiatrictimes.com/dsm/content/article/10168/1522341/. Accessed 25 February 2014.
17. Leckart B. DSM-5: assessing psych disability in PI and WC Cases. October 17, 2013. Available at: https://ww3.workcompcentral.com/columns/show/id/53e90d8c65fc3cee6f44d6cb441f8a82j. Accessed 30 May 2014.
18. Colorado Department of Labor and Employment, Division of Worker's Compensation. Workers' compensation rules of procedure: rule 12-permanent impairment rating guidelines. Available at: http://www.colorado.gov/cs/Satellite?blobcol=urldata&blobheader=application%2Fpdf&blobkey=id&blobtable=-MungoBlobs&blobwhere=1251894631025&ssbinary=true. Accessed 30 May 2014.
19. Americans with Disabilities Act, Pub. L. No. 101-336 (1990).
20. 29 CFR §1630 2(h((2)).
21. US Equal Employment Opportunity Commission, US Department of Justice, Civil Rights Division. EEOC enforcement guidance: the Americans with Disabilities Act and Psychiatric Disabilities. EEOC Notice No. 915.002; 1997. Available at: http//www.eeoc.gov/policy/docs/psych.html. Accessed 27 May 2014.

22. Scott CL. The Americans with Disabilities Act of 2008: implications for the forensic psychiatrist. *J Am Acad Psychiatry Law* 2010; 38:95–99.
23. Gold LH, Shuman DW. *Evaluating Mental Health Disability in the Workplace: Model, Process and Analysis*. New York, NY: Springer Publishing C; 2009.
24. Questions & answers about persons with intellectual disabilities in the workplace and the Americans with Disabilities Act (ADA). EEOC Web site. Available at: http://www.eeoc.gov/laws/types/intellectual_disabilities.cfm. Accessed 27 May 2014.
25. Definition of intellectual disability. AAIDD Web site. Available at: http://aaidd.org/intellectual-disability/definition#.U20-MijFkbA. Accessed 27 May 2014.
26. EEOC sues BAE systems for Disability Discrimination [press release]. Washington, DC: EEOC; September 27, 2011.
27. Illegal use of drugs and alcohol, 42 USC §12114(a) (1994).
28. Equal Employment Opportunity Commission, Technical Assistance Manual on the Employment Provisions (Title 1) of the Americans with Disabilities Act. Washington, DC: EEOC (1992).
29. Age Discrimination in Employment Act of 1967, 29 USC § 621-634 (1967).
30. U.S. Equal Employment Opportunity Commission, U.S. Department of Justice, Civil Rights Division. Regulations to implement the equal employment provision of the Americans with Disabilities Act, as amended, 29 C.F.R. Part 1630, RIN 3046-AA85. *Fed Regist* 2011; 76:16978–17017.
31. Social Security Administration. Disability benefits. Revised May 2014. Available at: http://www.ssa.gov/pubs/EN-05-10029.pdf. Accessed 30 May 2014.
32. Williams CD. Social Security Disability Income claims: treating mental health clinicians and consultative mental health examiners. In: Gold L, Vanderpool DL, eds. *Clinical Guide to Mental Disability Evaluations*. New York, NY: Springer; 2013: pp 185–213.
33. Revised medical criteria for evaluating mental disorders. *Fed Regist* 2003; 68:12639–12641. To be codified at 20 CFR §404 and §416.
34. Change in terminology: "mental retardation" to "intellectual disability." *Fed Regist* 2013; 78:46499–46501. Codified at 20 CFR §404 and §416.
35. The current use of GAF scores by the Social Security. Law offices of Tony Farmer and John Dreisser web site. Available at: http://farmerdreiser.wordpress.com/2013/10/26/the-current-use-of-gaf-scores-by-the-social-security/. Updated October 26, 2013. Accessed 30 May 2014.

CHAPTER 10
DSM-5 and Education Evaluations in School-Aged Children

INTRODUCTION

Education for children with disabilities has changed drastically over the past several decades. Today, more than six million children aged 3–21 with disabilities receive special education (approximately 13% of total enrollment). In stark comparison, as recently as 1970, only one in five children with disabilities was educated in U.S. schools. Numerous states had laws that specifically excluded certain students from public education, such as those who were emotionally disturbed, mentally retarded, deaf, or blind. As a result, many children and adults with disabilities were housed in state institutions where they were accommodated rather than thoroughly assessed or educated. Families were often not involved in the education process, and resources were not generally available to provide education within a disabled individual's community [1].

In 1975, Congress enacted the Individuals with Disabilities Education Act (IDEA), which fundamentally changed the landscape of education within the United States. The legislation guaranteed free, appropriate public education to each child with a disability in every state and local community across the country. The IDEA aimed to improve efforts to identify students with disabilities, educate these individuals appropriately, evaluate the success of these efforts, provide due process protection to children and their families, and provide financial resources for these programs and services. Since 1975, key amendments made to the IDEA have strengthened special education in the United States. Notable amendments have resulted in mandated extension of programs and services from birth to age 21, required transition plans and referrals as students transition out of the education system to postsecondary school enrollment or employment, increased neighborhood school involvement, increased partnership between schools and families as a result of more culturally relevant instruction, and improved quality of special education teachers and specialists. The accomplishments made as a result of the IDEA have been tremendous including the sheer number of individuals with disabilities who have received appropriate education, the significant improvement in graduation rates for those with disabilities, and the ongoing success of many individuals with disabilities in postsecondary school enrollment and employment [1].

FEDERAL AND STATE STATUTES

Individuals with Disabilities Education Act

At the federal level, the IDEA mandates that schools provide a free appropriate public education (FAPE) in the least restrictive environment (LRE) to all eligible students with disabilities. States are left to interpret these mandates and federal regulations and issue their own regulations on implementation. Individual school districts then develop plans for the delivery of special education to students with disabilities.

There are currently 13 disability categories for special education eligibility under the IDEA. The disability categories (as labeled by the IDEA) that are particularly relevant to the forensic evaluator when considering whether a mental health disorder impacts the student's functioning in the school setting include autism, emotional disturbance, mental retardation, other health impairments (which includes disorders such as Attention-Deficit/Hyperactivity Disorder (ADHD) and Tourette syndrome), specific learning disability, speech or language impairment, and traumatic brain injury.

KEY DSM-5 DIAGNOSTIC CHANGES AND IMPACT ON EDUCATIONAL EVALUATIONS

VIGNETTE

Alex is a 9-year-old boy previously diagnosed under the DSM-IV-TR with Asperger's Disorder. He is currently receiving special education services after satisfying the eligibility criteria of the Individuals with Disabilities Education Act (IDEA) under the category of Autism. He is currently in a regular class with a full-time aide who provides assistance particularly with his episodes of acting out in response to certain triggers. Initially, Alex functioned better between his episodic outbursts with an aide present. However, now his symptoms of inattention, hyperactivity, and impulsivity have led to continual disruptions to his class. His parents request an Individualized Education Plan (IEP) meeting because his grades have slipped from A's and B's to C's and D's. Under the DSM-IV-TR, Alex could not be diagnosed with both ADHD and Asperger's Disorder, which resulted in the school maintaining Asperger's Disorder as his sole diagnosis. More recently, Alex's parents have learned from other parents that there has been a significant change in how Asperger's Disorder is diagnosed, and they are concerned Alex may lose services under the new criteria. How might DSM-5 impact Alex's diagnosis and his eligibility for continued services?

With the publication of the Diagnostic and Statistical Manual of Mental Disorders, Fifth Edition (DSM-5) in 2013, mental health professionals, forensic evaluators, and educational professionals must address numerous changes from the DSM-IV, many of which are particularly relevant to children and adolescents. Notable DSM-5 changes that may affect educational evaluations include the diagnoses of autism spectrum disorder, intellectual disability, communication disorders, attention-deficit/hyperactivity disorder, specific learning disorder, depressive disorders, posttraumatic stress disorder ([PTSD] within trauma- and stressor-related disorders), and neurocognitive disorders (NCDs). Although these disorders are highlighted in this chapter due to significant changes in their diagnostic criteria, many other diagnoses (e.g., bipolar disorder, major depressive disorder, schizophrenia, and anxiety disorders) remain relevant to children and adolescents in an educational evaluation.

Autism spectrum disorder

Autism spectrum disorder (ASD) reflects one of the most significant DSM-5 diagnostic changes to DSM-IV-TR. DSM-IV-TR [2] had four distinct pervasive developmental disorders: Autistic Disorder, Asperger's Disorder, Childhood Disintegrative Disorder, and Pervasive Developmental Disorder Not Otherwise Specified (PDD NOS). In DSM-IV, the diagnosis of Autistic Disorder included three separate criterion required to make the diagnosis: (1) problems that involve social interchanges with others, (2) problems communicating with others (such as a having a language delay), and (3) "restricted repetitive and stereotyped patterns of behavior, interests, and activities" (RRBs) [2 (p75)]. In contrast, Asperger's Disorder required only two of these three descriptive criteria to make the diagnosis: problems interacting with others and RRBs. As a result, if someone had problems interacting with others and exhibited RRBs but *not* communication impairments, they would not qualify for a diagnosis of Autistic Disorder but would qualify for a diagnosis of Asperger's Disorder. DSM-5 provides one unifying diagnosis, autism spectrum disorder (ASD), which identifies deficits in "social communication and interaction" and "restricted, repetitive patterns of behavior" as the two major criteria categories [3 (p50)]. Although DSM-5 specifically notes that ASD encompasses disorders "previously referred to as early infantile autism, pervasive developmental disorder not otherwise specified, childhood disintegrative disorder, and Asperger's disorder" [3 (p53)], concerns have been raised that some children previously diagnosed under DSM-IV-TR with a PDD NOS or Asperger's Disorder will no longer be eligible for a neurodevelopmental disorder diagnosis under DSM-5. In the largest and most recent study to date, Huerta et al. [4] found that 91% of children with DSM-IV PDD diagnoses were diagnosed with ASD using the DSM-5, suggesting that ASD captures a substantial portion of the PDD population.

Critics of DSM-5's definition of ASD note several problems with this new diagnosis [5]. First, some of the DSM-5 language used to diagnose ASD is unclear. For example, Criterion A lists three examples of deficits in social communication and social interaction and instructs that such deficits are "manifested by the following, currently or by history" [3 (p50)]. However, this instruction does not indicate whether an individual requires symptoms from one, two, or all three domains of deficits to meet Criterion A requirements. In addition, Criterion A also notes that these examples are "illustrative not exhaustive" [3 (p50)], suggesting that examiners may use their own interpretation of what symptoms or behaviors qualify. Examining the requirements used to establish diagnostic criteria in field trials provides clarification on how Criterion A should be satisfied to make a DSM-5 diagnosis of ASD. In recent studies comparing DSM-5 criteria for ASD with DSM-IV criteria for the pervasive developmental disorders, researchers required at least one symptom from each of the three social communication and social interaction subdomains to be present [4, 6, 7]. Therefore, clinicians and forensic evaluators should require the same threshold of at least one symptom per social communication and social interaction domain to meet Criterion A for ASD to maintain consistency with how ASD has been diagnosed in research studies.

DSM-5 also describes that symptoms must be present in the "early developmental period" [3 (p50)], language that is again open to interpretation because development could arguably include a wide range of ages. The full DSM-5 text description of the development and course of ASD indicates more specifically that symptoms are typically recognized between 12 and 24 months of age (or later if symptoms are not obvious), and some features are evident at least in "early childhood" [3 (p55)]. The full text specifies that the presentation of autism spectrum disorder is most prominent during early childhood [3 (p56)]. For individuals who present for their first diagnosis of ASD in adulthood, the DSM-5 text indicates that the adult individual may be diagnosed if their clinical presentation is consistent with the diagnosis even if there is no evidence of impaired social and communication skills in childhood. A third challenge to the new wording used in DSM-5 for ASD is the notation that "individuals with a *well-established* DSM-IV diagnosis of autistic disorder, Asperger's disorder, or pervasive developmental disorder not otherwise specified should be given the diagnosis of autism spectrum disorder" [3 (p51)] (emphasis added). Concern has been raised that this language allows the clinician to decide whether to use either the DSM-IV-TR or DSM-5 to diagnose ASD [5, 8]. Of equal concern is the possibility that children with a well-established diagnosis of Asperger's Disorder prior to the publication of DSM-5 will be eligible for ASD, whereas children who would meet criteria for Asperger's Disorder after the publication of DSM-5 will not qualify because their Asperger's diagnosis is not "well- established." In Alex's case, he could be diagnosed with ASD based on the DSM-5 language that references inclusion of a prior diagnosis of Asperger's disorder.

Implications for DSM-5's definition of ASD remain unclear. A significant question involves whether the new diagnostic ASD criteria will impact the number of individuals eligible for special education services under the IDEA. The most important link allowing for disability eligibility under the IDEA is the direct impairment in learning and achievement as a result of an individual's autism or ASD. However, individuals with an autism diagnosis generally have an easier time establishing eligibility for disability under the IDEA [9]. Because some school districts limit eligibility for students diagnosed with Asperger's disorder or PDD NOS, having a unified diagnosis of ASD may increase eligibility for these affected individuals. Conversely, eligibility may decline for the individuals who would have met PDD NOS criteria but no longer meet criteria for ASD under DSM-5. Evidence suggests that those no longer meeting ASD criteria disproportionately met criteria for PDD NOS [8, 10, 11]. Many of these individuals may be reclassified into social communication disorder (see below), for which disability eligibility remains uncertain [12].

Diagnoses that DSM-5 notes are now included under the umbrella of ASD are listed in Table 10-1.

Table 10-1. DIAGNOSES INCLUDED UNDER AUTISM SPECTRUM DISORDER

Early infantile autism
Childhood autism
Kanner's autism
High-functioning autism
Atypical autism
Pervasive developmental disorder not otherwise specified
Childhood disintegrative disorder
Asperger's disorder

Intellectual disability

The DSM-5 diagnosis of intellectual disability replaces the DSM-IV-TR diagnosis of Mental Retardation. This DSM-5 change in terminology is reflective of terminology currently used by the World Health Organization's International Classification of Diseases, the American Association on Intellectual and Developmental Disabilities, and the U.S. Department of Education. A 2010 federal statute (Rosa's Law or Public Law 111-256) [13] replaces the term Mental Retardation with intellectual disability including within the language of IDEA. A significant change that comes with intellectual disability, as defined in DSM-5, is the new criterion that establishes the diagnosis and severity based primarily on adaptive functioning rather than the IQ test scores, although verification by both clinical assessment and individualized, standardized intelligence testing is still required. Intellectual disability is characterized by impairments of general mental abilities that affect adaptive functioning as defined in three domains (conceptual, social, and practical), and these impairments must begin in the developmental period (i.e., childhood and adolescence).

The new DSM-5 definition and emphasis on an individual's level of functioning is more in line with the IDEA definition of intellectual disability, which can only be established if the disability affects educational functioning. However, the new DSM-5 criteria may pose challenges for the evaluation. In particular, DSM-5 provides less guidance on intelligence test score ranges that qualify for a diagnosis of intellectual disability when compared with DSM-IV-TR's provision of specific IQ score ranges. Instead of an IQ level of 50–55 to approximately 70 to qualify for the DSM-IV-TR diagnosis of mental retardation, DSM-5 notes that individuals with intellectual disability have scores of approximately two standard deviations or more below the population mean. This language indicates that varying measures of IQ may result in varying IQ scores deemed by varying evaluators to qualify as intellectual deficits. DSM-5 further emphasizes that clinical training and judgment are required to interpret intelligence test results giving additional leeway to the examiner to determine whether intelligence testing deficits are alone sufficient to meet criteria for intellectual disability. In contrast to the DSM-IV-TR, the examiner rates whether the person meets criteria for intellectual disability and the severity of their intellectual disability (e.g., mild, moderate, severe, or profound) based primarily on the person's adaptive functioning. This important change in focus raises the following question: how should evaluators assess adaptive impairment within an educational setting?

DSM-5 gives some guidance on how to answer this question in a table included within the text. This table provides general examples of deficits for four severity levels of intellectual disability in conceptual, social, and practical domains. DSM-5 does not require any specific measure of adaptive functioning. Instead, the DSM-5 text indicates that adaptive functioning is assessed using "both clinical evaluation and individualized, culturally appropriate, psychometrically sound measures" [3 (p37)]. The American Academy of Child and Adolescent Psychiatry (AACAP) practice parameters for mental retardation note that there are standardized measures of adaptive functioning, such as the Vineland Adaptive Behavior Scale and the American Association for Mental Deficiency (AAMD) Adaptive Behavior Scales [14], but these instruments do not completely parallel the DSM-5 functional domains of impairment.

Communication disorders

Social (pragmatic) communication disorder (SCD) is a completely new DSM-5 diagnosis. The previous communication disorders included in the DSM-IV-TR were expressive language disorder, mixed receptive-expressive language disorder, phonological disorder, stuttering, and communication disorder not otherwise specified. The essential features of SCD involve ongoing problems in the "social use of verbal and nonverbal communication" in four areas: social communication; problems with changing how one communicates based on the unique aspects of the listener; problems adhering to basic conversational principles (such as waiting one's turn to speak); or difficulties in making inferences or understanding vague nuances of language [3 (p47–48)]. Like ASD, SCD requires impairment in social communication. Unlike ASD, SCD does not include restricted, repetitive patterns of behavior, interests or activities, and excludes the diagnosis of SCD if any evidence of restricted, repetitive patterns of behavior, interests or activities exist.

The new diagnosis of SCD may present potential challenges to the forensic evaluator. First, the language used to define the four categories of verbal and nonverbal communication is relatively vague with potentially wide ranging interpretations resulting. For example, Criterion A1 involves problems interacting socially with difficulties appropriately meeting others or volunteering information. Under a broad interpretation of this criterion, an oppositionally defiant child who does not politely greet his teacher when entering his classroom might be assessed by some as having difficulties in greeting and sharing information in accordance with the A1 SCD criterion. Likewise, social and pragmatic deficits are also common in other mental disorders, such as ADHD or conduct disorder [12]. To illustrate, individuals with ADHD are described as having difficulties taking turns or interrupting others, which overlaps with the SCD criterion A3 that reads, "difficulty for following rules for conversation and storytelling" [3 (p47)].

It is unclear whether the new SCD diagnosis will increase or decrease the number of children eligible for educational services. Those children who would have been diagnosed with PDD NOS under DSM-IV-TR may now meet the diagnosis of SCD. As a result, autism-related services that may have been provided to those with a PDD NOS diagnosis may not be deemed appropriate for those diagnosed with SCD. Instead, individuals with SCD may be eligible for special education services under the category of speech or language impairment. The IDEA defines speech or language impairment as, "a communication disorder, such as stuttering, impaired articulation, a language impairment, or a voice impairment, that adversely affects a child's educational performance" [15]. This definition does not specify issues in social pragmatic language, and whether or not individuals with SCD will now be classified in this category is important because of service-related interventions. In particular, evidence suggests that individuals eligible for disability under autism receive more robust services than those eligible under a speech or language impairment [12]. Alternatively, adding SCD to DSM-5 brings a sense of legitimacy to the diagnosis and may lead to increased awareness of an impairing disability and the need for more focused and effective treatments as well as individualized educational support. Effective treatments for SCD deficits and impaired pragmatic language skills [16] have been described [12], and the educational evaluator will play an important role in identifying this potentially treatable disorder and making appropriate recommendations.

Attention-deficit/hyperactivity disorder

ADHD is an important diagnosis to discuss because it is so frequently identified as an IDEA disability under the "other health impairment" category. Although the symptoms of inattention and hyperactivity-impulsivity remain the same, DSM-5 includes several important changes from DSM-IV-TR criteria for ADHD. Using DSM-5, symptoms must be present before the age of 12 years rather than 7 years as defined by DSM-IV-TR. DSM-5 lowers the threshold of symptoms (five instead of six) when diagnosed in adults, an important change reflecting research showing that ADHD symptoms can continue throughout adulthood for some individuals. Finally, DSM-5 no longer excludes individuals with ASD from being diagnosed with ADHD. Under the new criteria, Alex could now be diagnosed with both ASD and ADHD.

Significant concern has been raised that increasing the maximum age of symptom onset and lowering the threshold of symptoms for an adult ADHD diagnosis will increase the risk of overdiagnosis, potentially raising the prevalence of individuals who would qualify for special education services. For example, Thomas et al. [17] note that the DSM-5 changes to ADHD increase the risk that normal developmental processes, such as restlessness during puberty, will be confused with ADHD. However, in their study of 2232

British children, Polanczyk et al. [18] found that the prevalence of ADHD was increased by only 0.1% when the age of onset was increased from seven to 12 years.

Even if additional students are more accurately identified with ADHD using DSM-5 criteria, an increase in numbers could have a significant impact on access to special education services for children, older adolescents, and adults in educational settings. Likewise, DSM-5's formal recognition that individuals can have both ASD and ADHD may enhance service eligibility for those individuals who are functionally impaired by both conditions.

Specific learning disorder

Specific learning disorder is the most common disability in individuals who receive special education [19]. In DSM-5, the definition is broadened, unifying all learning disabilities under the diagnosis of specific learning disorder, rather than identifying three separate disorders of reading disorder, mathematics disorder, and disorder of written expression, as diagnosed under the DSM-IV-TR. Under DSM-5's specific learning disorder diagnosis, detailed specifiers distinguish between impairment in the areas of reading, mathematics, and written expression. Specific learning disorder is also characterized by persistent difficulties in reading, writing, arithmetic, or mathematical reasoning skills during formal years of school, and academic skills are substantially and quantifiably below those expected for the individual's chronological age.

Some changes to DSM-5's diagnosis of specific learning disorder are more similar to the IDEA definition. For example, specific learning disorder now specifies that the learning difficulties are not better accounted for by other disorders (such as intellectual disabilities, problems with hearing or seeing, lack of education, poverty, or any other mental or neurological disorder) [3 (p67)], which is congruent with the IDEA definition of specific learning disability. In addition, the DSM-5 no longer requires an aptitude (IQ)-achievement discrepancy, a change from the DSM-IV-TR that is much more in line with current research regarding methods of diagnosis for learning disorders [20]. However, DSM-5's requirement that learning deficits must be confirmed by individually administered standardized achievement measures and comprehensive clinical assessment for those age 16 or younger is stricter than the IDEA's definition of specific learning disorder.

Of note, the 2004 IDEA amendments expanded methods to identify students with specific learning disorders and no longer require demonstration of severe discrepancy between ability and achievement. Instead, the 2004 amendments to the IDEA encourage use of a response to intervention

(RTI) framework to identify students with specific learning disabilities and evaluate individual responses to increasingly intensive, scientific, and research-based interventions. However, RTI models remain widely variable, and the evaluator may find it helpful to be aware of the model [21]. The evaluator may also note that, although no longer required by either DSM-5 or the IDEA definition, IQ-achievement discrepancy is the most typically used method to identify children with learning disorder, particularly those with average achievement [22].

Depressive disorders

DSM-5 introduces a new diagnosis, disruptive mood dysregulation disorder (DMDD), which is relevant to the educational evaluator. DMDD characterizes the chronically irritable and temperamental child with severe and recurrent temper outbursts that go far beyond typical temper tantrums. DSM-5 specifies that the diagnosis should not be made for the first time prior to age six or after age 18, and symptoms appear before age 10. Although similarities exist between DMDD and oppositional defiant disorder (ODD) or bipolar disorder, DSM-5 attempts to distinguish these diagnoses. The full text description of DMDD explains that DMDD was added to DSM-5 to address concern about children presenting with chronic and persistent irritability versus the episodic mood symptoms of bipolar disorder [3 (p156–159)]. Given the alarming increase in bipolar diagnoses over the past couple decades [23], the inclusion of DMDD has the potential to lessen the frequency in which childhood bipolar disorder diagnoses are made.

Making the distinction between DMDD and ODD will likely be more challenging for the forensic or educational evaluator, and the DSM-5 DMDD criteria specify that these two diagnoses cannot coexist. If overlap occurs, DSM-5 instructs the evaluator or clinician to diagnose DMDD only. Whereas ODD describes a pattern of disobedience and defiant behavior towards authority figures, DMDD is considered more severe and requires a higher symptom threshold. However, what constitutes higher severity of DMDD from ODD is not clear from the diagnostic criteria. The Axelson et al. [24] 2012 study of 706 children could not distinguish a difference between DMDD and ODD or conduct disorder. Distinguishing between symptoms such as "severe recurrent temper outbursts" and "persistently irritable or angry" of DMDD [3 (p256)] from ODD symptoms such as "often loses temper," "is often touchy or easily annoyed," and "is often angry and resentful" [3 (p462)] relies on the subjective interpretation of the examiner. Copeland et al. [25] found that because primary DMDD symptoms are common, DMDD becomes a distinctive disorder only after frequency, duration, and cross-context criteria are applied. Therefore, the educational evaluator may more accurately diagnose DMDD using DSM-5 criteria for symptom frequency, duration, and cross-context criteria. For example, DMDD requires three or more temper outbursts per week, irritability nearly every day, a duration of 12 or more months, and the presence of symptoms in at least two of three settings. In contrast, ODD may only present in one setting, and symptoms need only occur once per week, "often," and over a period of at least six months. Unlike DMDD, conduct disorder requires only behavioral symptoms and does not require the presence of mood symptoms, such as irritability, to make the diagnosis.

Children and adolescents with DMDD may qualify for special education services through the IDEA if the disorder adversely affects the child's educational performance. The DMDD diagnosis would likely fall under the category of emotional disturbance, which includes presentations marked by "a general pervasive mood of unhappiness or depression" and "inappropriate types of behavior of feelings under normal circumstances" [15]. Although the prevalence of DMDD in a school environment (with resulting potential increase in special education services) is unknown, Copeland et al. [25] suggested a prevalence of DMDD close to 1%. Because children with conduct disorder alone may not be eligible for special education services as opposed to those with DMDD, evaluators will need to carefully distinguish between the two disorders to help determine those most appropriate special education services.

Posttraumatic stress disorder (within trauma- and stressor-related disorders)

Changes to the diagnosis of PTSD reflected in DSM-5 are relevant to all mental health professionals evaluating children and adolescents. In DSM-5, PTSD has been moved out of its prior inclusion under anxiety disorders and into its own category of trauma- and stressor-related disorders, highlighting the significant differences of trauma-related disorders from other disorders. To qualify for a PTSD diagnosis, the individual must be exposed to a traumatic event (including actual or threatened death, serious injury, or sexual violation), similarly to the DSM-IV-TR. However, the exposure can now include learning that the traumatic event occurred to a close family member or close friend. Another significant change is that children six years and younger are distinguished in DSM-5 with a detailed description and set of corresponding criteria. Notably, children six years and younger are required to have four listed symptoms versus six total symptoms as defined in DSM-5 for individuals older than six years and in DSM-IV-TR for all individuals [3 (p273)]. Also, symptoms are distributed slightly differently across clusters, indicating significant algorithmic differences between DSM-5 and DSM-IV-TR.

Evidence suggests that PTSD has been underdiagnosed in young children because the language and criteria used in DSM-IV-TR does not account for developmental differences in presentation [26]. For example, Scheeringa et al. [27] found that when DSM-IV and DSM-5 diagnostic criteria sets were applied to children ages three to six, the use of DSM-IV criteria led to significantly fewer PTSD cases compared with those diagnosed with DSM-5 criteria (13% versus 44%), and misclassified individuals were still highly symptomatic. Because an individual diagnosed with PTSD may qualify for special education, generally under the category of emotional disturbance or possibly other heath impairment ("heightened alertness to environmental stimuli"), the expanded DSM-5 PTSD diagnosis may lead to a significant increase in special education eligibility and request for services.

Neurocognitive disorders

Major or mild neurocognitive disorder due to traumatic brain injury is worth briefly describing due to its relevance to special education eligibility under the category of traumatic brain injury. Major neurocognitive disorder in DSM-5 replaces dementia in DSM-IV-TR, and it is similar in construct and definition. Mild neurocognitive disorder has been added to DSM-5 with the proviso by the American Psychiatric Association [3] that it may provide opportunities for early detection and treatment of cognitive decline before deficits progress. Although NCDs generally present much later than childhood or adolescence, major or mild neurocognitive disorder due to traumatic brain injury may present in childhood or adolescence if the traumatic brain injury was acquired during that time period. The inclusion of mild neurocognitive disorder and the language used to describe diagnostic criteria may present challenges to the forensic or educational evaluator. Although major neurocognitive disorder requires evidence of "significant cognitive decline," concern for "significant decline in cognitive function," "substantial impairment in cognitive performance," and interference with "independence in everyday activities" [3 (p602)], mild NCD requires only evidence of "modest cognitive decline," concern for "mild decline in cognitive function," "modest impairment in cognitive performance," and deficits that "do not interfere with capacity for independence in everyday activities" [3 (p605)]. This broad language used to describe mild NCD may leave evaluators uncertain as to how to best quantify these milder neurocognitive impairments. DSM-5 includes a table of neurocognitive domains with examples of symptoms, observations, and assessments that evaluators may find useful. However, no specific test or testing approach is required, although the text does describe that those individuals who qualify for mild NCD typically perform between 1 and 2 standard deviations below appropriate testing norms. The diagnosis of mild NCD does not require the level of cognitive deficits to interfere with the capacity for independence in everyday activities. In contrast, the IDEA-defined brain injury does require that the condition "adversely affects a child's educational performance" [15]. Therefore, do youth with mild NCD not qualify for services under IDEA? The answer to this question is uncertain.

Impact of DSM-5 on disability qualification and education accommodation

The overall impact of DSM-5 on disability qualification and education accommodations may have both positive and negative consequences. Disability qualification under the IDEA continues to be based on an individual's impairment in learning and achievement as directly linked to their disability. Therefore, individuals who currently receive special education services because of this educational impairment should continue to be eligible to receive special educational services. However, with many broadened diagnoses and several additional diagnoses to the DSM-5, more students with disabilities may be identified and deemed eligible for special education. In addition, more inclusive diagnoses with more subjective criteria may lead to inappropriate over diagnosing with inappropriate disability eligibility resulting.

Potentially positive impacts of DSM-5 as applied to students with disabilities are also important to consider. If new and changed diagnoses that are more relevant to children and adolescents are found over time to be more accurate, more individuals with functionally impairing disabilities may be identified and receive appropriate special education services. Greater accuracy of diagnosis may translate into more targeted and effective treatments and educational accommodations, which may have an overall positive effect on educational services. Treatments and accommodations that are more effective have the potential to ultimately decrease service need in some disabilities if the individual improves over time, requiring less educational and therapeutic services.

THE REHABILITATION ACT AND THE AMERICANS WITH DISABILITIES ACT

Although not the focus of this chapter, the educational evaluator should have a basic understanding of additional legislation relevant to students with disabilities. Whereas the IDEA is the education legislation that serves as the main vehicle for obtaining special education services, Section 504 of the Rehabilitation Act of 1973 [28] and Title II of the Americans with Disabilities Act of 1990 (Title II) [29] are civil rights statutes that protect individuals with disabilities. Section 504 applies to all federally funded schools and agencies, and it prohibits discrimination on the basis of disability in these settings. Title II of the ADA extends this prohibition of discrimination on the basis of disability to the full range of state and local government services, programs, and activities regardless of whether they receive federal funds. Section 504 serves to ensure that students with disabilities have equal access to educational services, programs, and activities as their nondisabled peers. Practically, Section 504 can be used to obtain reasonable school or classroom accommodations that would prevent discrimination within the school setting. Like the IDEA, Section 504 also requires school districts to provide a FAPE to qualified students. Unlike the IDEA, Section 504 does not allot for federal funds and is therefore not the primary statute used to obtain special education services. However, those students with disabilities who are not eligible for special education services under the IDEA may still be eligible for accommodations through Section 504.

SUMMARY

DSM-5 made substantial changes to prior DSM-IV-TR mental disorders and added new mental disorders. These changes are relevant to the educational evaluations of children and adolescents. Key summary points from this chapter include the following:

- The Individuals with Disabilities Education Act (IDEA), the main vehicle used for special education, mandates that schools provide a free appropriate public education (FAPE) in the least restrictive environment (LRE) to all eligible students with disabilities.
- Autism spectrum disorder reflects one of the most significant changes in the DSM-5 and has substantial implications for special education.
- Intellectual disability presents a new challenge in how to evaluate adaptive functioning.
- New diagnoses such as social communication disorder, disruptive mood dysregulation disorder, and mild neurocognitive disorder, as well as broadened criteria such as for ADHD and PTSD, raise questions of disability eligibility and concern that some children and adolescents may be over diagnosed.

REFERENCES

1. US Department of Education, Office of Special Education and Rehabilitative Services. *Thirty-five Years of Progress in Educating Children with Disabilities*

Through IDEA. Washington, DC: US Department of Education, Office of Special Education and Rehabilitative Services; 2010.

2. American Psychiatric Association. *Diagnostic and Statistical Manual of Mental Disorders, Fourth Edition*, Text Revision. Arlington, VA: American Psychiatric Association; 2000.
3. American Psychiatric Association. *Diagnostic and Statistical Manual of Mental Disorders, Fifth Edition*. Arlington, VA: American Psychiatric Association; 2013.
4. Huerta M, Bishop SL, Duncan A, et al. Application of DSM-5 criteria for autism spectrum disorder to three samples of children with DSM-IV diagnoses of pervasive developmental disorders. *Am J Psychiatry* 2012; 169:1056–1064.
5. Frances A. DSM-5 badly flunks the writing test. *Psychiatric Times*. Available at: http://www.psychiatrictimes.com/ dsm-5-badly-flunks-writing-test. Published June 11, 2013. Accessed 9 January 2014.
6. McPartland JC, Reichow B, Volkmar FR. Sensitivity and specificity of proposed DSM-5 diagnostic criteria for autism spectrum disorder. *J Am Acad Child Adolesc Psychiatry* 2012; 51:368–383.
7. Frazier TW, Youngstrom EA, Speer L, et al. Validation of proposed DSM-5 criteria for autism spectrum disorder. *J Am Acad Child Adolesc Psychiatry* 2012; 51:28–40.
8. Volkmar FR, McPartland JC. From Kanner to DSM-5: autism as an evolving diagnostic concept. *Annu Rev Clin Psychol* 2014; 10:8.1–8.20.
9. Ne'eman A, Kapp S. What are the stakes? An analysis of the impact of the DSM-5 draft autism criteria on law, policy and service provision. *Autistic Self Advocacy Network, Policy Brief.* 2012; 1–11. Available at: http://autisticadvocacy.org/wp-content/uploads/2012/06/DSM-5_Policy_Brief_ASAN_final.pdf. Accessed 12 May 2014.
10. Frances A. Will the DSM-5 reduce rates of autism? *Psychology Today*. 2012; Available at: http://www.psychologytoday.com/blog/dsm5-reduce-rates-autism. Published November 20, 2012. Accessed 8 January 2014.
11. Kulage KM, Smaldone AM, Cohn EG. How will DSM-5 affect autism diagnosis? A systematic literature review and meta-analysis. *J Autism Dev Disord* 2014; 44:1918–32.
12. Norbury CF. Practitioner review: social (pragmatic) communication disorder conceptualization, evidence and clinical implications. *J Child Psychol Psychiatry* 2014; 55:204–216.
13. Rosa's Law, Pub L No. 111-256, 124 stat. 2643 (2010).
14. Szymanski L, King BH. Practice parameters for the assessment and treatment of children, adolescents, and adults with mental retardation and comorbid mental disorders. *J Am Acad Child Adolesc Psychiatry* 1999; 38(12 Suppl):5S–31S.
15. Individuals with Disabilities Education Act, 20 USC §1400 *et seq.* (2004).
16. Volkmar F, Siegel M, Woodbury-Smith M, et al. Practice parameters for the assessment and treatment of children and adolescents with autism spectrum disorder. *J Am Acad Child Adolesc Psychiatry* 2014; 53:237–257.
17. Thomas R, Mitchell GK, Batstra L. Attention-deficit/hyperactivity disorder: are we helping or harming? *BMJ* 2013; 347(f6172):1–7.
18. Polanczyk G, Caspi A, Houts R, et al. Implications of extending the ADHD age-of-onset criterion to age 12: results from a prospectively studied birth cohert. *J Am Acad Child Adolesc Psychiatry* 2010; 49:210–216.

19. Snyder TD, Dillow SA. Digest of education statistics 2011 (NCES 2012-001). National Center for Education Statistics, Institute of Education Sciences, U.S. Department of Education. Washington, DC; 2012.
20. Scanlon D. Specific learning disability and its newest definition: which is comprehensive? and which is insufficient? *J Learn Disabil* 2013; 46:26–33.
21. Wishner J. Evaluations for special education. In: Benedek EP, Ash P, Scott CL, eds. *Principles and Practice of Child and Adolescent Forensic Mental Health.* Arlington, VA: American Psychiatric Publishing; 2010: pp 445–461.
22. Tannock R. Rethinking ADHD and LD in DSM-5: proposed changes in diagnostic criteria. *J Learn Disabil* 2013; 46:5–25.
23. Blader JC, Carlson GA. Increased rates of bipolar diagnoses among U.S. child, adolescent, and adult inpatients, 1996–2004. *Biol Psychiatry* 2007; 62:107–114.
24. Axelson D, Findling RL, Fristad MA, et al. Examining the proposed disruptive mood dysregulation disorder diagnosis in children in the longitudinal assessment of manic symptoms study. *J Clin Psychiatry* 2012; 73:1342–1350.
25. Copeland WE, Angold A, Costello EJ, Egger H. Prevalence, comorbidity, and correlates of DSM-5 proposed disruptive mood dysregulation disorder. *Am J Psychiatry* 2013; 170:173–179.
26. Nemeroff CB, Weinberger D, Rutter M, et al. DSM-5: a collection of psychiatrist views on the changes, controversies, and future directions. *BMC Med* 2013; 11:202–221.
27. Scheeringa MS, Myers L, Putnam FW, Zeanah CH. Diagnosing PTSD in early childhood: an empirical assessment of four approaches. *J Trauma Stress* 2012; 25:359–367.
28. Section 504 of the Rehabilitation Act of 1973, 29 USC §794 (2002).
29. Americans with Disabilities Act of 1990, 42 USC §12101 (2004).

CHAPTER 11
DSM-5 and Malingering

INTRODUCTION

The assessment of malingering is a critical component of a forensic evaluation, where external incentives can be substantial. To the chagrin of many in the legal and medical professions, malingering was removed from the index in DSM-5. However, in the text of the manual, the criteria for when to consider malingering remain unchanged. In the now-familiar wording, DSM-5 guidelines for when to suspect malingering include the presence of any two of the following: (1) assessments that occur during criminal or civil litigation; (2) when the person's reported symptoms or impairment are not consistent with collateral information or testing; (3) when the individual is uncooperative with the evaluation or prescribed treatments; and (4) co-occurring antisocial personality disorder [1 (p727)]. In a companion book titled "The Pocket Guide to the DSM-5 Diagnostic Exam," Nussbaum [2] provides six steps for arriving at a differential diagnosis. Step 1 is to "Always consider if a patient is intentionally producing findings" [2 (p199)]. This chapter covers the changes made to those DSM diagnoses that may increase the likelihood of feigning, with recommendations provided for the use of structured assessments of malingering, if available.

With all psychiatric disorders, clinicians rely on the self-report of their patients to accurately diagnose and subsequently treat such disorders. When patients misrepresent their symptoms–either consciously or unconsciously–clinician's jobs become substantially more challenging. Malingering is one such circumstance. The American Heritage Dictionary of the English Language defines malingering as "to feign illness or other incapacity in order to avoid duty or work." The American Psychiatric Association provides a more specific definition: malingering is "the intentional production of false or grossly exaggerated physical or psychological symptoms motivated by external incentives" [1 (p726)], a definition left unchanged from DSM-IV TR [3]. In the psychiatric setting, that external incentive can include the procurement of financial compensation (legal settlements, worker's compensation, disability benefits); the obtainment of prescription medications; access to a hospital bed; or avoidance of incarceration.

MALINGERING AND DSM-5 SOMATOFORM DISORDERS

Malingering was most prominent in the differential of somatic disorders, where physical symptoms were the primary presentation. In DSM-IV-TR, malingering was included in the differential of four (of the seven) somatoform disorders: somatization disorder, undifferentiated somatoform disorder, conversion disorder, and pain disorder. In each of these diagnoses, one criterion was that the symptoms were not intentionally produced. For factitious disorder, a separate category in DSM-IV-TR, the clinician was required to determine whether an external incentive existed in order to distinguish this diagnosis from malingering. The motivation for factitious disorder was "to assume the sick role" [(3 p517)], requiring the clinician to delve into the unconscious. In 2001, Feldman et al. [4] suggested that somatoform disorders, factitious disorder, and malingering should be viewed as lying on a continuum, rather than representing discrete entities. They proposed using the concept of factitious illness behavior, which others call abnormal illness-affirming behavior. Factitious illness behavior is defined as "sick role behavior that is not motivated by the desire to maintain or restore physical or mental health" [4 (p130)]. Feldman et al. [4] suggests that there is no scientific basis for attempting to determine whether a symptom is consciously or unconsciously produced and whether or not the motive is for external gain. He suggests that such behavior should be viewed as related to cognitive and motivational factors. This proposal may be one reason the motivational criterion for most somatic disorders was removed from DSM-5.

Enter DSM-5: somatoform disorders disappeared, replaced by "somatic symptom and related disorders," one of which is factitious disorder. No longer afforded its own category, factitious disorder is distinguished from other somatic symptom disorders by the criterion that *deception* is present absent external incentives. Motivations are no longer a part of any of the somatic symptom disorders, and there is no expectation that the clinician distinguish conscious from unconscious motivations. Somatic symptom disorder replaces somatization disorder and undifferentiated somatoform disorder, although the criteria are substantially different. In somatization disorder, the criteria were based on a history of numerous physical complaints (eight from four different categories), as well as the criterion that the symptoms could not be explained by a known medical condition. The criteria for somatic symptom disorder are that the symptom is distressing and/or disruptive and the individual thinks about the symptom excessively.

Malingering was removed from the differential, and the criterion that symptoms were not intentionally produced disappeared. Illness anxiety disorder, new to DSM-5, appears to replace hypochondriasis, because preoccupation and anxiety about seemingly imagined symptoms are the primary criteria. As in somatic symptom disorder, malingering is not included in the differential. However, the text states, that the majority of people who would have been diagnosed with Hypochondriasis under DSM-IV will be diagnosed with somatic symptom disorder under DSM-5 [1 (p315)]. In confusing contrast to this, in the section "Highlights of changes from DSM-IV to DSM-5," the text describes that hypochondriasis is now most often diagnosed as illness anxiety disorder; somatization disorder is now most often diagnosed as somatic symptom disorder [1 (p813)]. It is unclear which statement is accurate, and it appears that the only difference between somatic symptom disorder and illness anxiety disorder is the degree of actual symptoms.

Conversion disorder remains in DSM-5, but removed is the criterion that psychological factors are associated with the symptom. Although not in the criteria, malingering and factitious disorder are specifically mentioned in the differential diagnoses section. In particular, the DSM-5 texts cautions that the evaluator is not required to prove that the individual is *not* feigning symptoms because of the inherent unreliability in substantiating an individual's conscious intent. However, the text also notes that definite feigning likely indicates that the person is either malingering (when there is an established secondary gain) or has factitious disorder (when there is evidence that the person is seeking the attention of healthcare providers) [1 (p321)]. Thus, only in this text is there reference to the motivation for factitious disorder.

According to DSM-5, only two disorders involve the *intentional* production of symptoms: malingering and factitious disorder. DSM-5 states that factitious disorder focuses primarily on the production of medical symptoms without attributing any assumptions about the individual's reason for faking their illness [1 (p326)]. It further notes that unlike malingering, factitious disorder occurs when there is no clear secondary gain for the feigned symptoms [1 (p326)]. In the DSM, factitious disorder is a mental disorder, whereas malingering is classified as a "V-code"–other conditions that may be the focus of clinical attention, which the DSM emphasizes are *not* mental disorders. In addition, whereas the DSM-5 definition of mental disorders emphasizes the association of some type of resulting life impairment [1 (p20)], this criterion is absent from factitious disorder. For both factitious disorder and malingering the distinction is clear: one involves the intentional production of symptoms for external gain (malingering); and the other (factitious disorder) requires only deception, with reference to unconscious motivations removed, except in the above-noted text. Distress and/or disability have never been included in the diagnostic criteria for factitious disorder. Interestingly, DSM-5 now includes in the differential diagnosis of factitious disorder the diagnosis of borderline personality disorder, noting that the distinction between the two is the *deception* involved in the production of symptoms. Table 11-1 provides an overview of changes in somatoform disorders and factitious disorder from DSM-IV to DSM-5.

Clearly, the somatoform disorders have undergone substantial revisions. With one exception, malingering has been removed from the differential diagnosis of these disorders. It is unclear why motivations for these disorders were removed from the criteria, although the previously cited text (assessment of conscious intention is not reliable) indicates that this may have been an effort to improve reliability. With the de-emphasis on malingering found throughout the DSM-5, one wonders if the omission of malingering from the index may have been intentional rather than an oversight.

MALINGERING AND OTHER DSM-5 DISORDERS

The somatoform disorders are not the only diagnoses that have undergone substantial changes in DSM-5. In some diagnoses, the criteria have become so broad that feigning symptoms are likely to occur with increasing frequency. For example, the criteria for posttraumatic stress disorder (PTSD) have changed such that some believe that the number of people who could receive this diagnosis will substantially increase, with a comparable increase in the number who attempt to feign the disorder [5]. Mental retardation has been replaced with intellectual disability, and severity level is based on functional deficits, not measured intelligence, which may or may not be more easily feigned. Strategies for the detection of feigning would necessarily be different depending on whether the clinician is assessing the presence of symptoms versus the absence of deficits. For example, in PTSD, feigning involves the endorsement of a wide range of symptoms; in intellectual disability, feigning would require endorsing an *absence* of functioning. The text below is a brief discussion of the suggested components of a forensic interview, including a discussion of the strategies for the detection of feigning and examples of assessments for each strategy.

THE MALINGERING EVALUATION

To accurately diagnose malingering, a comprehensive evaluation is required to verify that feigning is occurring and an external incentive exists. This evaluation must consist of extensive interviewing, contact with collateral informants, and adjunctive psychological testing. Psychological testing can provide valuable information regarding effort and any response bias adopted

Table 11-1. CHANGES IN SOMATOFORM DISORDERS FROM DSM-IV TR TO DSM-5

DSM-IV TR Category	DSM-IV TR Diagnosis and Code	Intentional Symptom Production in DSM-IV TR Criteria	Malingering in DSM-IV TR Differential	DSM-5 Category	DSM-5 Diagnosis	Intentional Symptom Production in DSM-5 Criteria	Malingering in DSM-5 Differential
Somatoform disorders	Somatization Disorder 300.81	Yes	Yes	Somatic symptom and related disorders	Somatic symptom disorder 300.82	No	No
	Undifferentiated Somatoform Disorder 300.82	Yes	Yes		Somatic symptom disorder 300.82	No	No
	Conversion Disorder 300.11	Yes	Yes		Conversion Disorder 300.11	No	Yes
	Pain Disorder 307.80/307.89	Yes	Yes		Somatic symptom disorder with predominant pain specifier 300.82		
	Hypochondriasis 300.7	No	No		Illness Anxiety Disorder 300.7	No	No
	Body Dysmorphic Disorder 300.7	No	No		No comparable diagnosis		
	Somatoform Disorder NOS 300.82	No	No		Possibly Somatic symptom disorder		
					Psychological Factors Affection Other Medical Conditions 316	No	No
Factitious Disorder	Factitious Disorder 300.16/300.19	Yes	Yes		Factitious Disorder 300.19	Yes	Yes
					Other specified somatic symptom and related disorder 300.89		
					Unspecified somatic symptom and related disorder		

by the examinee. McGrath et al. [6] provide an informative review of response bias, defined as the patient responding in a manner that is unrelated to the item content. One type of response bias most relevant for malingering is negative impression management, which he defines as "responding in an excessively aberrant manner" [6 (p451)]. However, response bias can include styles that are independent of intentional effort. For example, inconsistent (or random) responding, acquiescence or negativism (yay or nay-saying) are examples of response biases that may not necessarily be purposeful. A final type of response bias not often seen in forensic evaluations, with the notable exception of custody evaluations, is positive impression management, which McGrath [6] describes as "the failure to report aberrant tendencies" [6 (p451)]. There are several methods of evaluating response bias with psychological testing, as summarized in part by Larrabee [7] and outlined below. Each of these methods will be discussed in general. Specific usage of each type of assessment will be provided in the discussions of the diagnostic changes in DSM-5 that might lead to an increased incidence of malingering.

Testing strategies

Ombudsmen tests of psychological functioning

Perhaps the most researched strategy in the detection of response bias is to use self-report tests of general psychological functioning that also include validity scales. The two instruments most often used in this regard are the most recent version of the Minnesota Multiphasic Personality Inventory (MMPI) [8], the MMPI-2 [9], and the Personality Assessment Inventory (PAI) [10].

The MMPI-2 is a 567-item self-report instrument designed as a measure of general psychopathology. It has been cited as being "the mostly widely administered objective personality test in forensic evaluations" [11 (p1)] largely because of the extensive research conducted on its ability to detect response bias via the embedded validity scales. The three original validity scales from the MMPI included the Lie scale (L), the Infrequency scale (F), and the Defensiveness scale (K). Various configurations of these scales were extensively researched to detect both positive and negative impression management [12]. Further research with the MMPI led to the development of many more validity scales, including VRIN (variable response inconsistency), the tendency to respond inconsistently to item content); TRIN (true response inconsistency), the tendency to respond mostly true (or false) to items regardless of content); Fb (Back Infrequency), the infrequency items contained on the latter half of the test; and Fp (Infrequency psychopathology scale), items rarely endorsed by psychiatric patients.

As Larrabee [13] describes, the MMPI-2 is efficient at measuring at least two types of feigning: feigned severe psychopathology (e.g., psychosis) and feigned somatic/neurocognitive complaints. Severe psychopathology is most often revealed in a pattern of elevations on the family of F scales (F, Fb and Fp) and is often associated with, for example, the feigning of psychosis in criminal cases. The feigning of somatic and/or neurocognitive complaints, often seen in civil litigation, has led to the development of other composite validity scales including the Fake Bad Scale (FBS) [14] and the Response Bias Scale (RBS) [15]. Larrabee [16] describes the FBS as a measure of "somatic malingering," although others have described it as a measure of general maladjustment. The majority of items on the FBS assess physical functioning and overlap with Scales 1 (hypochondriasis) and 3 (hysteria). In contrast, the RBS was developed empirically by examining the endorsement of items in individuals both passing and failing cognitive symptom validity tests. The authors suggest that the RBS improves accuracy in detecting feigned cognitive impairment above the F scales or the FBS [11].

The PAI is a 344-item self-report instrument designed to assess general psychopathology. As with the MMPI, inclusion of validity scales to assess response bias was a critical component of its development. The original validity scales included the ICN (Inconsistency, pairs of items with similar content), INF (Infrequency, items expected to be answered by both clinical and non-clinical populations in a similar fashion), NIM (Negative impression management, the endorsement of bizarre or unlikely symptoms), and PIM (Positive impression management, items that are rarely endorsed by both clinical and nonclinical respondents but frequently endorsed by those attempting to place themselves in a positive light). A supplementary validity scale was added later: DEF (Defensiveness, designed to detect underreporting) [17]. More recently, two additional scales have shown promise in the detection of malingering. The Malingering Index (MAL) [18] was constructed based on profile characteristics often associated with the feigning of psychiatric disorders. The Rogers Discriminant Function (RDF) [19] was constructed using three groups: a clinical group (patients with schizophrenia, major depression, and generalized anxiety disorder) and nonclinical participants categorized as either naïve or sophisticated. The results of the discriminant analysis indicated that the weighted combination of scales produced a hit rate (the rate of accurately detecting feigning) of 92%. Furthermore, the RDF performed well even with the "sophisticated" malingerers, with a hit rate of 73%.

Floor effect

The concept known as the "floor effect" involves the incorporation of extremely easy questions or tasks in the testing methodology. Such items generally involve over-learned information or simple skills that are easily retained, even in individuals with limited intellectual functioning.

Examples of such items include requests to perform simple arithmetic calculations (i.e., 2 + 2 = ?), questions about basic common information (ie, Who is President of the United States?), queries regarding basic autographical information (such as one's age or birthday), requests to complete a simple sequence (i.e., a, b, _; 3, 4, _), or instructions to copy or recall simple diagrams or designs. The Rey 15-item Test (FIT) [20] is an example of such an assessment. This test requires that individuals remember a set of 15 letters, numbers, and geometric shapes that are in fact quite simple because of their redundancy. Various cut scores have been suggested, although any score less than 10 is generally accepted as indicating a lack of effort. A meta-analysis of the FIT indicated that its specificity was much higher than its sensitivity (92% compared with 43%) with an overall hit rate of 70% [21]. In an effort to improve the sensitivity in particular, Griffin et al. [22] modified the FIT by increasing its redundancy, providing standardized administration instructions, and outlining a method of qualitative scoring. In a clinical population and using the qualitative scoring, he estimated the sensitivity at 71%, although the specificity dropped to 75% with this scoring system.

Symptom validity testing

Pankratz [23] initially discussed the concept of symptom validity testing (SVT) in the context of the assessment of sensory loss. He described a procedure wherein the individual is presented with a stimulus and instructed to guess whether or not the stimulus was present. Over a number of trials, if the individual performed worse than chance, it was presumed that he/she actually knew the correct response and chose not to report it. In a two-alternative forced-choice task, below chance performance is less than 50%, although exact probabilities can be obtained using the normal approximation to the binomial theorem [7]. In assessments of feigning, most SVT assessments incorporate feedback regarding the accuracy of the response.

Multiple assessments of feigned memory and cognitive deficits have been developed using this paradigm, often coupled with the floor-effect paradigm. One example is the Test of Memory Malingering [24] (TOMM). The TOMM is a visual recognition test that involves presenting an individual with 50 different picture drawings. Two learning trials are presented followed by a retention trial. Scores below chance or based on criteria developed from head injured or cognitively impaired individuals are indicative of feigned memory impairment.

Performance curve analysis

The performance curve analysis strategy, used to detect feigned cognitive deficits, is less widely used in psychological tests developed to assess malingering, perhaps in part because of the complexity of the development of such assessments. This strategy is based on the supposition that malingerers do not distinguish between easy and difficult items when providing inaccurate responses. With nonmalingering individuals, there is an expectation that accuracy of responses will decrease as item difficulty increases. Individuals exhibiting a lack of effort or random responding are as likely to respond inaccurately to easy as well as to difficult items. One test that uses this strategy, coupled with SVT, is the Validity Indicator Profile [25] (VIP). The VIP consists of verbal and nonverbal subtests, both utilizing a two-alternative forced choice paradigm. Item difficulty is randomly distributed throughout the test to prevent the test-taker from adopting a strategy of answering easy items accurately. After scoring, response styles are categorized as compliant, careless, irrelevant, and malingered. One concern with the VIP is that in order to be classified as malingering, the examinee has to exert effort; otherwise, responses are classified as either careless or irrelevant.

Unusual patterns of responses

Several psychological tests evaluate whether the examinee is providing atypical responses to questions about mental health symptoms. Examples of such atypical responses include symptoms rarely presented by those with a genuine mental disorder, an unusual combination of symptoms, highly improbable or absurd symptoms, or an inconsistency in reported symptoms compared with actual behavior observed during the evaluation. The most widely used assessment for the detection of feigned psychiatric symptoms using this paradigm is the Structured Interview of Reported Symptoms [26] (SIRS). The SIRS was developed to assess a broad range of strategies in the detection of feigning. It is a 172-item structured interview that takes approximately 30 to 45 minutes to administer. The original SIRS contained eight primary and five supplementary scales. The supplementary scales were used only if the respondent did not endorse symptoms in sufficient quantity to make a definitive determination. Responses on the primary scales were classified as honest, indeterminate, probable, or definite. An individual was considered to be feigning psychiatric symptoms if he/she scored in the definite range on at least one primary subscale or in the probable range on three or more primary subscales. Studies indicated that these criteria optimized both sensitivity and specificity [26]. The SIRS has been shown to be both a valid and reliable method for detecting malingering [27, 28] with very low false-positive rates [29], although others have found the false-positive rate to be extremely high [30]. Despite this criticism, the SIRS has been reported to have general acceptance among forensic experts in evaluations [31] and is often cited as the "gold standard" [32] or "benchmark" [33] in the detection of feigned psychiatric symptoms. The SIRS has recently been revised [34] (SIRS-2), although the primary scales remain unchanged. A new supplementary scale was added, which was developed to assess feigned cognitive deficits. The SIRS-2 provides an algorithm for decision making that includes the use of composite scores as well as the primary scales. No information has yet been provided on the likelihood of feigning based on this algorithm. Table 11-2 provides a list of structured assessments developed to assess the feigning of psychiatric symptoms and cognitive deficits for each described method.

MALINGERING OF SPECIFIC DSM-5 DISORDERS

The above strategies may all be useful in detecting feigning of various types of disorders. For example, if a patient is feigning cognitive deficits, an assessment of feigned psychosis is unlikely to provide useful information. In the discussion of each diagnosis, suggestions will be provided, as appropriate, for the use of structured assessments in the detection of malingering.

Malingered posttraumatic stress disorder

PTSD is especially easy to malinger because the diagnosis is almost exclusively based on the person's self-report. Unfortunately, information about PTSD criteria is readily available, as more than six million citations describing PTSD were noted in a recent Google search [35]. Furthermore, many of the standard instruments to assess PTSD use a structured interview format with questions that are obviously directed toward possible PTSD symptoms. Questioning in this suggestive manner may actually teach specific PTSD symptoms to the examinee, thereby enhancing the possibility of successful feigning. The changes made to the diagnosis in DSM-5 may alter the frequency with which the disorder is feigned. For DSM-IV TR, estimates of feigning ranged from 14% to 30% for individuals in the military seeking disability benefits [36, 37]. In DSM-IV-TR, the clinician was warned to consider malingering when evaluating for the presence of PTSD [3 (p467)]. In DSM-5, this warning was removed for unknown reasons, although the removal of malingering from the differential of other disorders suggests a de-emphasis on the construct as a whole.

Table 11-2. STRATEGIES FOR DETECTING MALINGERING WITH EXAMPLE TESTS

Name	Content
Floor Effect Tests	
Rey 15-item Test (FIT)	15 redundant items grouped 3 in 5 rows Score less than 9 = probable malingering
The b test	Circle all lowercase b's in a 15-page booklet, requires distinguishing between q's, p's, and d's
Coin-in hand test	Show coin in hand for 2 seconds Close eyes count backward 10–1 Clench both hands Tap hand with coin 10 trials, random hand
Symptom Validity Testing	
Test of Memory Malingering (TOMM)	2 alternative forced choice, 50 target pictures, recognize from 50 presentations of 2 pictures
Word Memory Test (WMT)	20 linked word lists; oral and computerized version
Validity Indicator Profile (also performance curve analysis strategy)	100 problems assessing nonverbal abstraction; 78 word problems; 2 alternative forced choice
Unusual Patterns of Responses	
Structured Interview of Reported Symptoms (SIRS)	172-item structured interview Scores classified as Honest, Indeterminate, Probable, Definite Eight Primary Scales: Rare Symptoms, Symptom Combinations, Improbable/Absurd Symptoms, Blatant Symptoms, Subtle Symptoms, Selectivity of Symptoms, Severity of Symptoms, Reported versus Observed Symptoms One or more in definite, three or more in probable = malingering
Structured Interview of Reported Symptoms—Revised (SIRS-2)	Scores classified as Genuine, Indeterminate, Probable, Definite Primary scales the same, new Supplementary Scale to assess feigned cognitive deficits (Improbable Failure) Algorithm to determine if malingering
Miller Forensic Assessment of Symptoms Test (M-FAST)	25-item structured interview Total score greater than or equal to 6 suggestive of malingering

The criteria for PTSD have changed so substantially, it is unclear whether it will be more or less likely to be successfully feigned. For example, DSM-5 has narrowed the criteria for what constitutes a trauma: only threatened death (or exposure to actual death), serious injury, or sexual violence are included. A threat to one's integrity has been removed, although repeated exposure to trauma that occurs with, for example, first responders has been added (with the caveat that this exposure is *not* through electronic media unless the exposure is work-related). However, no longer is experiencing or witnessing the traumatic event necessary: learning of traumas to close family or friends also constitutes a circumstance under which one could develop PTSD. Number 3 of Criterion A emphasizes that nonaccidental causes of death to a close friend or family member do *not* qualify as a traumatic stressor but violent or accidental stressors can qualify [1 (p271)]. As a result, this criterion may include other types of trauma experienced by family and friends (e.g., serious injury, sexual violence). One author believes that including this criterion (learning about a traumatic event) "will open a forensic quagmire in determining who is entitled to compensatory damages in civil suits" [38]. An individual's emotional reaction to the trauma was removed from the exposure criterion. DSM-5 states the emotional reaction requirement was eliminated because individuals react differently to trauma, and some individuals may not demonstrate any emotional reaction at the time of the traumatic event [1 (p274)].

Although the number of symptoms required to arrive at the diagnosis is unchanged, avoidance and negative cognitions/mood are two distinct criteria in DSM-5. Although avoidance was a criterion in DSM-IV, negative affect was subsumed under this criterion, and the individual had to meet only three (of the seven) criteria, only two of which were related to avoidance. Avoidance is now required in DSM-5: avoidance of "memories, thoughts or feelings," or avoidance of "external reminders" (one or both) [1 (p271)]. "Negative alterations in cognitions and mood" [1 (p271)] are now afforded their own criterion (D), of which two are required to make the diagnosis. Not dissimilar to the other criteria, these rely solely on patient report. Only with some of these criteria would collateral information be helpful. Under intrusive symptoms, the description of flashbacks has broadened, as DSM-5 notes that there can be a range of flashback presentations, with more severe flashbacks resulting in an individual's inability to appreciate their current circumstances [1 (p274)]. Validating the more subtle form of a flashback could present challenges, although flashbacks are not required for a PTSD diagnosis.

Strategies for the detection of feigned PTSD are problematic due to the broadness of the criteria. Although the definition of trauma has narrowed, the remaining criteria have not. In addition, as with most psychiatric diagnoses, the criteria rely on accurate self-report. The ombudsmen tests of psychological functioning have proved to be the most fruitful in detecting malingering of PTSD in the past and with some exceptions are likely to be the most effective with the DSM-5. The MMPI-2 in particular has evidenced some utility in detecting feigned PTSD. However, the detection of malingered PTSD is complicated by the fact that individuals with genuine PTSD can experience substantial distress and may legitimately elevate some MMPI-2 validity scales. In a study of veterans seeking disability compensation who were instructed to feign, the family of F scales, most notably F, Fb, and Fp, were most effective in discriminating between honest reporters and feigners [39]. Fp in particular was superior in discriminating the two groups. The authors suggest using a cut score of Fp greater than 99 (t score) for identifying individuals feigning PTSD. The FBS has shown promise in identifying malingered PTSD in personal injury claims [40], although further research was mixed in this regard [39, 41, 42].

Elhai et al. [43] developed a scale specifically to detect feigned PTSD-Fptsd (Infrequency posttraumatic stress disorder scale), which includes items that were infrequently endorsed by veterans with legitimate PTSD. In the development sample, this scale was found to improve the accuracy of detection of feigned PTSD above other F scales, although subsequent research failed to replicate that finding. They also note that the Fptsd scale did not improve the accuracy of detection (above the traditional F scales) and that the FBS scale "produced unacceptable positive predictive power" and should not be used [44].

The Morel Emotional Numbing Test (MENT) [45] has been described as a SVT specific to PTSD. This instrument assesses affect recognition in a two-alternative forced-choice format. Although many of the SVT's commonly used are measures of malingered memory deficits, the MENT assesses primarily malingered PTSD. Using a two-alternative format, the MENT is designed to give the test taker the impression that deficits in affect recognition are pathognomonic of PTSD. The evaluee is told "Some individuals with PTSD may have difficulty recognizing facial expressions," and they are then asked to note the emotion associated with the facial expressions they are shown. In brief, the MENT consists of 20 photographs of 10 facial expressions for both genders. Three trials are presented; in the first trial, one photo is presented with two words. The subject is asked to circle the word that describes the emotion. In the second trial, two photos are shown with one word; the subject is asked to select the photo that matches the word. In the third and final trial, two photos and two words are presented, and the task is to match the appropriate photo with the word. According to Morel [45], any adult who puts forth a reasonable amount of effort (except for the visually impaired or those with less than a 3rd grade reading level) can complete the task with 90%–100% accuracy even if they have PTSD, recommending that more than nine errors is suggestive of malingering. In a study investigating the use of the MENT with Croatian war veterans (who have been shown to evidence symptom overreporting when seeking compensation), using a cut score of nine produced a sensitivity of 92% and specificity of 96% [46].

This finding suggests that the MENT may be useful as one component of an assessment of malingered PTSD.

The Atypical Response (ATR) scale of the Trauma Symptom Inventory-2nd edition (TSI-2) [47] has also been described as useful in distinguishing genuine symptoms of PTSD from simulated PTSD. In their study of 75 undergraduate students trained to simulate PTSD and 49 undergraduate students with genuine PTSD, Gray et al. [48] determined that the ATR correctly classified 75% of genuinely distressed individuals and 74% of PTSD simulators. This scale is a revised version of the ATR from the original TSI, which had evidenced unimpressive classification rates [41, 49].

PTSD VIGNETTE

Mary Jane is a 43-year-old woman who is seeking compensation from a school district related to the sexual assault of her 13-year-old cognitively impaired daughter, Sue. Records indicate that Sue was forced to orally copulate two older and more functional (although also impaired) boys while in school. In addition to damages sought in her daughter's behalf, Mary Jane is also seeking compensation for herself. She is alleging that since she learned of the incident, she has developed symptoms consistent with PTSD, for which she has sought treatment. Symptoms include recurrent distressing dreams in which her daughter is sexually assaulted, recurrent, intrusive redepictions of the event when awake, avoidance of the school and the neighborhood in which the school is located (Mary Jane removed Sue from the school and has retained a private educator expert in tutoring special needs children), persistent self-blame regarding the incident, impaired relationship with her husband, irritability, and insomnia. Mary Jane ultimately quit her job because of her inability to concentrate on her work. The psychiatrist diagnosed Mary Jane with PTSD and is providing pharmacologic treatment. He has also suggested Mary Jane begin individual therapy.

Mary Jane is referred for a forensic evaluation to determine whether her PTSD is feigned. The first question to be answered is does the event that happened with her daughter qualify as a trauma to Mary Jane under DSM-5? Although the criterion states "In cases of actual or threatened death of a family member or friend, the event(s) must have been violent or accidental," it seems that sexual violence would qualify. The assessment tool most effective in detecting feigned PTSD is the MMPI-2, and this instrument should be part of the forensic evaluation of Mary Jane. The TSI-2 may be useful, as well as extensive collateral interviewing to aid in describing Mary Jane's reaction to her daughter's assault.

Intellectual disability

DSM-5 has eliminated the diagnosis of mental retardation, consistent with Rosa's Law (Public Law 111-256) [50], in favor of the diagnosis intellectual disability. Although the criteria are essentially unchanged, the focus shifted from intelligence to adaptive skills and level of support necessary resulting from skills deficits. According to the DSM-5, the following three criteria are required to be diagnosed with an intellectual disability: impairment in intellectual functioning verified by clinical evaluation and standardized testing; limitations in adaptive functioning requiring ongoing support in one or more activities of daily living (removed requirement of deficits in two areas); and onset during the developmental period (removed onset before 18, although the text notes that 'developmental period' means childhood and adolescence) [1 (33)].

In contrast to DSM-IV-TR, where severity was based on the IQ assessment, in DSM-5 severity is based on functioning in three domains: conceptual (problem solving, reasoning ability; most likely to be associated with lower levels of intelligence), social (social and communicative behavior), and practical (self-care). DSM-5 defines four categories: mild, moderate, severe, and profound based on the extent of deficits in the above domains, noting that adaptive skills deficits dictate the level of support needed and that measured IQs in the lower levels are less accurate. According to the text, deficits need only be identified in one of the three domains. It is unclear whether conceptual deficits—the domain most associated with lowered intelligence—are adequate in making the diagnosis of intellectual disability.

DSM-5 recommends the use of the World Health Organization Disability Assessment Schedule 2.0 (WHODAS 2.0) [51] as an assessment of functional deficits, a self-report instrument (although a "knowledgeable informant" is an acceptable substitute). The WHO-DAS assesses individuals in six domains: understanding and communicating, getting around, self-care, getting along with people, life activities—household, life activities—school/work, and participation in society. The individual rates themselves on a scale from 1 (no deficits) to 5 (cannot do at all). There are other adaptive skills instruments available, most notably the Vineland Adaptive Behavior Scales [52], which provides a comprehensive evaluation of skills and deficits across four domains: communication, daily living skills, socialization, and motor skills, seemingly more consistent with the three domains in the DSM-5.

Unfortunately, there are no assessment strategies for determining whether an individual is feigning deficits in adaptive skills, and most structured assessments of such are based on self-report. However, because such deficits must be present throughout childhood and into adulthood, a careful review of collateral information would be critical in making this determination. An individual with a lower measured intelligence who has functioned relatively well throughout childhood and has lived independently as an adult would not be diagnosed with intellectual disability. Likewise, an individual with low measured intelligence who self-reports deficits in adaptive functioning that are inconsistent with collateral reports also would not be diagnosed with intellectual disability.

Detecting feigned low intelligence—still required as one criterion for the diagnosis—can be problematic, because most assessments of feigned cognitive deficits are related to attention and memory. The structure of standardized assessments of intelligence requires effort in order to obtain a valid IQ. If the evaluee responds "I don't know" to all questions, no accurate assessment of IQ can be obtained. Unfortunately, there are few effort tests or validity scales embedded in intelligence assessment instruments. One exception to this is the Reliable Digit Span (RDS), which uses the digit span subscale on the Wechsler Adult Intelligence Scale (WAIS). Developed from the WAIS-R, the RDS is calculated by summing the longest string of digits without error in both the forward and backward conditions [53]. In a recent meta-analysis, the RDS was found to distinguish individuals exhibiting appropriate effort from those who appear to not be providing adequate effort [54]. However, a more recent study indicated that the specificity for certain groups was unacceptably low, including those with low measured intelligence [55]. Of particular concern, individuals with intellectual disabilities may be falsely identified as not providing adequate effort on many of the effort tests commonly used to assess feigned cognitive impairment [56]. Evaluators should use caution in incorporating the same symptom validity tests and neurocognitive test indicators for malingering utilized for reported cognitive dysfunction when evaluating individuals with intellectual disabilities. Research also has shown that individuals can successfully feign deficits on tests designed to measure intelligence. For example, Graue et al. [57] showed that community volunteers were able to feign a lowered IQ on the WAIS-III when instructed to do so, and embedded tests of malingering (Digit Span Scaled Score and RDS) did not reliably identify such feigning. Likewise, measures of adaptive behavior are also susceptible to manipulation [58]. In their survey of 50 forensic psychology diplomats, Victor and Boone [56] determined that 64% reported using the TOMM, 50% reported used the Validity Indicator Profile, and 44% reported using the FIT to assess malingered intellectual disabilities, only one of which is a measure of feigned intellectual deficits (VIP).

Under DSM-5, Donald would meet criteria for intellectual disability, although he has been denied services in the past. As a forensic examiner, you intend to administer the most recent version of the WAIS, recognizing

VIGNETTE

Donald is a 28-year-old male who had lived with his mother his entire life until her recent death. He was placed in special education classes in the 3rd grade, where he remained until he dropped out of school in the 9th grade. Donald was tested using the Wechsler Intelligence Scale for Children while in the 6th grade, on which he achieved a full scale IQ score of 73, which did not allow him to receive services from the local developmentally disabled agency (IQ too high, did not qualify as mentally retarded). He received SSDI since the age of 10 for learning disabilities, which his mother managed (she was the payee). Donald was never able to obtain employment, although he performed odd jobs (e.g., lawn mowing) for neighbors. Although Donald was able to perform self-care adequately, his mother provided a home and meals for him. Donald had very few friends and preferred spending his days at home watching TV when not performing the above-noted odd jobs. Upon mother's death, Donald's older, more functional brother moved in to the home and replaced mother as payee and caretaker. Within two months of his mother's death, Donald was arrested and charged with petty theft, his first arrest. He was instructed by his older brother to steal a six-pack of beer from the local convenience store. Although Donald recognized that to do so was wrong, he wanted to please his brother and "fit in" with his brother's friends, and his brother was his sole source of support. His attorney expressed concerns about Donald's judgment and intelligence and requests a competence to stand trial evaluation. You are the forensic examiner and understand that malingering should always be considered in such evaluations.

that the embedded effort tests are inaccurate for individuals with intellectual deficits. Therefore, collateral information such as school records and information from neighbors and/or brother would be crucial in documenting adaptive skills deficits.

Mild neurocognitive disorder

Mild Neurocognitive Disorder, new to DSM-5, was classified as a diagnosis for further study in DSM-IV TR. The criteria include evidence of "modest cognitive decline" [1 (p605)] that does not interfere with independent functioning, documented by self-report *and* cognitive testing (both are required). The suspected etiology may be specified but is not required. In his critique of DSM-5, Frances [38] notes that the criteria for this disorder are "so impossibly vague that it includes me, my wife, and most of our friends" [38 (p2)]. Detecting feigned mild cognitive decline is comparable to the detection of mild traumatic brain injuries, and many similar procedures will be used.

In contrast to the *production* of psychiatric symptoms, feigning cognitive impairments requires a demonstration of *absence* of functioning. Slick et al. [59] coined the term "Malingering of Neurocognitive Dysfunction" (MND), which they note is characterized by the intentional exaggeration or fabrication of cognitive dysfunction for the purpose of obtaining some external incentive or avoiding responsibility. They provided guidelines regarding when to suspect this type of malingering, which includes four criteria, designated as Criteria A through D. Criterion A is the presence of financial incentive. Criterion B includes evidence of exaggeration on neuropsychological tests. Criterion C includes evidence of false or exaggerated self-report, and Criterion D is that both criteria B and C cannot be accounted for by psychiatric, neurological, or developmental factors. An individual can be considered a "probable malingerer" when Criterion A is met and two or more items (of a list of six) are met from Criterion B or one from B and one from C (of a list of five). Possible malingering is defined as the presence of Criterion A plus two (or more) items from Criterion C. More simply put, these investigators believe that self-report evidence (other than an admission of malingering) is only suggestive of malingering; evidence of malingering on standard neuropsychological testing is necessary to be more definitive.

The National Academy of Neuropsychology (NAN) issued similar guidelines regarding possible feigned performance on neurocognitive tests as outlined below [60]:

1. Inconsistencies in various domains (e.g., symptoms inconsistent with known pattern of brain function)
2. Performance on neuropsychological assessments
3. Evidence of exaggeration on psychological testing
4. Poor performance on symptom validity testing
5. Below-chance performance on forced-choices assessments

Clearly the use of structured, standardized assessments is a critical component when evaluating the validity of neurocognitive dysfunction. In a meta-analysis of 32 studies of the most commonly used testing, Vickery et al. [21] found that individuals feigning cognitive deficits achieved scores more than one standard deviation below honest responders. In a survey of neuropsychologists who consistently practice in the area of compensation claims [61], more than 45% indicated that they routinely use the TOMM [24], and more than 33% indicated that they use the FIT [20].

There is substantial literature indicating high rates of exaggeration of cognitive impairment in patients with mild head injury (MHI) seeking compensation. Binder [62] found that 33% of patients with MHIs exaggerated deficits on the Portland Digit Recognition Test. Greiffenstein and Baker [63] found a 37% base rate of malingering in individuals with MHI who were seeking compensation of some sort. Larrabee [64], in a review of 11 studies, found a prevalence rate of malingering of 40% in 1363 patients who were seeking compensation for an MHI. Larrabee [65] opined that the incidence of exaggeration of deficits in MHI patients seeking compensation was 10 times higher than the base rate for actual deficits. In support of this finding, Green et al. [66] found that the evaluee's effort explained 53% of the variability seen on neuropsychological testing of head-injured patients. The evaluee's level of education explained only 11% of the variance and age explained only 4%. Patients with MHIs scored significantly lower on effort tests than patients with more severe injuries. When the MHI patients who demonstrated no effort were removed from the study sample, however, scores on neuropsychological testing for this group (MHIs) were higher than for patients with severe head injuries, as expected. It is highly likely that a similar pattern of results would be found for individuals feigning mild neurocognitive disorder. Determining the external incentive would be essential in deciding that this disorder is malingered.

Dissociative identity disorder

The basic criteria for dissociative identity disorder (DID) are essentially unchanged. However, Criterion A in DSM-5 includes possession experiences in addition to the "two or more distinct personality states" [1 (p292)] found in DSM-IV TR. DSM-5 describes that DID possession states commonly present as if a spirit or supernatural force has taken over the individual, and as a result the individual talks or behaves in an obviously different manner than usual [1 (293)]. DSM-5 is very clear that culture is a critical aspect of this type of dissociation and is likely not relevant in most U.S. cultures, suggesting that an effort to feign this disorder by claiming feeling possessed is unlikely to be successful. DSM-5 also has clearly specified that the symptoms cause distress or impairment in functioning (Criterion C), absent in DSM-IV TR.

In an interesting break from the seeming lack of acknowledgment of malingering in other disorders commonly feigned, the text for dissociative identity disorder (DID) provides guidelines for distinguishing feigned from "legitimate" DID. In the Differential Diagnosis section, DSM-5 cautions examiners to consider factitious disorder or malingering, as did DSM-IV

TR. However, DSM-5 provides specific examples, suggesting that individuals who feign DID report well known symptoms, such a memory loss, while not reporting less common symptoms, such as depression [1 (p297)]. Furthermore, DSM-5 indicates that individuals feigning DID "seem to enjoy 'having' the disorder" [1 (p297)]—in stark contrast to Criterion C, which requires clinically significant distress or impairment. The final paragraph describes that individual who are malingering DID often present with an "all good" or "all bad" identity, sometimes with feigned memory loss, as a means to obtain a particular goal (e.g., avoidance of criminal punishment) [1 (p297)]. As in all malingering, establishing an external incentive is critical.

Unfortunately, aside from providing these guidelines, literature on detecting malingered DID is lacking and draws mostly from detecting feigned PTSD. The Structured Interview of Reported Symptoms and the Personality Assessment Inventory both have been found to overclassify DID patients as malingering [67–69]. Previous research with the MMPI and feigned DID met with similar results [70, 71]. However, one recent study examining the MMPI-2 and feigned DID found that, consistent with feigned PTSD, the Fp scale was most useful and evidenced the highest sensitivity and specificity [72]. They also found a unique pattern of differences in the Dissociative Experiences Scale (DES) [73]. The DES is a 28-item questionnaire that lists dissociative experiences and instructs the examinee to estimate the percentage of time each one occurs, on a scale from 0 to 100. The instrument is scored by summing the percentages and dividing by 28. In contrast to most other assessments of malingered psychiatric symptoms, where detection strategies are based on over-reporting, these authors found that individuals malingering DID *under*-reported on the DES. Individuals with nonfeigned DID scored an average of 46.79 on the DES; coached and uncoached participants instructed to feign scored 7.42 and 11.49, respectively.

Non-rapid eye movement sleep arousal disorders

In DSM-5 sleepwalking and sleep terrors are classified as Non-Rapid Eye Movement (NREM) Sleep Arousal Disorders. The criteria for both remain essentially unchanged and include little to no memory of dreams, amnesia for the episode, and episodes cause distress or impairment. However, in sleepwalking the specifier, "with sleep-related sexual behavior" (sexsomnia) has been added [1 (p399)]. DSM-5 specifically notes that a range of sexual behaviors (e.g., groping, sexual intercourse, or masturbation) may be observed in individuals suffering from sexsomnia and as a result, the individual may become involved in legal trouble [1 (p400)]. Although malingering remains in the differential, the text refers to a diagnosis that no longer exists in DSM-5 , i.e., dissociative fugue. Furthermore, the text explaining how to differentiate non-rapid eye movement sleep arousal disorders (to include sexsomnia) from malingering or a dissociative fugue is confusing and reads, "As with dissociative fugue, malingering or other voluntary behavior occurring during wakefulness arises from wakefulness" [1 (p403)].

Historically, sleepwalking used in a criminal defense challenges the *actus reus* requirement: that the action was under voluntary control [74]. In the United States, the defense has utilized three legal arguments: automatism, unconsciousness, and insanity [75, 76]. Because the defense has been raised so infrequently, the courts have been inconsistent in how this defense is viewed. According to Horn [76], the distinction between the automatism and unconsciousness defense has lessened and are now considered essentially equivalent. More interesting is the use of sleepwalking as an insanity defense. The Supreme Courts in three states (North Carolina, Wyoming, and Indiana) all opined that the insanity defense was inappropriate, because sleepwalking is not a mental disease or defect that requires mental health treatment [74].

As with many other mental disorders, when sleepwalking and/or sexsomnia are mounted as a criminal defense, malingering should be carefully considered. Unfortunately, the science regarding the detection of feigned sleep disorders is not well developed. Although sleep studies may be useful and should be performed, polysomnograms may not detect such a rare event. More critical is a thorough psychological/psychiatric evaluation that includes an assessment of the individual's sleep history, as well as family members' sleep history. Sleepwalking very rarely develops in adulthood and often is clustered in families.

Collateral information, especially if the individual has a bed partner, to corroborate past incidents of sleepwalking would be important. Although ombudsman tests of personality functioning may be useful in detecting feigned psychopathology, there is no consistent psychopathology found in individuals with somnambulism [77]. Amnesia for the episode is one criterion for the diagnosis, although the use of memory testing may suggest an exaggeration of memory deficits not associated with the episode. Finally, determining the external incentive is critical.

SUMMARY

Although malingering was removed from the DSM-5 index, malingering remains as a V code. Although DSM-5 emphasizes that malingering is not a mental disorder, forensic evaluators routinely evaluate for malingering in both civil and criminal litigation. Important summary points from this chapter include the following:

- Malingering has been removed from the differential of all but one of the somatic symptom and related disorders.
- The somatoform disorders underwent substantial revision in an apparent effort to improve reliability of the diagnoses, as implied by the statement that distinguishing conscious from unconscious motivations is unreliable.
- The revision of PTSD to include "learned of" trauma is likely to greatly increase the number of individuals meeting diagnostic criteria as well as the number attempting to feign the disorder.
- The criteria for intellectual disability are impossibly confusing such that both of the following are true:
  - One could receive the diagnosis with a low average IQ with deficits in one domain.
  - One could receive the diagnosis with a low IQ with deficits only in the conceptual domain.
- It is unknown whether the changes to diagnosing intellectual disability will lead to an increase in the incidence of malingering, because adaptive skills may be more easily feigned.
- In dissociative identity disorder, examples are given to aid in distinguishing genuine from feigned disorder.
- Adding "sexsomnia" as a specifier to sleepwalking may increase the incidence of malingering as a defense against a sex offense.

REFERENCES

1. American Psychiatric Association. *Diagnostic and Statistical Manual of Mental Disorders, 5th edition*. Arlington, VA: American Psychiatric Publishing; 2013
2. Nussbaum AM. *The pocket Guide to the DSM-5 Diagnostic Exam*. Arlington, VA: American Psychiatric Publishing; 2013.
3. American Psychiatric Association. *Diagnostic and Statistical Manual of Mental Disorders, 4th Edition,* Text Revision. Washington, DC: American Psychiatric Association; 2000.
4. Feldman M, Hamilton J, Deemer H. Factitious disorder. In: Phillips KA, ed. *Somatoform and Factitious Disorders*. Washington, DC: American Psychiatric Association; 2001: pp 129–166.
5. First MB. The PTSD stressor criterion as a barrier to malingering: DSM-5 draft commentaries. *Psychol Inj Law* 2010; 3:255–259.
6. McGrath RE, Mitchell M, Kim BH, et al. Evidence for response bias as a source of error variance in applied assessment. *Psychol Bull* 2010; 136:450–470.
7. Larrabee GJ. Assessment of malingering. In: Larrabee GJ, editor. *Forensic Neuropsychology: A Scientific Approach*. Oxford: University Press; 2011: pp 116–159.

8. Hathaway SR, McKinley JC. *MMPI Manual*. New York: Psychological Corporation; 1967.
9. Butcher JN, Dahlstrom WG, Graham JR, et al. *MMPI-2: Manual for Administration and Scoring*. Minneapolis: University of Minnesota Press; 1989.
10. Morey LC. *Personality Assessment Inventory: Professional manual*. Odessa, FL: Psychological Assessment Resources, 1991.
11. Wygant DB, Sellbom M, Gervais RO, et al. Further validation of the MMPI-2 and MMPI-2-RF Response Bias Scale: findings from disability and criminal forensic settings. *Psychol Assess* 2010; 22:745–756.
12. Greene RL. *The MMPI: An Interpretive Manual*. New York: Grune & Stratton, Inc.; 1980.
13. Larrabee GJ. *Forensic Neuropsychology*. New York: Oxford University Press, 2005.
14. Lees-Haley PR, English LT, Glenn, WJ. A fake bad scale for the MMPI-2 for personal injury claimants. *Psychol Rep* 1991; 68:203–210.
15. Gervais RO, Ben-Porath YS, Wygant DB, et al. Development and validation of a Response Bias Scale (RBS) for the MMPI-2. *Assessment* 2007; 14:196–208.
16. Larrabee G. Somatic malingering on the MMPI and MMPI-2 in litigating subjects. *Clin Neuropsychol* 1998; 12:179–188.
17. Morey LC. Defensiveness and malingering indices for the PAI. Paper presented at the meeting of the American Psychological Association, Toronto, Ontario, Canada, August 1993.
18. Morey LC. *An Interpretive Guide to the Personality Assessment Inventory (PAI)*. Odessa, FL: Psychological Assessment Resources, 1996.
19. Rogers R, Gillard ND, Wooley CN, et al. The detection of feigned disabilities: the effectiveness of the Personality Assessment Inventory in a traumatized inpatient sample. *Assessment* 1996; 19:77–88.
20. Rey A. *L'examen Clinique en Psychologie [The Clinical Examination in Psychology]*. Paris: Presses Universitaire de France, 1964.
21. Vickery CD, Berry DT, Inman TH, et al. Detection of inadequate effort on neuropsychological testing: a meta-analytic review of selected procedures. *Arch Clin Neuropsychol* 2001; 16:45–73.
22. Griffin GA, Glassmire DM, Henderson EA, et al. Rey II: redesigning the Rey screening test of malingering. *J Clin Psychol* 1997; 53:757–766.
23. Pankratz L. Symptom validity testing and symptom retraining: procedures for the assessment and treatment of functional sensory deficits. *J Consult Clin Psychol* 1979; 47:409–410.
24. Tombaugh TN. *Test of Memory Malingering (TOMM)*. New York: Multi-Health Systems; 1996.
25. Frederick RI, Foster HG. *The Validity Indicator Profile*. Minneapolis: National Computer Systems; 1997.
26. Rogers R, Bagby RM, Dickens SE. *Structured Interview of Reported Symptoms: Professional Manual*. Odessa, FL: Psychological Assessment Resources, 1992.
27. Gothard S, Viglione DJ, Meloy JR, et al. Detection of malingering in competency to stand trial evaluations. *Law Hum Behav* 1995; 19:493–505.
28. Hayes JS, Hale DB, Gouvier WD. Malingering detection in a mentally retarded forensic population. *Appl Neuropsychol* 1998; 5:33–36.
29. Rogers R. *Handbook of Diagnostic and Structured Interviewing*. New York: Guilford Press, 2001.
30. Pollock PH. A cautionary note on the determination of malingering in offenders. *Psychology, Crime and Law* 1996; 3:97–110.

31. Lally SJ. What tests are acceptable for use in forensic evaluations? A survey of experts. *Prof Psychol Res Pr* 2003; 34:491–498.
32. Green D, Rosenfeld B. Evaluating the gold standard: a review and meta-analysis of the structured interview of reported symptoms. *Psychol Assess* 2011; 23:95–107.
33. Kocsis RN. The structured interview of reported symptoms 2nd edition (SIRS-2): the new benchmark towards the assessment of malingering. *Journal of Forensic Psychology Practice* 2011; 11:73–81.
34. Rogers R, Sewell KW, Gillard ND. *Structured Interview of Reported Symptoms Professional Manual (2nd Edition)*. Odessa, FL: Psychological Assessment Resources, 2010.
35. https://www.google.com/search?q=PTSD&ie=utf-8&oe=utf-8&aq=t&rls=org.mozilla:en-US:official&client=firefox-a. Accessed 9 May 2014.
36. Frueh BC, Hammer MB, Cahill SP, et al. Apparent symptom overreporting in combat veterans evaluated for PTSD. *Clin Psychol Rev* 2000; 20:853–885.
37. Gold PB, Frueh BC. Compensation-seeking and extreme exaggeration of psychopathology among combat veterans evaluated for PTSD. *J Nerv Ment Dis* 1999; 187:680–684.
38. Frances A. DSM 5 writing mistakes will cause great confusion. Available at: http://www.psychologytoday.com/blog/saving-normal/201306/dsm-5-writing-mistakes-will-cause-great-confusion. Accessed 9 May 2014.
39. Arbisi PA, Ben-Porath YS, McNulty J. The ability of the MMPI-2 to detect feigned PTSD within the context of compensation seeking. *Psychol Serv* 2006; 3:249–261.
40. Lees-Haley PR. Efficacy of MMPI-2 validity scales and MCMI-II modifier scales for detecting spurious PTSD claims: F, F-K, Fake Bad scale, Ego Strength, Subtle-Obvious subscales, DIS and DEB. *J Clin Psychol* 1992; 48:681–689.
41. Efendov AE, Sellbom M, Bagby RM. The utility and comparative incremental validity of the MMPI–2 and trauma symptom inventory validity scales in the detection of feigned PTSD. *Psychol Assess* 2008; 20:317–326.
42. Elhai JD, Gold SN, Sellers AH, Dorfman WI. The detection of malingered Posttraumatic Stress Disorder with MMPI-2 fake bad indices. *Assessment* 2001; 8:221–236.
43. Elhai JD, Ruggiero KJ, Frueh BC, et al. The Infrequency-Posttraumatic Stress Disorder scale (Fptsd) for the MMPI-2: development and initial validation with veterans presenting with combat-related PTSD. *J Pers Assess* 2002; 79:531–549.
44. Elhai JD, Naifeh JA, Zucker IS, et al. Discriminating malingered from genuine civilian Posttraumatic Stress Disorder: a validation of three MMPI-2 infrequency scales (F, Fp, and Fptsd). *Assessment* 2004; 11:139–144.
45. Morel KR. Development and preliminary validation of a forced-choice test of response bias for Posttraumatic Stress Disorder. *J Pers Assess* 1998; 70:299–314.
46. Geraerts E, Kozaric-Kovacic C, Merckelbach H. Detecting deception of war-related posttraumatic stress disorder. *J Forens Psychiatry Psychol* 2009; 20:278–285.
47. Briere J. *Trauma Symptom Inventory, 2nd ed. (TSI-2) Professional Manual.* Odessa, FL: Psychological Assessment Resources, 2010.
48. Gray MJ, Elhai JD, Briere J. Evaluation of the Atypical Response scale of the Trauma Symptom Inventory-2 in detecting simulated posttraumatic stress disorder. *J Anxiety Disord* 2010; 24:447–451.

49. Elhai JD, Gray MJ, Naifeh JA, et al. Utility of the Trauma Symptom Inventory's Atypical Response Scale in detecting malingered post-traumatic stress disorder. *Assessment* 2005; 12:210–219.
50. Rosa's Law: Public Law 111 – 256 - OCT. 5, 2010.
51. WHODAS 2.0. World Health Organization Disability Assessment Schedule 2.0. Available at: http://who.int/classifications/icf/WHODAS2.0_12itemsINTERVIEW.pdf. Accessed 9 May 2014.
52. Sparrow S, Balla DA, Cicchetti DV. *Vineland Adaptive Behavior Scales: Survey Form Manual.* Circle Pines, Minnesota: American Guidance Service, 1984.
53. Greiffenstein MF, Baker WJ, Gola T. Validation of malingered amnesia measures with a large clinical sample. *Psychol Assess* 1994; 6:218–224.
54. Jasinski LJ, Berry DT, Shandera AL, Clark JA. Use of the Wechsler Adult Intelligence Scale Digit Span subtest for malingering detection: a meta-analytic review. *J Clin Exp Neuropsychol* 2011; 33:300–314.
55. Schroeder RW, Twumasi-Ankrah P, Baade LE, Marshall PS. Reliable digit span: a systematic review and cross-validation study. *Assessment* 2012; 19:21–30.
56. Victor TL, Boone KB. Identification of feigned mental retardation. In K. B. Boone (Editor.), *Assessment of Feigned Cognitive Impairment: A Neuropsychological Perspective*. New York: Guilford Press. 2007; pp 310–345.
57. Graue LO, Berry DT, Clark JA, et al. Identification of feigned mental retardation using the new generation of malingering instruments: preliminary findings. *Clin Neuropsychol* 2007; 21:929–942.
58. Doane B, Salekin KL. Susceptibility of current adaptive behavior measures to feigned deficits. *Law Hum Behav* 2009; 33:329–343.
59. Slick DJ, Sherman EM, Iverson GL. Diagnostic criteria for malingered neurocognitive dysfunction: proposed standards for clinical practice and research. *Clin Neuropsychol* 1999; 13:545–561.
60. Bush SS, Ruff RM, Troster AI, et al. Symptom validity assessment: Practice issues and medical necessity NAN Policy & Planning Committee. *Arch Clin Neuropsychol* 2005; 20:419–426.
61. Slick DJ, Tan JE, Strauss EH, et al. Detecting malingering: a survey of experts' practices. *Arch Clin Neuropsychol* 2004; 19:465–473.
62. Binder LM. Assessment of malingering after mild head trauma with the Portland digit recognition test. *J Clin Exp Neuropsychol* 1993; 15:170–182.
63. Greiffenstein MF, Baker WJ. Miller was (mostly) right: head injury severity inversely related to simulation. *Legal and Criminological Psychology* 2006; 11:131–145.
64. Larrabee GJ. Detection of malingering using atypical performance patterns on standard neuropsychological tests. *Clin Neuropsychol* 2003; 17:410–425.
65. Larrabee GJ. Forensic neuropsychological assessment. In: Vanderploeg AD, ed. *Clinician's Guide to Neuropsychological Assessment.* 2nd ed. Malwah, NJ: Lawrence Erlbaum; 2000; pp 301–305.
66. Green P, Rohling ML, Lees-Haley PR, et al. Effort has a greater effect on test scores than severe brain injury in compensation claims. *Brain Inj* 2001; 15:1045–1060.
67. Brand BL, McNary SW, Loewenstein RJ, et al. Assessment of genuine and simulated dissociative identity disorder on the Structured Interview of Reported Symptoms. *J Trauma Dissociation* 2006; 7:63–85.

68. Stadnik R, Brand B, Savoca A. Personality Assessment Inventory profile and predictors of elevations among dissociative disorder patients. *J Trauma Dissociation* 2013; 14:546–561.
69. Brand BL, Turisch M, Tzall D, Loewenstein RJ. Utility of the SIRS-2 in distinguishing genuine from simulated dissociative identity disorder. *Psychol Trauma* 2014; 6(5):308–317.
70. Coons PM, Milstein V. Factitious or malingered multiple personality disorder: eleven cases. *Dissociation: Progress in the Dissociative Disorders* 1994; 7:81–85.
71. Welburn KR, Fraser GA, Jordan SA, et al. Discriminating dissociative identity disorder from schizophrenia and feigned dissociation on psychological tests and structured interview. *J Trauma Dissociation* 2003; 4:109–130.
72. Brand BL, Chasson GS. Distinguishing simulated from genuine dissociative identity disorder on the MMPI-2. *Psychol Trauma* 2014; doi: 101037/a0035181.
73. Bernstein EM, Putnam FW. Development, reliability, and validity of a dissociation scale. J Nerv Ment Dis 1986; 174:727–735.
74. Weiss KJ, Watson C, Makkov D, et al. Parasomnias, violence and the law. *J Psychiatry Law* 2011; 39:249–286.
75. Bourget D, Whitehurst L. Amnesia and crime. *J Am Acad Psychiatry Law* 2007; 35:469–480.
76. Horn M. A rude awakening: what to do with the sleepwalking defense? *Boston Coll Law Rev* 2004; 46:149–182.
77. Atay T, Karacan I. A retrospective study of sleepwalking in 22 patients: Clinical and polysomnographic findings. *Sleep Hypn* 2000; 2:112–119.

INDEX

Page numbers followed by *f* or *t* indicate figures or tables, respectively.

CPSIA information can be obtained
at www.ICGtesting.com
Printed in the USA
BVHW08s1323200918
527979BV00002B/74/P

9 780199 368464